Ultrasonography for the Upper Limb Surgeon

Thomas Apard • Jean Louis Brasseur
Editors

Ultrasonography for the Upper Limb Surgeon

Springer

Editors
Thomas Apard
Centre d'échochirurgie de la main
Hôpital Privé de Versailles
Versailles, France

Jean Louis Brasseur
Radio-diagnostic
Pitié-Salpêtrière Hospital
Paris, France

Translation from the French language edition: L'échographie pour le chirurgien du membre supérieur by Thomas Apard, and Jean Louis Brasseur, © Sauramps Medical, Montpellier, France, 2019. Published by Sauramps Medical. All Rights Reserved.

Original French edition published by Sauramps Medical, Montpellier, France, 2019

ISBN 978-3-030-84233-8 ISBN 978-3-030-84234-5 (eBook)
https://doi.org/10.1007/978-3-030-84234-5

This Springer imprint is published by the registered company Springer Nature Switzerland AG
The registered company address is: Gewerbestrasse 11, 6330 Cham, Switzerland

Special thanks to Dr. Melissa Odoemene for her help in this translation of the original French.

Foreword

Ultrasound is a rapidly expanding imaging tool. Initially reserved for radiologists only, it was gradually adopted by other specialties: anesthetists, rheumatologists, general practitioners. The noninvasive, nonradiant, portable, and dynamic real-time imaging character makes this tool a real extension of the practitioner's senses.

In recent years, surgeons of the upper limb, whether they are plastic surgeons or orthopedists, have more and more become aware of the potential of this tool. Some classical techniques have already been converted under ultrasound control, such as the release of the median nerve to the carpal canal or the cure of the trigger finger. The term ultrasonosurgery has thus been consecrated. Much remains to be discovered and codified, though.

The future of upper limb ultrasound surgery now depends on the research and teaching of this transversal discipline requiring long learning. This is how the interuniversity diploma (IUD) in ultrasonosurgery saw its creation in 2012, which has gathered a growing number of practitioners, ranging from the intern to experienced senior surgeon. In the same logic, Thomas Apard and Jean Louis Brasseur offer us, in this book, an already existing knowledge base in ultrasound, as well as various ways of development. This book is probably just the beginning of a long and exciting story that remains to be written.

Marc Soubeyrand
Conservative and Traumatological
Surgeon Service, Bicêtre Hospital
Le Kremlin-Bicêtre, France

Preface

Ultrasonography is one of the best examinations to explore upper limb disorders from the shoulder to the digit. It is the only dynamic and comparative tool easily accessible for the surgeon without side effects.

Indeed, ultrasonography is actually available in all the departments of your hospital: in the operating room with the anesthesiologists, in the hospitalization area thanks to the radiologists, and in the emergency room with the traumatologists.

Recent innovations permit to see superficially (high-frequency probes), precisely (smaller probes), and with greater software for an effective Mode B or Doppler mode. The screens are smaller and more convenient as in the past in order to propose a better panel of machines for the practitioner from the pocket scan to the big machine with rollers.

All these evolutions involve a good exploration and as the result, a relevant education: it is the purpose of this book to unify all these talented ultrasound practitioners to teach you how to get the better of the machines for your patients.

Versailles, France — Thomas Apard
Paris, France — Jean Louis Brasseur

Contents

Part I

Shoulder

Ultrasound in the Pathology of the Rotator Cuff

1

Jean Louis Brasseur

1.1 Introduction

Performing the ultrasound of the shoulder can only be done after a clinical examination directed toward a pathology of the rotator cuff, because in case of instability or articular pathology, the role of ultrasound examination is much less important.

It should also never be forgotten that in case of pain evoking a damage to the cuff, the aim of imaging investigations is to determine the cause of this pain, which is not always easy, and the big mistake is to stop at the first pathological picture discovered, forgetting that the majority of the lesions are asymptomatic (e.g., ruptures and calcifications) [1, 2].

In this diagnostic approach, several elements must be taken into account, inflammatory or mechanical character, sudden and progressive onset, but also the age of the patient, because the prevalence of symptomatic but above all asymptomatic ruptures increases progressively to become very frequent after the age of 65 years [3, 4].

The evolutionary stage of discovery is also decisive in the analysis of pain since calcification causes a hyperalgesic crisis when it disappears [5], whereas a rupture leads to symptomatology when the tendon tears and becomes the most asymptomatic afterwards [1].

Finally, the various pathologies of the tendons and their sheath are sometimes multiple, which further complicates the determination of the pain factor; thus the hypertrophic character of an enthesopathy may cause an anterosuperior impingement itself which generates bursitis.

The etiological assessment of cuff pain is therefore not only the search for a rupture or a preoperative assessment, it is much more complex if one wishes to perform a correct analysis of painful pathologies to guide the treatment satisfactorily.

Let's see how far ultrasound is able to bring certain elements of response to the only important question: what is the cause of the patient's pain?

1.2 Why Use Ultrasound?

After the clinical examination, the diagnostic strategy, in case of a painful shoulder, first uses standard X-ray images, but this combination (clinic + XR) is rarely sufficient to analyze the different painful etiologies of the cuff [6–8].

Clinically, the differentiation of these pathologies is difficult because, even if some elements are specific, the same lesion often has a very dif-

J. L. Brasseur (✉)
G.H. Pitié-Salpêtrière, Service de Radiologie, Paris, France
e-mail: jlbrasseur@impf.fr

T. Apard, J. L. Brasseur (eds.), *Ultrasonography for the Upper Limb Surgeon*,
https://doi.org/10.1007/978-3-030-84234-5_1

ferent symptomatology from one patient to another, and on the other hand, the anatomical layering of the elements of the cuff limits the clinical discrimination because painful palpation can correspond to either bursitis or tendinopathy [1, 9–11].

Standard X-ray shots are essential to see joint spacing and eliminate underlying pathology, but in the case of cuff lesions they show only two important elements:

- The thinning of the subacromial space which testifies to a large image of ancient transfixing rupture [7]
- The blurred and fragmented appearance of the contours of a calcification oriented toward its "active" character [8]

For the remainder, these are indirect signs pointing to a pathology of the cuff that are present:

- Irregularity of facets and subacromial densification [8, 11]
- Importance of the frontal overhang of the acromion since a very overlapping acromion favors lesions of the cuff [12]

Then, in order to choose an imagery to properly explore a cuff, some prerequisites are indispensable because the technique used must be capable of:

- Differentiating the different anatomical elements between the insertion facets and the deltoid
- Visualizing the two sides (joint and bursal) of the cuff
- Showing the very structure of the tendons

Only two techniques meet these requirements: ultrasound and MRI (or arthro-MRI).

In addition to the noninvasive and nonirradiant nature, the advantages of ultrasound are well known:

- The availability
- The *cost* (ten times cheaper!)

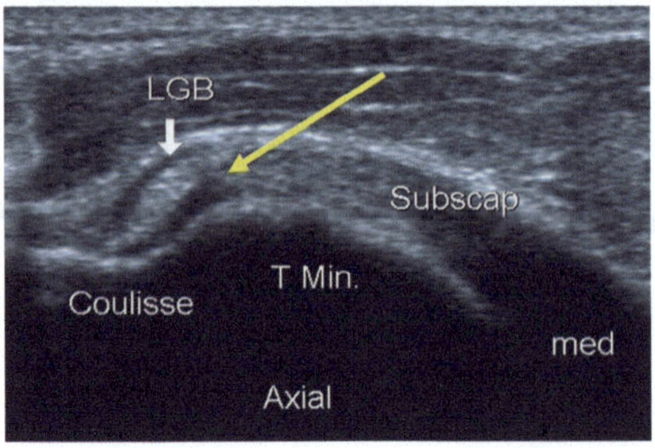

Fig. 1.1 Spatial resolution of the ultrasound allowing to analyze the different tendon "layers"

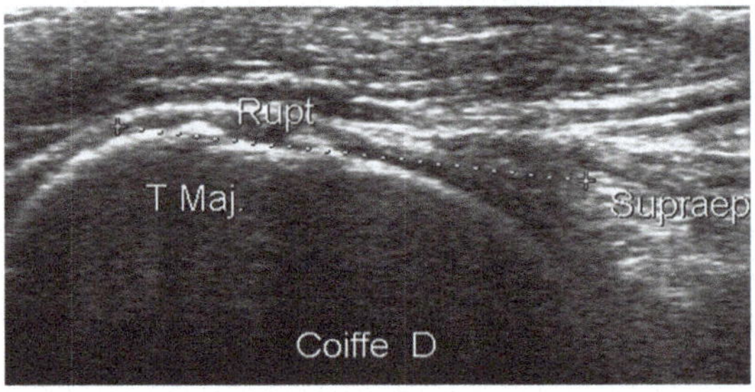

Fig. 1.2 Asymptomatic rupture (perforation) of the supraspinatus cuff

But it is also necessary to add in connection with these cuff lesions

- The importance of its *spatial resolution* (Fig. 1.1).
- Its *dynamic character* very useful in the study of this mobility articulation.
- The possibility of systematic comparison on the opposite side given the numerous asymptomatic lesions (Fig. 1.2) [1–4] requiring *bilateral examination*. This last point is crucial, often unknown, and if only one cuff is examined, it is often the first anomalous image discovered that makes the diagnosis and not the true painful etiology.

The main pitfall of ultrasound is its great difficulty at the root of its reputation as an operator-dependent examination. It requires a long learning curve and the use of a high-performance machine; these two elements are fundamental, and their lack of knowledge is at the root of many disillusionments [13, 14].

For these reasons, the other limitations mentioned are most often problems of operator confidence and understanding of the images; this distrust is reinforced by the numerous errors encountered.

It should also be borne in mind that ultrasound of the shoulder never makes a comprehensive assessment of this joint and that its isolated use is dangerous and reprehensible. It is useful, after standard X-rays, when the clinical examination suspects a pathology of the cuff and has much less interest in instability, a little more in the case of articular pathology [15].

1.3 How Do You Do an Ultrasound of the Cuff?

It must be repeated; it is a difficult examination which, in order to be effective, requires a long apprenticeship and the use of efficient equipment [14, 16].

It is therefore essential, first of all, to learn how to do this ultrasound on many asymptomatic people of varying age and different morphology before considering examining a patient; the many variants must be known before approaching the pathology because it is impossible without this prerequisite: to assert that an image is abnormal.

For the same reason, it is better to start the examination with the supposedly healthy shoulder to visualize how non-painful anatomical structures are in this patient. Bursaries can be thick, effusions are visible in a non-negligible number of people, and there are many asymptomatic calcifications (Fig. 1.3).

In addition, acromioclavicular changes and irregularities of entheses are usually present after 35 years in patients with significant sports or manual activity. There is also a high number of asymptomatic, partial, or transfixative ruptures, the percentage of which increases with age [1, 2].

Regardless of the painful topography and the presumed clinical diagnosis, the examination must be systematic, carried out always in the same way to be complete and not stop at the first

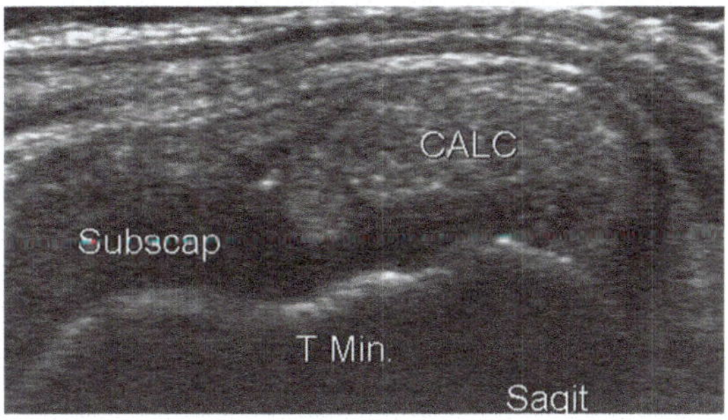

Fig. 1.3 Voluminous calcification of the subscapularis in an asymptomatic patient on this side

abnormal picture encountered; the biggest mistake in ultrasound is to directly put the probe on the painful area.

Keyframes must always be identical, well documented, understandable by all, and capable of being reread. The number of these images may be limited, but all the pathological elements relevant to the diagnosis should be included. It is necessary to be able to report the examination solely on the basis of the documents given to the patient; indeed, even within a dynamic sequence, it is always possible to identify the instructive shot, and the ultrasound shots must be reread as in other techniques of imaging.

The use of a high-performance device is also essential. The quality of the resources is increasing, but the differences remain important.

In this context, it should never be forgotten, when choosing an ultrasound device, that the reflexogenous appearance of the subcutaneous tissue progresses significantly depending on the age of the patient and the essentially fat thickness of the tissue. The beautiful images made on the models are therefore of no interest because they are not the ones we get in real life. It is necessary to try the devices on elderly people and preferably obese!

The best criterion for choosing a machine for a rotator cuff study is to differentiate in all patients (and therefore mainly in obese and elderly patients) the boundary between the superficial slope of the supraspinatus and the subacromiodeltoid bursa (SADB). This differentiation is crucial because it is one of the main elements of the orientation of therapy (see below).

1.4 Analysis of Painful Etiologies

After these indispensable elements:

- Clinical suspicion of damage to the cuff
- Standard X-rays performed
- Competent operator
- Conducting a bilateral review
- Using high-performance equipment

Let's see how far ultrasound can differentiate different symptomatic etiologies.

It is necessary first of all to separate acute pathologies from chronic ones because their ultrasound semiology differs fundamentally.

1.5 The Various Acute Disorders

Whether the acute lesion is posttraumatic, occurs "in a serene environment," or is the brutal aggravation of a chronic injury, clinical examination is often difficult, and the diagnostic contribution of ultrasound is very important. Different lesions can be found: tendon and bursal lesions are analyzed but also lesions of bone cortices and sometimes associated capsuloligamentous lesions, the detection of which complements the ultrasound assessment [16–18].

1.5.1 Bone and Osteoarticular Lesions

If the spongy bone and the joint intervals are not analyzable, the cortical lesions are perfectly seen by ultrasound, which shows the interrupting images very clearly, especially in the case of a fracture of the greater tubercle. These lesions are sometimes ignored by the radiographic assessment, which is often negative at the early stage in usual cases. Fracture is detected on ultrasound by an interruption of the hyperechogenic line of the cortex, sometimes accompanied by displacement and in the overwhelming majority of cases a neighboring hypoechogenic zone (Fig. 1.4). It is important because it differentiates old and recent lesions [19]. These lesions are electively painful on an ultrasound palpation and are most often accompanied by a hematic bursal effusion with, in some cases, the disinsertion of peripheral fibers of the supraspinatus (Fig. 1.5). Sometimes, if the line reaches the joint side of the insertion, it will be an intra-articular effusion that will be observed.

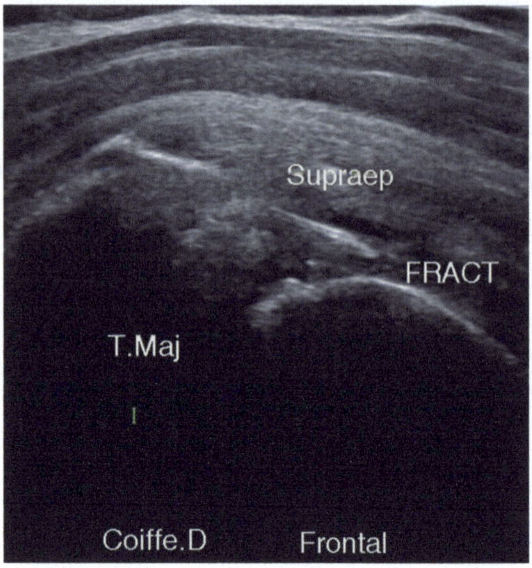

Fig. 1.4 Fracture of the greater tubercle. Interruption of the cortex and hypoechoic neighborhood remodeling

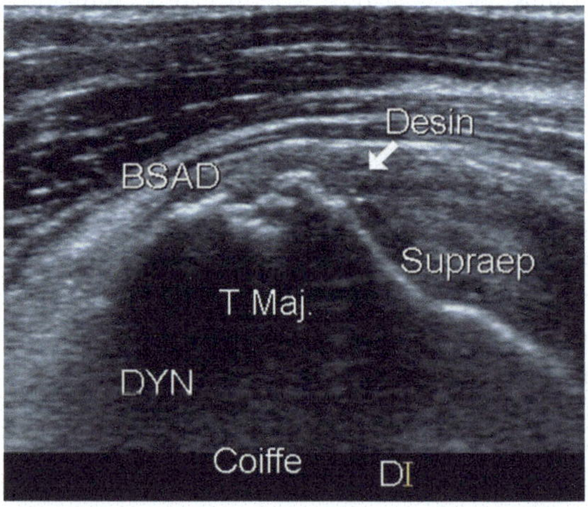

Fig. 1.5 Fracture of the greater tubercle with disinsertion of peripheral supraspinatus fibers and neighboring bursitis

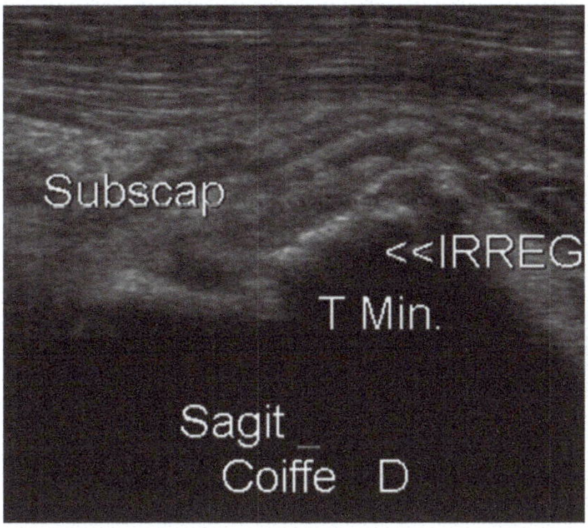

Fig. 1.6 Posttraumatic irregularity of lesser tubercle (bone edema through MRI) without cortical detachment

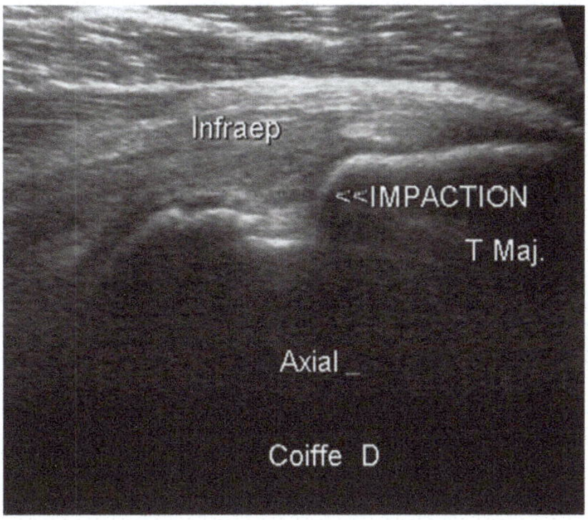

Fig. 1.7 Impaction on the posterior-superior side of the head after spontaneously reduced dislocation

However, in some cases, the fracture line is prolonged by cracking in the thickness of the tendon, and in this case no effusion accompanies the lesion.

A small irregularity of the cortex can also be observed with a small remodeling of the neighboring tendinous insertion expressing a bruise (Fig. 1.6), but some of them are only visible in MRI when they are not accompanied by any change in the periphery of the bone. Anamnesis helps to differentiate these lesions from degenerative irregularities.

Images of disinsertion of ossification nuclei can be found in adolescents, particularly at the subscapularis attachment; these lesions are detected by a hypoechogenic range detaching the nucleus from the superficial side of the cortex. Their consolidation is quick at this age if care is taken to prohibit any external rotational movement of the arm.

Impactions are correctly detected, especially those of the posterior side of the head after anteroinferior dislocation (Fig. 1.7). Their discovery is interesting to confirm a spontaneously reduced dislocation, but the role of ultrasound is primarily to check the integrity of the adjacent tendon. Ultrasonic examination, however, is in no way capable of making an overall assessment of an accident of instability because the damage to the labrum is only incompletely visualized, especially anterior; abnormal mobility is, on the other hand, well analyzed on a posterior axial section in dynamic ultrasound.

1.5.2 The Effusion and Bursitis

In ultrasound, effusions are indirect signs directing the diagnosis to either intra (effusion within a scapulohumeral recess) or periarticular (effusion within the SADB) pathology. Their recognition is imperative in acute pathology.

As the examination is performed in a sitting position, intra-articular effusion most often results in the occurrence of a distension from the bicipital recess leading to the appearance of an anechoic area surrounding the long biceps at its side. In some cases, the effusion is also visualized at the posterior part of the interval (mainly in external rotation) which lifts the deep slope of the infraspinatus [20].

Detection of periarticular effusions (in the subacromiodeltoid bursa) can be carried out at several levels. We know the classical image of the distended bursa facing the superficial slope of the supraspinatus and extending along the lateral slope of the humerus. However, some bursitis is also observed under the acromiocoracoid liga-

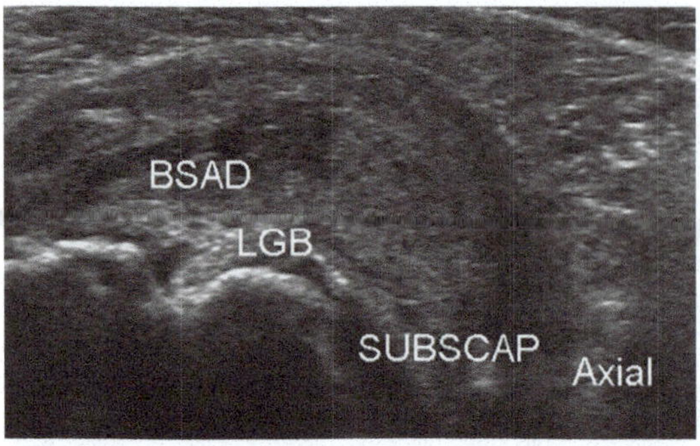

Fig. 1.8 Significant bursitis extending to the front of the subscapularis

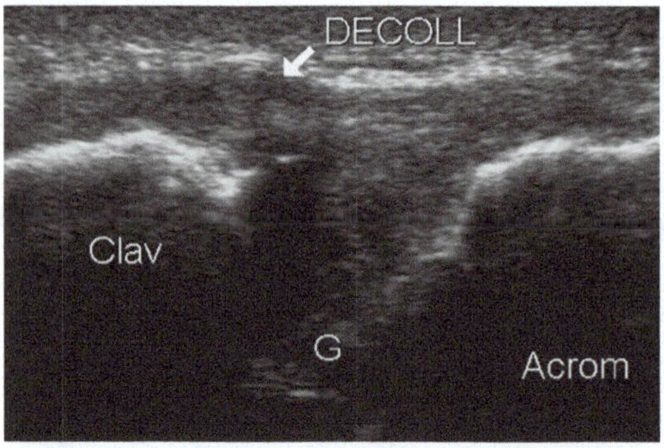

Fig. 1.10 Sprain of the acromioclavicular joint with painful removal of capsular insertion

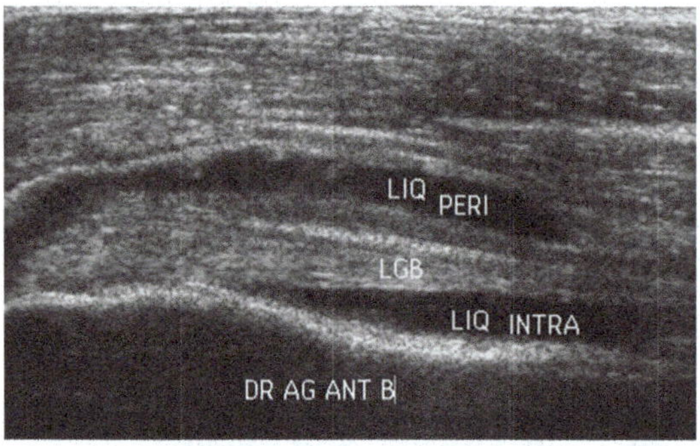

Fig. 1.9 Simultaneous intra- and periarticular effusion indicating, in acute form, a communication between the two compartments

ment or in front of the anterior surface of the subscapularis (the subscapular bursa communicates in most cases with the subacromial and subdeltoid bursas) (Fig. 1.8) [21].

In acute form, the presence of a double effusion (coexistence of an intra effusion and a periarticular effusion) is almost pathognomonic of transfixing lesion of the rotator cuff since the existence of this double effusion means either that there is a communication between the two compartments or a double pathology (Fig. 1.9) [22, 23].

In addition to its role as an indirect sign, post-traumatic bursitis can also be painful; pain usually appears in the night following an indirect trauma such as a fall on the wrist or elbow resulting in an impact between the humeral head and the underside of the acromion.

1.5.3 Capsuloligamentous Lesions

At the scapulohumeral level, ligamentous damage is only rarely detected during an ultrasound examination of the shoulder, and the glenohumeral ligaments are very poorly visualized. On the other hand, a lesion of the rotator interval may be detected by hypoechogenic thickening or disinsertion of the coracohumeral ligament at its attachments on the upper part of the bicipital groove with sometimes small bone avulsion surrounded by a hypoechogenic zone and lowering of the head (this is the aforementioned ligament of this head).

Subluxation of the tendon of the long biceps (LBT (long biceps tendon)), which then has a normal fibrillar structure, in front of the anterior surface of an intact subscapularis may be visible in the event of rupture of this coracohumeral ligament.

The capsuloligamentous lesions of the acromioclavicular interval are often clinically unknown and are well accessible to ultrasound. It is the capsular detachments at the origin of a hypoechogenic sleeve surrounding the extremity of the clavicle that cause the most severe pain (Fig. 1.10), but simple joint distension can be painful; these changes must be interpreted according to the clinic (pain on palpation by the probe) and compared to the opposed side given the large number of asymptomatic changes.

1.5.4 Tendon Pathologies

They are rare in posttraumatic conditions, and acute damage occurs most often on a "background" of chronic pain. They originate from significant lesions and from different locations, the detection and quantification of which are important at this stage in order not to delay the initiation of treatment.

1.6 Transfixing Ruptures

Posttraumatic damage on healthy tendon is rare but easy to detect because, in addition to a "double" effusion, a clear solution of continuity is often clearly visible.

But the most frequent acute lesions occur in case of aggravation of a preexisting lesion (interest of anamnesis). In these cases, a transfixative lesion is painful when it is formed, that is, when a partial lesion is aggravated or when it occurs on a field of chronic tendinopathy. These acute transfixing lesions of the supra and/or infraspinatus, which aggravate another lesion (tendinopathy and/or partial rupture), are difficult to visualize in ultrasound because the classical criteria (flat and/or tendon disappearance) are not present in the acute phase. The borders of a recent injury are often poorly defined, and there is usually a simple diffuse hypoechogenic swelling of the tendon within which the zone of interruption is not visible (Fig. 1.11). Stretching and compression maneuvers should be carried out in order to best unmask this rupture passing through the tendon and thus communicating the two joint compartments through an anechoic area rarely visible in this type of lesion [16].

It is therefore the indirect signs that are most important to spot, allowing to suspect this transfixing lesion:

- The presence of effusion on either side of the tendon, that is, both intra-articular and within the subacromiodeltoid bursa (sign of double effusion) [22, 23].
- The absence of a junction between the superficial slope of the supraspinatus and the lateral part of the insertion zone: this is the sign of absence of a crossing and the space then visible between the extremity of the facet and the upper surface of the tendon is filled by the SADB which extends, distended, to the lateral side of the humerus (Fig. 1.12).
- Another indirect sign is a highly reflexogenic cartilaginous surface ("too well seen" cartilage), which indicates the existence of a pathological tendon (too trans-sonic) often present in case of a recent transfixing rupture (Fig. 1.13).

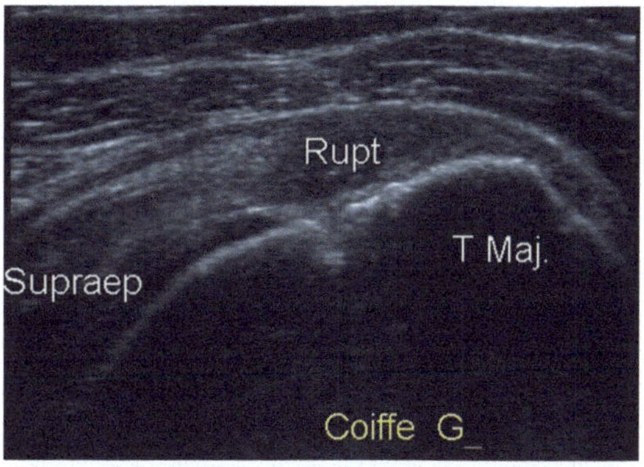

Fig. 1.11 Recent rupture of the supraspinatus with no visible "gap" between the borders of the rupture

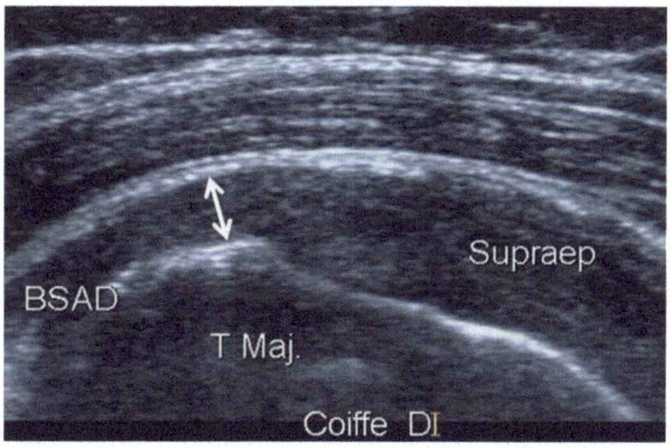

Fig. 1.12 Absence of crossing at the periphery of the insertion facet = indirect sign of recent rupture

1.7 Partial Ruptures

Partial damage visualized acutely can affect one of the two sides of the cuff (deep, articular or superficial, bursal) or even lead to an

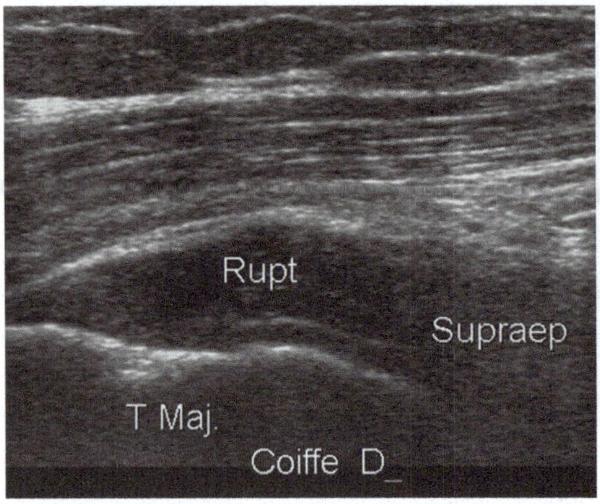

Fig. 1.13 Too clear visualization of cartilage surface = indirect sign of recent rupture

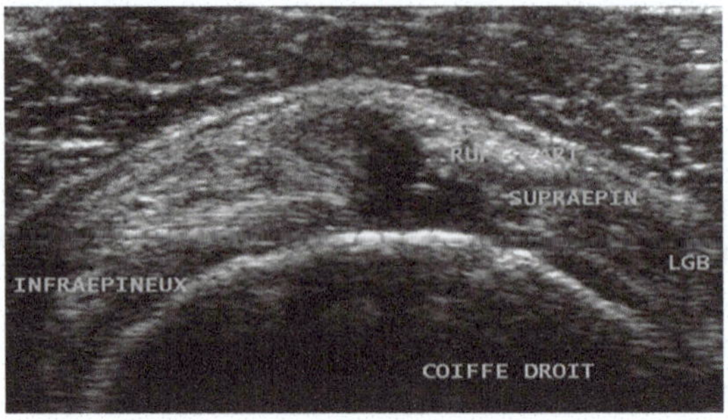

Fig. 1.14 Partial rupture of the deep surface of the supraspinatus

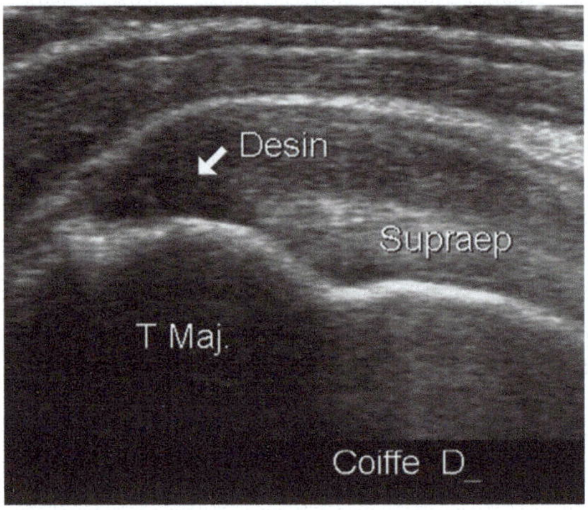

Fig. 1.15 Disinsertion of superficial, bursal, supraspinatus fibers

intratendinous cleavage not joining one of the two tendon surfaces [16, 24].

- On the deep, articular slope, the lesion is almost systematically located at the junction of the cephalic cartilage and the insertion zone; it is visible in the case of acute damage in the form of a poorly systematized hypoechogenic range associated with tendon thickening and tendon effusion localized only intra-articularly (i.e., most often in the bicipital recess). It undertakes the medial part of the insertion zone, and this topography makes it possible to differentiate it from the enthesopathies that reach the entire area of insertion. The hypoechoic zone does not pass through the tendon in any place, leaving a normal fibrillar contingent in the area of the tendon (Fig. 1.14).
- Partial ruptures affecting the superficial, bursal, side of the supraspinatus and resulting in the occurrence of an effusion in the SADB are disinsertions of peripheral fibers; this type of lesion is very common, aggravating enthesopathy; it occurs in isolation or, sometimes, in association with lateral contusion of the greater tubercle. It should be noted that these acute non-transfixing lesions of the peripheral slope are in fact disinsertions and not ruptures (Fig. 1.15).
- Purely intratendinous cleavages are rare in acute; they usually accompany a fracture of the greater tubercle, the cleavage extending the fracture line in some way. No effusion is detected in this type of lesion.

1.8 Disinsertions of the Subscapularis

Apart from the tearing of the apophyseal nucleus in adolescents (see above), the importance of the disinsertion of the subscapularis is often difficult to specify in ultrasound examination performed in the acute phase, only marked by heterogeneous and hypoechogenic swelling, poorly circumscribed, adjacent to the insertion facet of the minor tubercle. This disinsertion

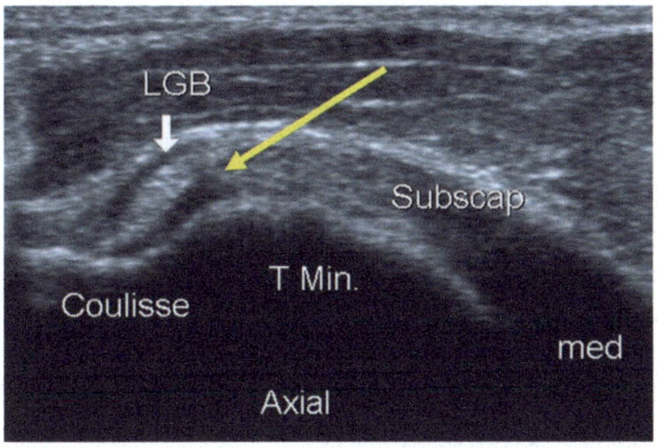

Fig. 1.16 Sign of the triangle. A hypoechogenic triangular zone (arrow) separating the LBT (long biceps tendon) from the medial side of the groove that attests to the normal position of this tendon

may be partial or complete, but as with other tendon lesions, swelling is observed at this stage, not a flat plane.

It is primarily the associated dislocation of the long head of the biceps that must be detected with the spread of the LBT (long biceps tendon) on the medial edge of the groove or subluxation in the thickness of the subscapularis. Note that a subluxation in front of the anterior surface of an intact subscapularis may accompany a lesion of the interval strap (see above).

It is therefore essential to check whether the tendon of the long head of the biceps is in place at the top of the groove and whether the subscapularis fits into its vicinity. The most important sign to look for is the presence of the hypoechogenic triangle on the medial side of the upper part of the groove. It consists of collagen tissue, as it forms the insertion of the coracohumeral ligament and disappears as soon as the tendon subluxes on the inner border of the groove. This sign of the triangle is therefore indispensable to affirm the correct position of the long head of the biceps in the groove (Fig. 1.16) [25].

1.8.1 SLAP (Superior Labrum Antero-Posterior)

The visualization of the insertion of the long head of the biceps on the upper bead can be difficult in the case of a posterior attachment, and the analysis of this region constitutes one of the limitations of the possibilities of the technique. The view of this insertion requires retropulsion of the arm and maximum external rotation to clear the upper pole of the head. Partial disinsertion of the head along the biceps (falling under SLAP) may be suspected if a hypoechoic image is visualized near its upper glenoid attachment knowing that ultrasound can only suspect such a lesion, which will be assessed by the Arthoscanner or Arthro-MRI. Ultrasound can, on the other hand, clear this junction if it is perfectly identified without hypoechogenic neighborhood remodeling.

1.9 The Dislocation of the Head Along the Biceps

This dislocation can be the cause of acute symptomatology.

As we have seen, it most often accompanies an injury to the subscapularis but can also occur during an isolated lesion of the ligament strap of the rotator interval. In this case, the tendon of the biceps is visualized on the anterior surface of the subscapularis, and there is no remodeling (Fig. 1.17) [26–28].

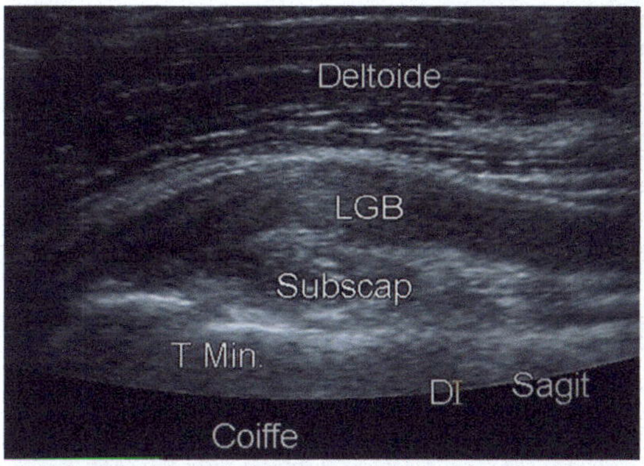

Fig. 1.17 Rupture of the rotator interval strap with the presence of LBT (long biceps tendon) in front of the intact subscapularis on this sagittal section

1.10 Calcification

It may be surprising to cite calcification in acute cases, but alteration of the crystalline structure of calcification or its migration results in, in some cases, a significant hyperalgesic reaction (pseudo-gout attack), and the patient presents ~~himself~~ urgently with a frozen shoulder, unexaminable.

The "active" character of a calcification is marked by its fragmented appearance, complemented by heterogeneous remodeling of the neighboring tendon. In addition, in case of migration, the superficial slope of the tendon is interrupted, and at least part of the calcification migrated into a thickened and heterogeneous SADB (Fig. 1.18). Hyperechogenic sludge (calcium milk) can even be found there as well as hypervascularization of bursal walls in the color Doppler study [29, 30]. More rarely, calcification migrates intra-articularly with calcium fragments in a distended recess, sometimes intraosseous with focal defect of the facet (often with a pseudo tumor image in MRI) or, in some cases, distal to the tendon near its myotendinous junction.

1.11 The Different Chronic Conditions

Apart from acute impairment, two clinical situations are observed each with a particular ultrasound semiology: pain due to overuse of the young subject and aggravation of a degenerative change in the older patient. In both cases, the most important point is whether the cause of the pain is of tendon (in general non-inflammatory) or bursal (inflammatory) origin, without forgetting the possibility of arthropathy or early capsulitis.

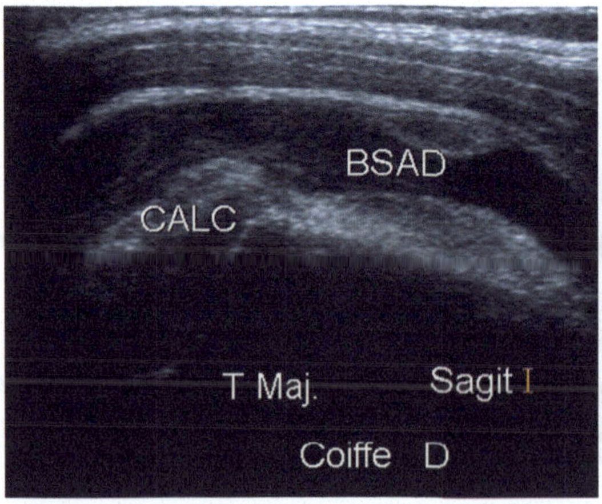

Fig. 1.18 Migration of supraspinatus calcification within BSAD (subacromiodeltoid bursa)

1.11.1 Enthesopathy

The involvement of the tendon insertion on the bone is common, mainly after 35 years in manual workers and sportsmen. The change always begins on the dominant side and is not always symptomatic. Enthesopathy essentially leads to hypoechogenic remodeling, sometimes hypertrophic, of the entire insertion zone, most often with no intra-articular effusion (Fig. 1.19); later, we observe the occurrence of fine curvilinear calcification, an irregularity of the facet, or small ossified spicules joining the cortex (often irregular in these cases) in the center of the enthesopathy zone (Fig. 1.20). This is the pathology of the

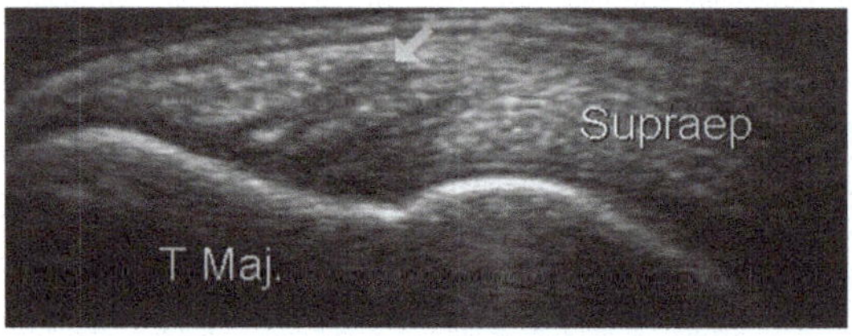

Fig. 1.19 Enthesopathy at the attachment of the supraspinatus on the facet of the greater tubercle

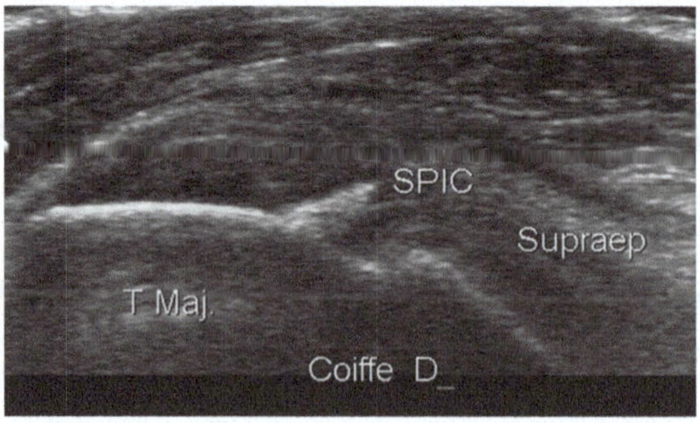

Fig. 1.20 Ossified spicule of enthesopathy at the attachment of the supraspinatus

overtrained young athlete, of the resumption of sport after a stop (pregnancy for example), but it is in fact extremely common after 35 years, especially among manual workers. Its symptomatic character can therefore be asserted only with great caution and after comparison with the opposite side [1, 16, 31].

This enthesopathy corresponds to a dissociation of collagen fibers which continues by a chondroid transformation of the insertion zone and therefore contains no inflammatory components.

There is, however, a continuum in histology and imaging between these enthesopathies and the more severe lesions: disinsertion and rupture. Small cracks lengthening of the spicules, or even partial disinsertions, aggravating enthesopathy, can be visualized, causing often painful progressive laceration of a tendon.

Another sign, a hyperechogenic line doubling the cortex (sign of the double line), is important to look for because it testifies to the disinsertion of calcified fibrocartilage from the enthesis, complicating enthesopathy (Fig. 1.21) [32].

1.11.2 Impingements

Three impingements are mainly found in the rotator cuff, and their detection is facilitated by the dynamic specificity of the ultrasound, which shows in this case the consequences of these impingements but also its exact location and origin.

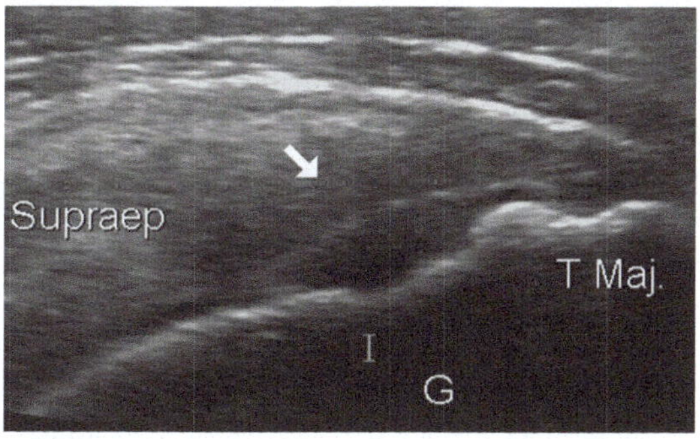

Fig. 1.21 "Detachment" of the calcified fibro-cartilage layer causing a "double line"

1.11.2.1 Anterosuperior

The most common impingements are the result of abnormal contact between the superficial side of the supraspinatus and the arch formed posterior to the acromion and anterior to the acromiocoracoid ligament. It leads to thickening of the walls of the subacromiodeltoid bursa often responsible for the painful symptomatology of the patient [16, 32, 33]. It is screened in dynamic ultrasound; the abduction maneuver internal rotation of the arm positioned in slight retropulsion shows deformation of the superficial side of the tendon with focal thickening of the walls of the SADB opposite the site of impingement (Fig. 1.22). A significant difference from the opposite side must be found in conjunction with these changes to assert that this impingement is indeed the cause of the painful symptomatology.

Conventionally, in addition to muscle dysfunction, this anterosuperior impingement may result from the prominent aspect of the lower slope of the acromion or the acromioclavicular interval coming from "aggression" on the superficial side of the tendon (interest of the cuff profile), but deformation of the facet or hypertrophy of the contents of the subacromial space and in particular hypertrophic calcification may also be the cause of this impingement.

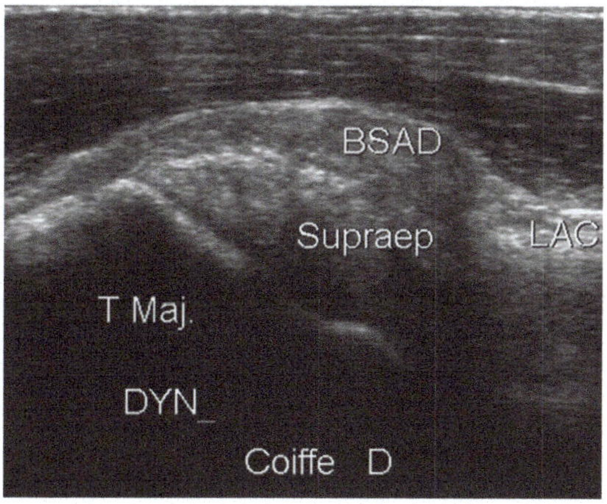

Fig. 1.22 Thickness of the BSAD (subacromiodeltoid bursa) during the dynamic test showing anterosuperior impingement

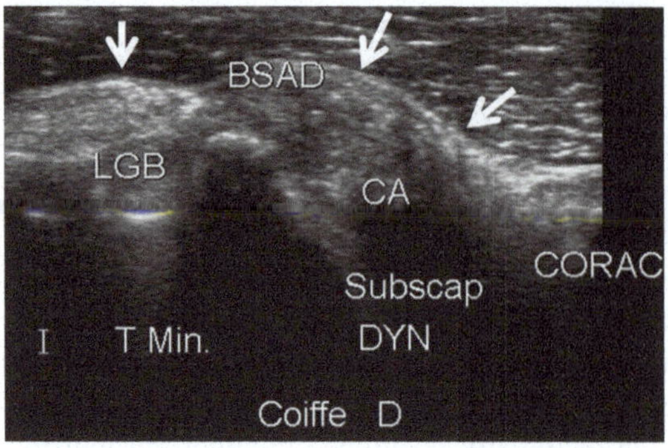

Fig. 1.23 Impingement anterior to the passage of the subscapularis, thickened by calcification, under the coracoid process

1.11.2.2 Anterior Impingement

Several anterior impingements have been described, but the most common is the cause of abnormal contact between the anterior side of the subscapularis and the coracoid, which is detected by internal rotation maneuver (Fig. 1.23). It is conventionally the result of a decrease in the space separating the coracoid tip from the humerus, but, in fact, in most cases, it is a hypertrophic calcifying tendinopathy of the upper part of the subscapularis tendon that constitutes the etiological factor of the impingement [16, 34]. Anterior subluxation of the head may also occur.

It is detected on an axial section by an internal rotation maneuver of the arm, sliding the subscapularis under the coracoid hook in search of tendon deformation and/or thickening of the bursa in front of the subscapularis. Any thickening or effusion within this bursa, however, is not a sign of anterior impingement given its frequent communication with the subdeltoid bursa.

1.12 Posterosuperior Impingement

This impingement described by Walch [35] is of different topography since it involves the joint slope of the posterior portion of the supraspinatus tendon and the upper part of the infraspinatus tendon. It occurs mainly in throwing sports, tennis and baseball, and results in non-transfixing damage to the joint side of the tendon associated with irregularity of the adjacent bone contour and often intra-articular effusion.

1.12.1 Tendon Ruptures

Tendon ruptures are very common, often bilateral and asymptomatic, especially after 50 years. It is known that it is mainly the formation and aggravation of the rupture that are painful as well as the associated lesions (LBT (long biceps tendon) and SADB). The challenge of imaging is to determine whether tendon perforation is the cause of the symptomatology of the patient. For this purpose, ultrasound analysis must detect these ruptures but above all carry out a global, comparative assessment, analyzing the main causes of pain in case of rupture, i.e., the walls of the SADB and the bicipital tendons [1, 13, 14, 16, 36–39].

Several studies have shown that the sensitivity and specificity of ultrasound are similar to that of MRI for the detection of transfixing ruptures [40–42].

1.13 The Transfixative Rupture

It is often well tolerated when it remains localized in the median and posterior parts of the supraspinatus, especially in patients with a satisfactory thickness of the deltoid. Indeed, in this type of limited rupture, the anterior portion of the supraspinatus, which is more important functionally, protects, by its thickness, the reflective area of the tendon of the long head of the biceps to the upper part of the groove. In addition, the anterior (subscapularis) and posterior (infraspinatus) shrouds are respected allowing for satisfactory stability of the head in the anteroposterior plane.

In the chronic stage, these ruptures are detected on ultrasound by a flat plane if the damage is small (Fig. 1.24) and by the disappearance of the tendon image replaced by a capsule bursa (sometimes with contact between the major process and the acromion) if the rupture is wide and the tendon is retracted (Fig. 1.25). This image must be differentiated from a tendon that is simply thinned but continuous as it is encountered in

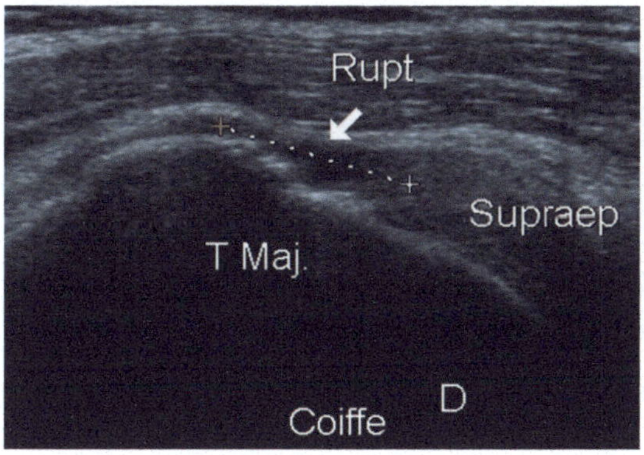

Fig. 1.24 Old transfixing rupture of small size with flat part of supraspinatus attachment

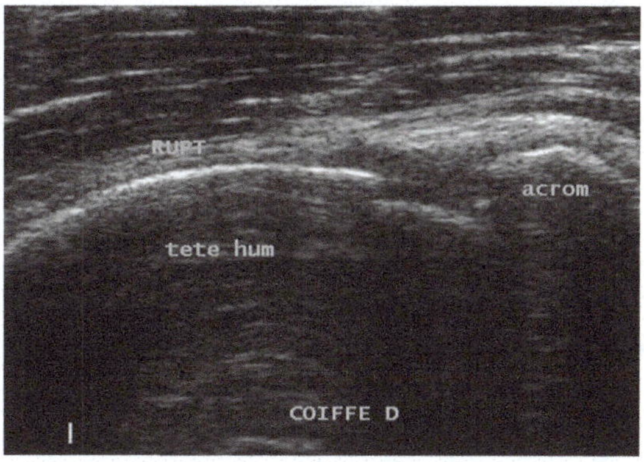

Fig. 1.25 Large transfixing rupture with disappearance of the cuff and ascent of the head that comes in contact with the underside of the acromion

polyarthritis but also after adhesive capsulitis and on any antero-inferior dislocation.

Recall that there is a continuum between the lesions of the cuff. Thus, enthesopathies or tendinopathies do not turn overnight into rupture or disinsertion; stages of passage exist.

The rupture usually occurs gradually, and this lesion in the process of being formed is painful because residual tendon fibers persist on which all the tensile forces arise (Fig. 1.26).

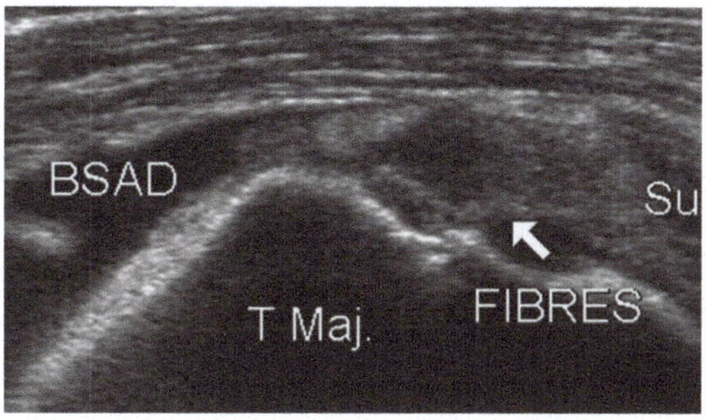

Fig. 1.26 Only a few residual fibers persist after partial lesions of the surface but also of the deep surface of the supraspinatus

However, when this rupture is formed, it is not the "hole" in the tendon that is painful but what is around the "perforation" (LBT (long biceps tendon), SADB), and it is these elements that are interesting to analyze to determine the causes of painful symptomatology. For this reason, as ruptures are frequently bilateral, it is the analysis of the opposite cuff that is the essential element of the workup because it is the difference between the two ruptures that will determine what is the factor causing the pain.

To perform a rupture check on ultrasound:

- It is measured in the frontal and anteroposterior plane.
- The number of lesioned tendons is determined; in order to determine whether the rupture extends to the infraspinatus, this is based on the angulation between the facets of the greater tubercle in the sagittal plane or a rupture size greater than 2 cm in this plane because this value corresponds to the width of the anteroposterior insertion of the supraspinatus.
- A preserved anterior supraspinatus fragment is detected, which is a favorable element because, by its thickness, it protects the long head of the biceps from contact with the lower slope of the acromion.
- Intra-articular effusion or bursitis is sought to explain the etiology of the painful symptomatology because these elements often accompany a mild rupture.
- There is also an associated tendinopathy of the long head of the biceps (another cause of mild damage in case of rupture), especially in relation to the upper pole of the humeral head (see chapter tendinopathy) as well as:
- The existence of a posterior cleavage in the thickness of the infraspinatus tendon to be sought in the external rotation of the arm so as not to collide the edges of this cleavage.

- An associated disinsertion of the subscapularis whose presence may alter the therapeutic strategy.
- Anteroposterior instability is detected by performing a rotational maneuver on a posterior axial section because an unstable humeral head in the anteroposterior plane is a sign of unfavorable evolution.
- Similarly, fatty degeneration of the fleshy bodies of the supra and infraspinatus, since significant damage (higher than grade 2 of the Bernageau and Goutallier classification) may cause a surgical repair to be rejected [43]. The lack of complete visualization of the subscapularis muscle is, on the other hand, a limiting factor of ultrasound and does not allow a complete assessment of the rupture when it has an earlier extension.

These transfixing ruptures rarely undertake the infraspinatus in isolation except after anteroinferior dislocation in relation to the impaction detected on the posterosuperior side of the humeral head. Ultrasound semiology is then similar to that described above. Damage to the myotendinous junction of this muscle is sometimes detected, especially after repeated infiltration.

Chronic disinsertions of the subscapularis, often asymptomatic, can occur in isolation, especially when a traumatic history (back fall, epileptic seizure, etc.) is found at the anamnesis. Most often, they prolong a rupture of the supraspinatus and rotator interval, which is an unfavorable prognosis because the long head of the biceps is affected as well as the anterior stability of the joint due to the loss of this anterior shroud. The ultrasound aspect of chronic lesion of the subscapularis is the disappearance of the tendon "stripping" the anterior facet of the lesser tubercle.

1.14 Partial Ruptures

Rupture of one of the sides of the supraspinatus, as well as partial disinsertion of the individual, is also frequently asymptomatic, and its frequency increases with the age of patients. In these cases

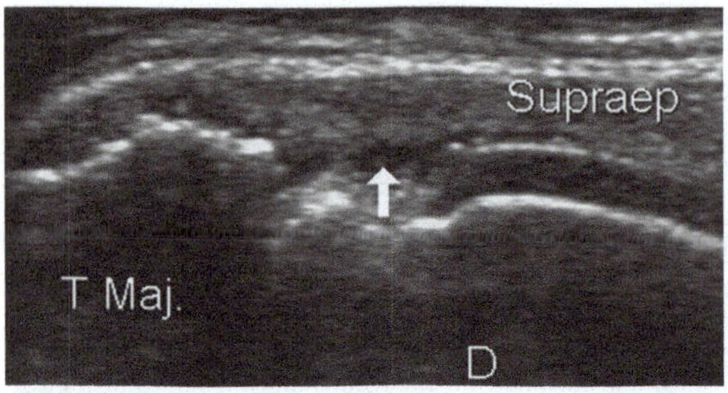

Fig. 1.27 Disinsertion of deep fibers with shrinkage and thinning of the insertion area

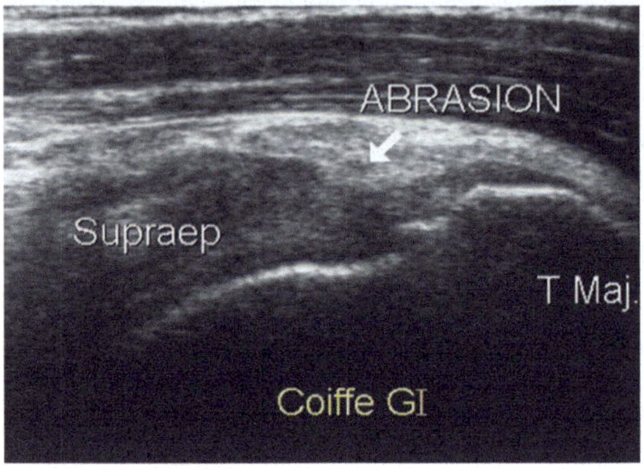

Fig. 1.28 Abrasion of the supraspinatus surface in chronic impingement

too, the effusion, associated signs, and comparison on the opposite side will make it possible to assert the symptomatic character of these ruptures [1, 16, 24].

Lesions of the articular side. In the chronic stage, this type of lesion leads to a thinning of the insertion zone with "bare" appearance of the medial portion of the facet (Fig. 1.27). A cleavage is often visible in the depth of the insertion area.

Lesions of the superficial slope are practically always located at the supraspinatus. Two types of ultrasound images can be visible, systematically accompanied by bursitis when the lesion is symptomatic:

- An irregularity, or even a digging zone, at a distance from the facet, in case of chronic anterosuperior impingement "abrading" the surface slope (Fig. 1.28).

Peripheral disinsertion similar to that described in acute lesions

These two types of lesions must be differentiated because the second (peripheral disinsertion) does not have any impingement during the dynamic test and its treatment is therefore different.

Both peripheral and deep damage can also be seen in the chronic stage. In some cases, only a few fibers persist, which explains the painful symptom because all the pulling forces concentrate on these few remaining fibers.

Purely intratendinous damage is visualized as a central hypoechogenic zone extending by an intratendinous fissure respecting the peripheral slopes of the tendon. This type of lesion is best detected when the tendon is relaxed with slight abduction. No effusion is added in these intratendinous cleavages, and their symptomatic character is therefore difficult to assert.

1.14.1 Calcifying Tendon Disease

Calcification images are frequently found on X-ray photographs; the predominance of female images is known, which mainly affect the shoulders of patients aged 30–60 years. Vascular origin is sometimes advanced to explain the occurrence of these calcifications, which in our experiment predominate (such as ruptures) in the posterior part of the supraspinatus. The existence of an evolutionary cycle has been proposed to explain the occurrence and disappearance of these calcifications which pass successively through a stage of formation followed by a state phase where calcification is stable to arrive at the stage of fragmentation allowing resorption of calcium deposits [5].

In addition to the often significant pain accompanying the resorption phase (see above), this calcification can be symptomatic in two different ways:

- By "irritating" the neighboring tendon that becomes hypoechogenic and sometimes hypervascular in power Doppler when calcification breaks and resorbs.

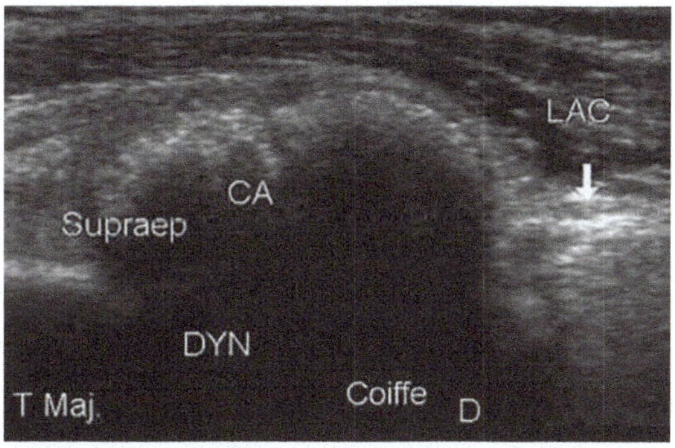

Fig. 1.29 Voluminous hypertrophic calcification causing an impingement resulting from tendon hypertrophy

- When calcification is hypertrophic causing anterosuperior impingement (Fig. 1.29).

Ultrasound is also used to guide a possible puncture/washout of this calcification [16, 28, 29, 44], the effectiveness of which is recognized by everyone to date.

1.14.2 Tendinopathy

Tendinopathy is mainly degenerative with several etiologies and should be discussed with caution in ultrasound. The term "tendinitis" must be banned because the inflammatory component is in fact virtually zero; it is above all the difference with the opposite side that allows us to discover an echostructure modification with disorganization of the fibrillar structure, sometimes hypertrophic and the presence of ranges hyper and hypoechogenic plaques at the origin distinctly heterogeneous in appearance [38, 44]. It must be differentiated from enthesopathy because tendinopathy takes the whole tendon and not just the enthesis.

We sometimes find a very hypoechogenic appearance of this tendon, which seems to us to constitute a stage of pre-rupture (Fig. 1.30).

Late, punctiform hyperechogenic calcifications, rarely interrupting the ultrasonic wave, may appear following an acidophilic necrosis reaction; they are associated with a very fragile stage of tendon degeneration. These calcifications should not be punctured, and this appear-

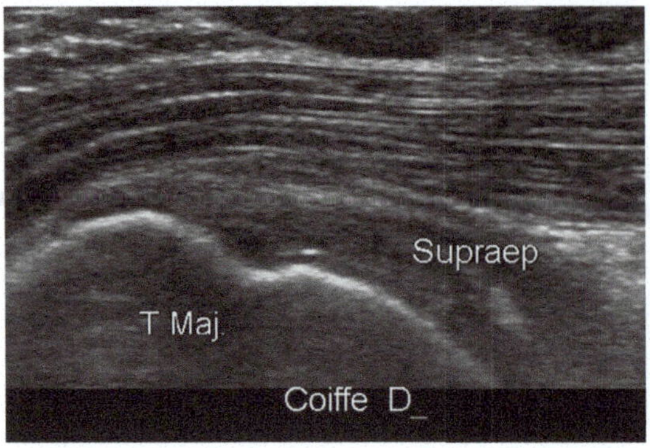

Fig. 1.30 Hypoechogenic tendinopathy corresponding to a pre-rupture stage

ance of calcium punctuation is completely different from the calcifying tendon disease described above.

Moreover, this hypertrophic character of the tendon in this case must be distinguished from a normal tendon covered with a thickened bursa as can be seen in case of impingement because the therapeutic direction is different; this tendinopathy does not involve an inflammatory lesion such as bursitis. The perfect visualization of the superficial side of the tendon is therefore extremely important to differentiate these two types of lesions (see technical chapter).

Bicipital tendinopathy often causes severe pain and needs to be identified.

LBT (long biceps tendon) tendinopathy is rarely an inflammatory process (less than 10%, according to Streit [45]) but most often a degenerative process. On the other hand, it is accompanied by peritendinous inflammatory damage, and, in the chronic phase, both are associated, especially since inflammation leads to fibrous degeneration, associated with a decrease in tendinoblastic capacity and an increase in pain mediators such as calcitonin gene-related peptide (CGRP) or substance P [46]. This tendinopathy can be complicated by fissures (well differentiated from duplication or ancillary insertion of the supraspinatus).

Partial and total ruptures are then observed.

Considering the severe pain caused by tendinopathy and the nonfunctional appearance of the "inflamed" tendon, this rupture is often considered as "saving" because, like the tendon section, it ends a long painful period.

In addition to glenoid insertion lesions (SLAP), this tendinopathy should be investigated along the entire length of the tendon. In ultrasound, the signs are [47, 48]:

- Loss of fibrillar structure.
- A decrease in anisotropy artifact.
- Hypoechogenic appearance of the tendon.
- Swelling at the level of the groove or upper pole of the head compared to the opposite side. Renoux showed in ultrasound that the maximum thickness of the tendon was 2.5 mm at the upper pole of the head [49]. When hypertrophy is important at the upper pole, the tendon may have an "hourglass" appearance and no longer mobilize correctly at the upper part of the groove because it "gets stuck" at this level due to its hypertrophy during abduction of the arm [50].
- Thinning can, paradoxically, also be a sign of tendinopathy (most often severe). Like the posterior tibial tendon that stretches in case of pre-rupture, thinning by "stretching" can be visualized in chronic tendinopathies as shown by Rasselet [51] (Fig. 1.31). This sign can be distinguished from flattening and is therefore valid only in the absence of compression of the LBT (long biceps tendon) on a hard base (caused by isolated retropulsion of the arm without external rotation for the upper part and by retropulsion of the elbow for the vertical part) because these positions can lead to a flattening especially in case of a pathological tendon (more deformable).
- A cleavage (longitudinal cracking) not to be confused with duplication or ancillary insertion [52] (Fig. 1.32).
- A synovial thickening (sometimes vascularized with Doppler) surrounding the tendon in its vertical portion (Fig. 1.33).

Other factors that may promote the development of LBT (long biceps tendon) tendinopathy should be investigated:

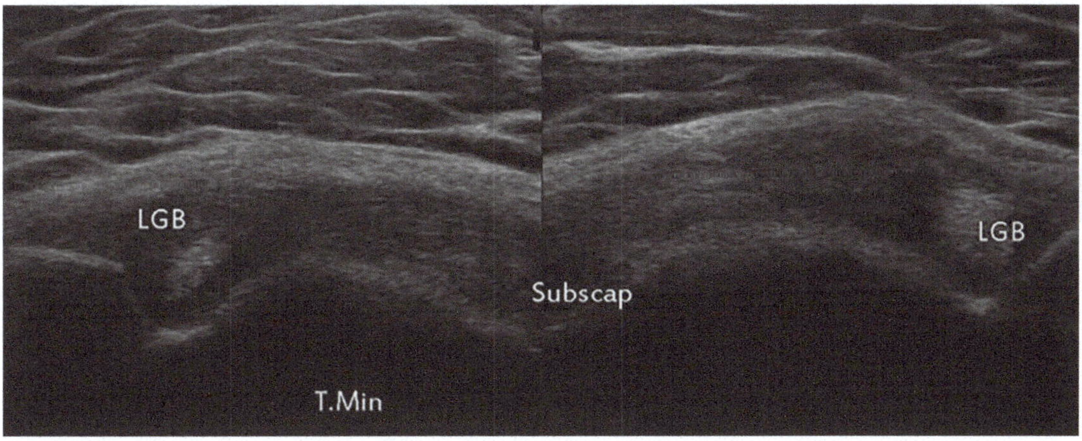

Fig. 1.31 Thinning of the right LGB (long biceps tendon) on this comparative axial section evoking stretching to be related to severe tendinopathy

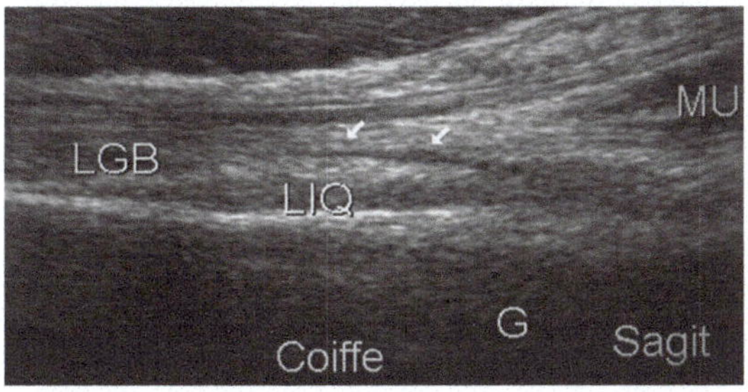

Fig. 1.32 Cracking of the LGB (long biceps tendon) close here to the myotendinous junction

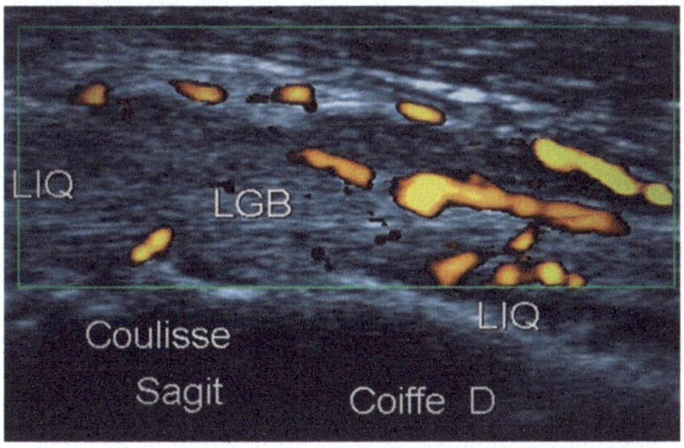

Fig. 1.33 Significant vascularized synovitis from the bicipital recess

- An osteochondromatous nodule incarcerated within the bicipital recess.
- A disinsertion of the subscapularis causing subluxation of the LBT (long biceps tendon)

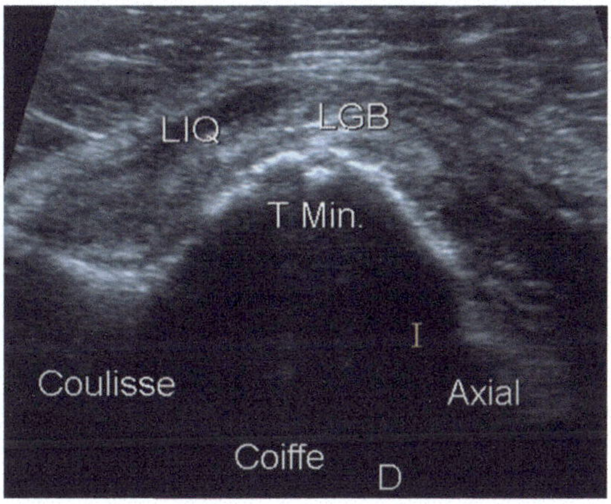

Fig. 1.34 LGB (long biceps tendon) tendinopathy spread over the medial edge of the groove due to partial disinsertion of the subscapularis

or its "spread" on the medial edge of the groove [53] (Fig. 1.34). In case of tendon malposition, the most important sign to look for is the disappearance of the hypoechogenic triangle normally present between the tendon and the medial side of the groove.
- A rupture of the cuff reaching the anterior portion of the supraspinatus because it often accommodates a disinsertion of the lateral bundle of the LCH, resulting in an impingement between the LBT (long biceps tendon) and the acromio-coracoidal ligament or even the underside of the acromion.

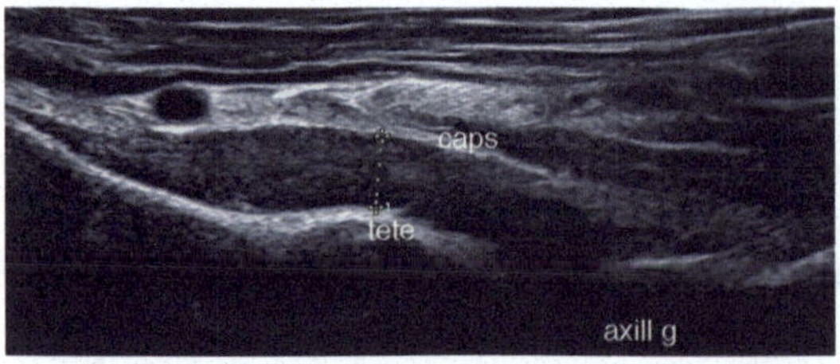

Fig. 1.35 Thickness of capsulosynovial folds on axillary view

1.14.3 Adhesive Capsulitis

Common in diabetics, but can also occur in other patients especially postoperatively, after trauma or after illness or emotional shock, capsulitis develops for about 2 years. It begins with an inflammatory phase affecting all shoulder structures (tendon, synovial, capsule bursa) during which the clinical symptomatology is often noisy, contrasting with the poverty of the signs detected on ultrasound:

- Discreet intra-articular effusion.
- Hypoechoic halo surrounding LBT (long biceps tendon).
- Greater vascularization of rotator interval and recess region under coracoid.
- Thickening of the axillary recess compared to the opposite side (Fig. 1.35).

These signs are inconsistent, and it is more the echoclinical disproportion that must attract attention and suggest the diagnosis that is important to make at this early inflammatory stage and to confirm it as soon as possible by arthro-infiltration, in order to reduce pain and thus facilitate rehabilitative treatment [16].

Then, the retraction phase sets in, and the diagnosis is purely clinical, only an important omarthrosis easily discovered on standard images can also be the cause of such painful retraction.

1.15 Conclusion

A difficult but highly performing examination, shoulder ultrasound is an ideal complement to standard radiological X-rays. It takes stock of tendon lesions and makes it possible to dismantle the catch-all term of scapulohumeral periarthritis because it often explains the exact cause of the painful symptomatology, allowing the treatment to be directed in a specific way. On the other hand, it requires great rigor, systematization in the conduct of the examination, and above all a high-end device that alone allows the reliable study of these pathologies.

References

1. Brasseur JL, Lucidarme O, Tardieu M, et al. Ultrasonographic rotator-cuff changes in veteran tennis players: the effect of hand dominance and comparison with clinical findings. Eur Radiol. 2004;14(5):857–64.
2. Sher JS, Uribe JW, Posada A, Murphy BJ, Zlatkin MB. Abnormal findings on magnetic resonance images of asymptomatic shoulders. J Bone Joint Surg Am. 1995;77:10–5.
3. Milgrom C, Schaffler M, Gilbert S, van Holsbeeck M. Rotator-cuff changes in asymptomatic adults. The effect of age, hand dominance and gender. J Bone Joint Surg Br. 1995;77:296–8.
4. Tempelhof S, Rupp S, Seil R. Age-related prevalence of rotator cuff tears in asymptomatic shoulders. J Shoulder Elbow Surg. 1999;8:296–9.
5. Uhthoff H, Sarkar K. Calcifying tendonitis. In: Rockwood CA, Matsen FA, editors. The shoulder. Philadelphia: WB Saunders; 1990. p. 774–90.
6. Leroux JL. Diagnostic and pre-therapeutic imaging (medical or surgical) in front of a soft shoulder with a sign of conflict. Reflect Rheumatol. 2001;5(35):13–9.
7. Railhac JJ, Sans N, Rigal A, et al. Radiography of the shoulder from the face of the shoulder in the supine position: interest in the assessment of ruptures of the rotator cuff. J Radiol. 2001;82(9):979–85.
8. Sintzoff S. Diagnostic value of simple X-rays in shoulder pathology (calcifications, tendinopathies, ruptures of the cuff, retractile capsulitis, instability, osteoarthritis)?: necessary and sufficient impact, cost, irradiation. Rev Rum. 1997;64(2bis):3S–10S.
9. Dinnes J, Loverman E, McIntyre L, Waugh N. The effectiveness of diagnostic tests for the assessment of shoulder pain due to soft tissue disorders: a systematic review. Health Technol Assess. 2003;7(29):iii.
10. Leroux JL, Thomas E, Bonnel F, Blotman F. Diagnostic value of clinical tests for shoulder impingement syndrome. Rev Rhum Engl Ed. 1995;62(6):423–8.
11. Naredo E, Aguado P, De Miguel E, et al. Painful shoulder: comparison of physical examination and ultrasonographic findings. Ann Rheum Dis. 2002;61(2):132–6.
12. Nyffeller RW, Werber C, Sukthankar A, Schmid MR, Gerber C. Association of a large lateral extension of

the acromion with rotator cuff tears. J Bone Joint Surg Am. 2006;88(4):800–5.
13. Allen GM, Wilson DJ. Ultrasound of the shoulder. Eur J Ultrasound. 2001;14(1):3–9.
14. Brewer JL. Value of ultrasonography in the pathology of the shoulder. Rev Rhum (Ed.Fr.). 1997:64(2bis):11–8.
15. Martinoli C, Bianchi S, Prato N, Pugliese F, Zamorani MP, Valle M, Derchi LE. US of the shoulder: non-rotator cuff disorders. Radiographics. 2003;23(2):381–401.
16. Brewer JL, Montagnon D, Hacquard B, Tardieu M. Osteo-articular ultrasound: shoulder. J Radiol. 2000;81(3 Suppl):330–45.
17. Farin PU, Jaroma H. Acute traumatic tears of the rotator cuff: value of sonography. Radiology. 1995;197:269–73.
18. Teefey SA, Middleton WD, Bauer GS, Hildebolt CF, Yamaguchi K. Sonographic differences in the appearance of acute and chronic full-thickness rotator cuff tears. J Ultrasound Med. 2000;19(6):377–8.
19. Wang CL, Shieh JY, Wang GT, Hsieh FJ. Sonographic detection of occult fractures in the foot and ankle. J Clin Ultrasound. 1999;27:421–5.
20. Schweitzer ME, Magbalon MJ, Fenlin JM, Frieman BG, Ehrlich S, Epstein RE. Effusion criteria and clinical importance of glenohumeral joint fluid: MR imaging evaluation. Radiology. 1995;194:821–4.
21. van Holsbeeck M, Strose PJ. Sonography of the shoulder: evaluation of the subacromial-subdeltoid bursa. AJR Am J Roentgen. 1993;160:561–4.
22. Hollister MS, Mack LA, Patten RM, Winter TC 3rd., Matsen FA 3rd., Veith RR. Association of sonographically detected subacromial/subdeltoid bursal effusion and intraarticular fluid with rotator cuff tear. AJR Am J Roentgen. 1995;165:605–8.
23. Arslan G, Apaydin A, Kabaalioglu A, Sindel T, Luleci E. Sonographically detected subacromial/subdeltoid bursal effusion and biceps tendon sheath fluid: reliable signs of rotator cuff tear. J Clin Ultrasound. 1999;27:335–9.
24. van Holsbeeck MT, Kolowich PA, Eyler WR, Craig JG, Shirazi KK, Habra GK, Vanderschueren GM, Buff JA. US depiction of partial-thickness tear of the rotator cuff. Radiology. 1995;19:443–6.
25. Azaïez-Mathari A, Lemary JB, Zeitoun-Eiss D, Brewer JL. Sono anatomy of the tendon of the head along the biceps. In: Brasseur JL, Zeitoun-Eiss D, Dion E, editors. News in ultrasound of the musculoskeletal system. Montpellier: Sauramps Medical; 2004. p. 229–45.
26. Ptasznik R, Hennessy O. Abnormalities of the biceps tendon of the shoulder: sonographic findings. AJR Am J Roentgen. 1995;164:409–14.
27. Zanetti M, Pfirrmann CW. Biceps tendon disorders: ultrasound, MR imaging and MR arthrography. Radiologe. 2004;44(6):591–6.
28. Farin PU, Jaroma H, Harju A, Soimakallio S. Medial displacement of the biceps brachii tendon: evaluation with dynamic sonographic during maximal external shoulder rotation. Radiology. 1995;195:845–8.
29. Sarrat P, Cohen M, Charasset S, Goddé J, Francheschi JP, Aswad R. Lithotrities focus on treating calcifying tendinopathies. J Radiol. 2004;85(10):1721–5.
30. Farin PU, Jaroma H. Sonographic findings or rotator cuff calcifications. J Ultrasound Med. 1995;14:7–14.
31. Zanetti M, Holder J. Imaging of degenerative and posttraumatic disease in the shoulder joint with ultrasound. Eur J Radiol. 2000;35:119–25.
32. Guerini H, Campagna R, Thévenin F, Vuillemin V, Demondion X, Morvan G, Drape JL. The sign of "double cortical" in small ruptures of the tendon of the supraspinatus. In: Brasseur JL, Mercy G, Massein A, Grenier P, editors. News in ultrasound of the musculoskeletal system, vol. 11. Montpellier: Sauramps Médical; 2014. p. 143–52.
33. Brewer JL, Lazennec JY, Tardieu M, Richard O, Roger B, Grenier P. Dynamic ultrasound of the shoulder in the antero-superior conflict. Rev Im Med. 1994;6:629–31.
34. Gerber C, Terrier F, Zehnder R, Ganz R. The subcoracoid space. An anatomic study. Clin Orthop. 1987;215:132–8.
35. Walch G, Liotard JP, Boileau P, Noël E. The postero-superior glenoid conflict: another shoulder conflict. Rev Chir Orthop. 1991;77:571–4.
36. Jacobson JA, Lancaster S, Prasad A, van Holsbeeck MT, Craig JG, Kolowich P. Full-thickness supraspinatus tendon tears: value of US signs in diagnosis. Radiology. 2004;230(1):234–42.
37. Teefey SA, Rubin DA, Middleton WD, Hildebolt CF, Leibold RA, Yamaguchi K. Detection and quantification of rotator cuff tears. Comparison of ultrasonographic, magnetic resonance imaging, and arthroscopic findings in threeseven consecutive cases. J Bone Joint Surg Am. 2004;86A(4):708–16.
38. van Moppes FI, Veldkamp O, Roorda J. Role of shoulder ultrasonography in the evaluation of the painful shoulder. Eur J Radiol. 1995;19:142–6.
39. Wohlwend JR, van Holsbeeck M, Craig J, Shirazi K, Habra G, Jacobsen G, Bouffard JA. The association between irregular greater tuberosities and rotator cuff tears: a sonographic study. Am J Roentgenol. 1998;171:229–33.
40. Bryant L, Shnier R, Bryant C, Murrell GA. A comparison of clinical estimation, ultrasonography, magnetic resonance imaging and arthroscopy in determining the size of the rotator cuff tears. J Shoulder Elbow Surg. 2002;11(3):219–24.
41. Kluger R, Mayrhofer R, Kroner A, et al. Sonographic versus magnetic resonance arthrographic evaluation of full-thickness rotator cuff tears in millimeters. J Shoulder Elbow Surg. 2003;12(2):110–6.
42. Swen WA, Jacobs JW, Algra PR, et al. Sonography and magnetic resonance imaging equivalent for assessment of full-thickness rotator cuff tears. Arthritis Rheum. 1999;42(1):2231–8.

43. Goutalier D, Postel JM, Lavau I, Bernageau J. The fat degeneration of the muscles of the broken ten-dineuse cuff of the shoulder. Rev Rhum. 1995;62:439–46.
44. Aina R, Cardinal E, Office NJ, Aubin P, Armband P. Calcific shoulder tendinitis: treatment with modified US-guided fine-needle technique. Radiology. 2001;221(2):455–61.
45. Streit JJ, Shishani Y, Rodgers Nakata W, Katou S, Fujita A, Nakata M, Lefor AT, Sugimoto H. Biceps pulley: normal anatomy and associated lesions at MR arthrography. Radiographics. 2011;31(3):791–810.
46. Murthi AM, Vosburgh CL, Neviaser TJ. The incidence of pathologic changes of the long head of the biceps tendon. J Shoulder Elbow Surg. 2000;9(5):382–5.
47. Brewer JL. The biceps tendons: from the top and from the bottom. J Ultrasound. 2012;15(1):29–38.
48. Renoux J, Mercy G, Brewer JL. The bicipital tendon in the interval and the slides. In: Vuillemin V, Lapège F, Collin P, et al., editors. The shoulder of the classic to the new. Montpellier: Sauramps Médical; 2016. p. 219–30.
49. Renoux J, Zeitoun-Eiss D, Brewer JL. Tendinopathy of the head along the biceps: imaging contribution. In: Brasseur JL, Zeitoun-Eiss D, Renoux J, Grenier P, editors. News in ultrasound of the musculoskeletal system, vol. 3. Montpellier: Sauramps Médical; 2006. p. 201–14.
50. Boileau P, Ahrens PM, Hatzidakis AM. Entrapment oft to the long head of the biceps tendon: the hourglass bicepsa cause pain and locking of the shoulder. J Shoulder Elbow Surg. 2004;13(3):249–57.
51. Rasselet B, Cyteval C. Ultrasound of the long biceps: correlation with arthroscopy. In: Brasseur JL, Mercy G, Monzani Q, Grenier P, editors. News in ultrasound of the musculoskeletal system, vol. 12. Montpellier: Medical Sauramps; 2015. p. 159–71.
52. Moser TP, Cardinal E, Bureau NJ, Guillin R, Lanneville P, Grabs D. The aponeurotic expansion of the supraspinatus tendon: anatomy and prevalence in a series of 150 shoulder MRI. Skeletal Radiol. 2015;44(2):223–31.
53. Walch G, Nové-Josserand L, Boileau P, Levigne C. Subluxations and dislocations of the tendon of the long head of the biceps. J Shoulder Elbow Surg. 1998;7(2):100–8.

Ultrasound of the Tendon of the Long Biceps Operated

2

H. Ghersi, O. Marès, R. Coulomb, A. Laborde, and L. Moscato

2.1 Biceps Brachial Muscle in Ultrasound

The biceps is inserted on the scapula proximally and on the forearm distally; the biceps brachial muscle has several tendons that exhibit several anatomical features making their ultrasound study very "varied." Proximally, the tendon of the short head of the biceps presents a straight path and inserts at coracoid level; no lesions are to our knowledge described at this level. The tendon of the long head of the biceps inserts on the upper slope of the glenoid, has a virtually horizontal path to the superior pole of the humeral head, and passes within the rotator intervals. Then, before entering the intertubercular bicipital groove, it has an angulation that results from the rotation of the humerus.

Distally, an Italian-Canadian study [1] showed that the distal tendon insertion on the radial tuberosity is bifid; thanks to the presence of a bursa allowing a harmonious sliding, it wraps around this tuberosity during prono-supination. In addition to this bifid tendon, there is a third structure distally, the lacertus fibrosus, aponeurotic lamina detached from the medial side of the tendon. It crosses over the humeral artery and the median nerve to insert into the superficial fascia of the flexor muscles.

Bridging the scapulohumeral joint and elbow joint, the biceps muscle, bi-articular, "passes" to the anterior side of the arm having only an aponeurotic attachment with the brachialis located on its deep slope. The ultrasound study can therefore be divided into nine areas of interest:

1. Long head's attachment on the glenoid
2. Passage to the upper pole of the head
3. Rotator interval
4. Reflection at the top of the bicipital groove
5. Behind the scenes
6. Upper myotendinous junction
7. Lower myotendinous junction
8. Distal tendon(s)
9. Lower enthesis

This article deals only with points 1–5.

2.2 Insertion of the Long Head of the Biceps to the Upper Pole of the Glenoid and on the Upper Labrum

This insertion has many anatomical variants; the most important for the ultrasound practitioner is its anterior or posterior topography, since only

H. Ghersi
CHU Nîmes, Nîmes, France

O. Marès (✉) · R. Coulomb · A. Laborde · L. Moscato
Department of Conservative and Traumatological Surgery, Spine Surgery, CHU Carémeau, Nîmes, France

T. Apard, J. L. Brasseur (eds.), *Ultrasonography for the Upper Limb Surgeon*,
https://doi.org/10.1007/978-3-030-84234-5_2

previous insertions are accessible to ultrasound by putting the arm in retropulsion and external rotation.

Thanks to Mathari [2], the relationship between the topography of this insertion and the depth of the bicipital groove was analyzed. The more posterior the insertion is, the deeper the groove. It is only possible to visualize the insertion of the supra-spinatus and subscapularis tendons surmounting a little groove with an anterior insertion with the probe at the anterior part of the shoulder.

Ultrasound is also very limited in this area, and no precise lesion diagnosis can be performed. Hypoechogenic swelling compared to the opposite side may be considered as an indirect sign of insertion pathology of the long head of the biceps (SLAP) justifying the use of another technique (Arthro-MRI or Arthro-CT in this case) to confirm the diagnosis [3].

2.3 Transition to the Upper Pole of the Head

With the arm in the same position (retropulsion and external rotation), a long perpendicular cut is performed at the height of the cephalic cartilage; this cut must be comparative. Renoux [4] showed that a tendon of more than 2.5 mm thick at this level is pathological (Fig. 2.1). This is a valuable sign because this type of bicipital tendinopathy is difficult to highlight.

Other ultrasound signs are pain when passing the probe and a clash of the tendon at the entrance to the bicipital groove, shown by Boileau [5], because the thickened tendon cannot fit into the groove when the arm is raised (hourglass effect).

2.4 Passage in the Interval of the Rotators

The long head then passes into the space separating the supraspinatus (posterolateral) from the subscapularis (anteromedial); this passage is covered by the coracohumeral ligament. The latter merges with the upper glenohumeral ligament to form a strap preventing the medial dislocation of the tendon (Fig. 2.1).

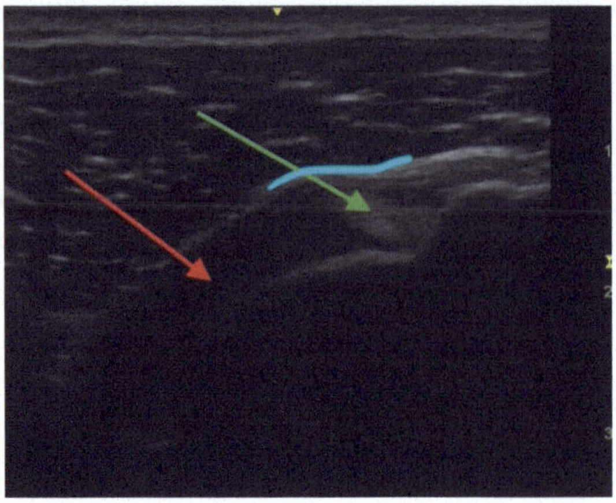

Fig. 2.1 Ligamentous strap holding the tendon of the long head within the interval. The strap is formed of the coracohumeral ligament (blue) in surface, biceps (green arrow), and subscapularis (red arrow)

Tendinopathies of the long head can be observed at this level mainly in case of rupture affecting the anterior part of the supraspinatus. This causes a retraction of the coracohumeral ligament, and the tendon directly conflicts with the lower slope of the acromion generating microtraumas inducing tendinopathy [6].

The tendon is thickened, hypoechoic, and its contours are less well defined (Fig. 2.4); this pathology is associated with inflammatory painful phenomena. A tendon rupture may result in a significant decrease in painful symptomatology but may cause an ascent of the head disrupting scapulohumeral mobility. In addition to tendinopathy and rupture, disinsertion or rupture of the coracohumeral ligament may also cause a dislocation of the long head of the biceps on the anterior part of the subscapularis (Fig. 2.2). Traumatic ligament lesions and calcifications can also generate pain in the area of the interval, and it should not be forgotten that an increase in the thickness of the coracohumeral ligament is an excellent indirect sign of adhesive capsulitis as we learned from Homsi [7].

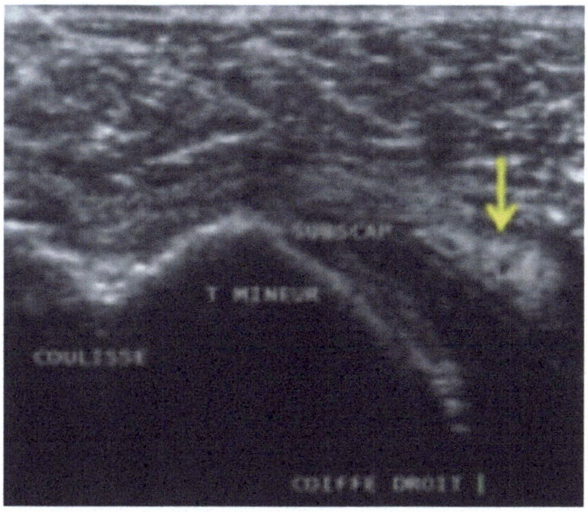

Fig. 2.2 Coracohumeral ligament rupture causing a dislocation of the long head of the biceps on the anterior slope of the subscapularis

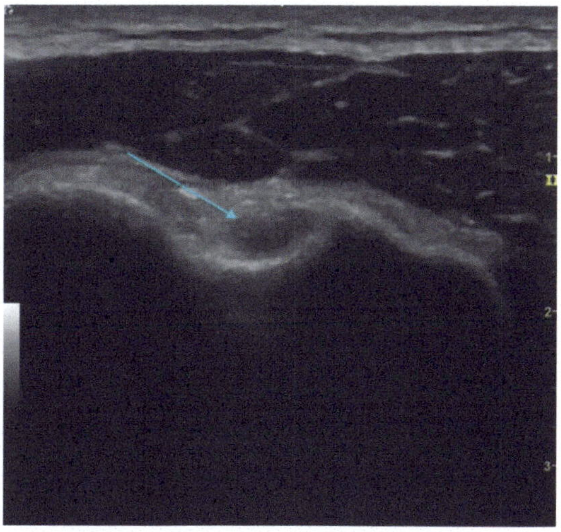

Fig. 2.3 Biceps in its groove: blue arrow

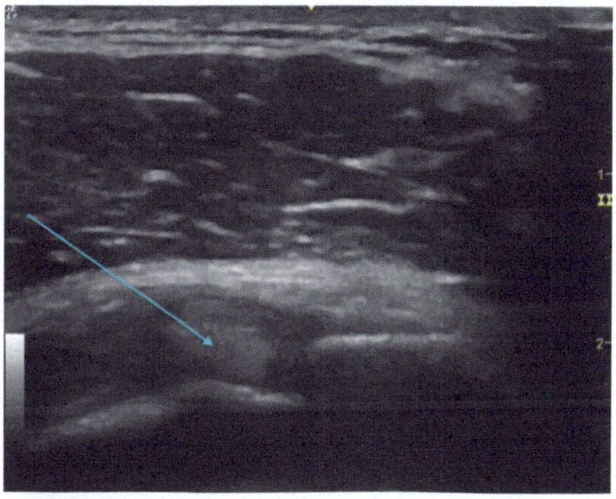

Fig. 2.4 Biceps subluxed: blue arrow

2.5 Reflection at the Top of the Groove

Tendon subluxation is the main pathological element to be sought at this level. It is favored by angulation of the tendon generating its attraction medially. The ligament strap of the interval is a holding element of the biceps, at the upper part of the groove. The integrity of the subscapularis, inserted on its medial side, is a major factor of stability, and its superficial fascia lines the groove and inserts into its lateral side; this expansion constitutes the transverse humeral ligament.

The depth of the groove is the other element of stability at this level [2]. The ultrasonographic element sought is the hypoechoic triangle, consisting of collagen histologically [2], between the tendon of the long head and the medial edge of the upper end of the bicipital groove. This triangle is present regardless of the depth of the groove. Its presence signs the correct position of the tendon of the head, and its disappearance is an excellent indirect sign of subluxation.

The disinsertion of the subscapularis is the other element to be sought; it is favored by the fasciculation of this tendon facilitating partial disinsertion, which often begins in front of the upper part of the groove and then extends downwards. The tendon of the long head then "spreads out" on the medial border, then subluxes itself on the anterior facet of the lesser tubercle, and finally dislocates intra-articularly [3] (Figs. 2.3 and 2.4). This results in bicipital tendinopathy. Partial disinsertion can be detected by dynamic analysis of the shoulder under ultrasound guidance by instructing the patient to perform an internal rotation agents resistance to detect instability at a minimum, especially in high-performance sports patients practicing throwing sports (handball, javelin) [8–10].

2.6 In the Background

Ultrasound visualization of the tendon is not always easy due to the anisotropic artifact and its oval section with a large oblique axis anteriorly and medially; in the longitudinal plane, the study plan must be sagittal oblique, and the tendon must be parallel to the probe requiring mobilization of the elbow forward. In the axial plane we look at the cross section surface and sharpness of the tendon contours, whereas in the longitudinal plane the fibrillar structure is the important element.

A peritendinous effusion, intra-articular, is often visible in the lower part of the bicipital recess since the examination is performed in a sitting position and the fluid mobilizes in a declining position. This is an indirect sign of joint, capsular, ligamentous, or capsulolabral pathology and sometimes bicipital tendinopathy.

This last point is absolutely not the rule because the tendon of the long head, enlarged by tendinopathy, can "occupy" the whole recess preventing the reactional effusion from collecting there. Signs of tendinopathy at this level are mainly the disappearance of the fibrillar structure in the longitudinal plane and the hypoechoic and heterogeneous thickening of the tendon in the axial plane; it often loses its oval section and becomes rounded (Fig. 2.5).

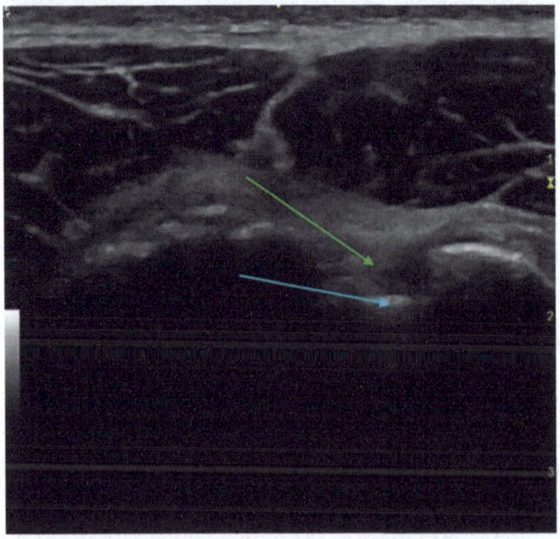

Fig. 2.5 Tenodesed biceps in its groove: biceps (green arrow), tenodesis anchor (blue arrow)

The causes of this bicipital tendinopathy are multiple: subluxation, foreign bodies, bone irregularities in the groove, sequelae of tenodesis, but also the presence of a cyst pushing back on the long head of the biceps.

2.7 Conclusion

The ultrasound-guided examination allows static and dynamic analysis of the biceps in its bicipital groove portion. Ultrasound also makes it possible to carry out ultrasound guidance infiltrations into the groove in case of localized inflammation and also to carry out tenotomy procedures with local anesthesia.

References

1. Tagliafico A, Michaud J, Capaccio E, Derchi LE, Martinoli C. Ultrasound demonstration of distal biceps tendon bifurcation: normal and abnormal findings. Eur Radiol. 2010;20(1):202–8.
2. Azaïez-Mathari A, Lemary JB, Zeitoun-Eiss D, Brewer JL. Sono anatomy of the tendon of the head along the biceps. In: Brasseur JL, Zeitoun-Eiss D, Dion E, editors. News in ultrasound of the musculoskeletal system. Montpellier: Sauramps Médical; 2004. p. 229–45.
3. Brewer JL. Input diagnosis of ultrasound in the pathology of the rotator cuff. In: Blum A, Tavernier T, Brasseur JL, Noël E, Walch G, Cotten A, Bard H, editors. The shoulder a multidisciplinary approach. Montpellier: Sauramps Médical; 2005. p. 149–70.
4. Renoux J, Zeitoun-Eiss D, Brewer JL. Tendinopathy of the head along the biceps: imaging contribution. In: Brasseur JL, Zeitoun-Eiss D, Renoux J, Grenier P, editors. News in ultrasound of the musculoskeletal system, vol. 3. Montpellier: Sauramps Médical; 2006. p. 201–14.
5. Boileau P, Ahrens PM, Hatzidakis AM. Entrapment oft to the long head of the biceps tendon: the hourglass bicepsa cause pain and locking of the shoulder. J Shoulder Elbow Surg. 2004;13(3):249–57.
6. Bianchi S, Martinoli C. Shoulder. In: Bianchi S, Carlo M, editors. Ultrasound of the musculoskeletal system. Berlin: Springer; 2009. p. 189–332.
7. Homsi C, Bordalo-Rodrigues M, da Silva JJ, Stump XM. Ultrasound in adhesive capsulitis of the shoulder: is the assessment of the coracohumeral

ligament a valuable diagnostic tool? Skelet Radiol. 2006;35(9):673–8.
8. Burkhart SS, Morgan CD, Kibler WB. Shoulder injuries in overhead athletes. Clin Sports Med. 2000;19(1):125–58.
9. Snyder SJ, Karzel RP, Del Pizzo W, Ferkel RD, Friedman MJ. SLAP lesions of the shoulder. Arthroscopy. 1990;6(4):274–9.
10. Ide J, Maeda S, Takagi K. Sports activity after arthroscopic superior labral repair using suture pulleys in overhead-throwing athletes. Am J Sports Med. 2005;33:507–14.

3 Ultrasound of Coracoid Process

A. Moraux

3.1 Introduction

The coracoid is a central structure of the anterior side of the shoulder involved in the acromioclavicular arch, acromioclavicular joint stability, and glenohumeral stability. It is the seat of many tendon and ligamentous insertions. While it is easily accessible to ultrasound over a whole part of its length, the coracoid process remains an unexplored element in routine ultrasound examination of the shoulder.

3.2 Anatomy

The coracoid is a bony, hook-shaped process developed at the expense of the anterior side of the scapula neck. It consists of a base, an ascending segment facing upwards and inwards, and a descending segment facing downwards and out (Fig. 3.1).

It is derived from two main ossification nuclei that merge around 15 years old with the scapula [1]. The angle and apex can be the seat of accessory ossification centers. Non-fusion should be differentiated from a pseudo-arthritis fracture [2]. The size and shape of the coracoid vary widely [3]. Anatomy and pathology can be segmented by the function:

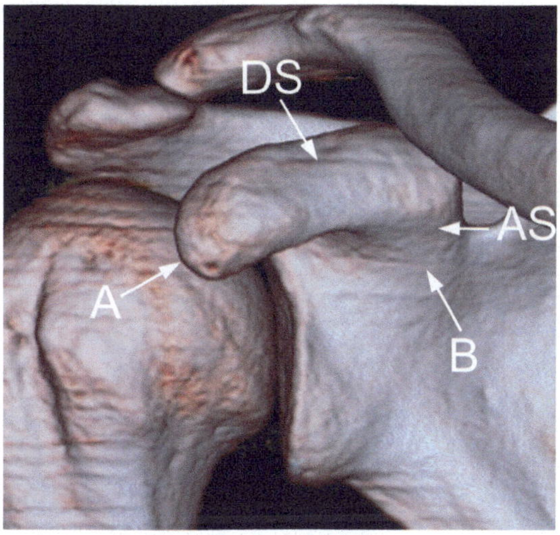

Fig. 3.1 Volume reconstruction of a shoulder scanner showing the different segments of the coracoid (*B* base, *As* ascending segment, *Ds* descending segment, *A* apex)

- Stabilization of the acromioclavicular joint on the upper side by coracoclavicular ligaments
- Stabilization of the glenohumeral joint by the coracohumeral ligament
- Procession under the coracoid on thc lower and deep slope
- Acromiodeltoid arch on the upper side with acromiocoracoid ligament
- Brachial muscle insertions: short head of the biceps (or coracobiceps), coracobrachialis, and pectoralis minor

A. Moraux (✉)
Medical Imaging Jacquemars Giélée, Lille, France

T. Apard, J. L. Brasseur (eds.), *Ultrasonography for the Upper Limb Surgeon*,
https://doi.org/10.1007/978-3-030-84234-5_3

3.3 Coracoid and Acromioclavicular Joint

3.3.1 Anatomy

On the upper and medial slope of the ascending segment of the coracoid, insert the extrinsic ligaments of the acromioclavicular joint, the trapezoid ligament outside, and the conoid ligament inside (Fig. 3.2) [4, 5]. At the clavicle, the trapezoid ligament is inserted on the trapezoid line, and the conoid ligament is inserted on the conoid tubercle. These ligaments form a fan with upper clavicular base and lower coracoid apex. They are responsible for the vertical and horizontal stability of the acromioclavicular joint.

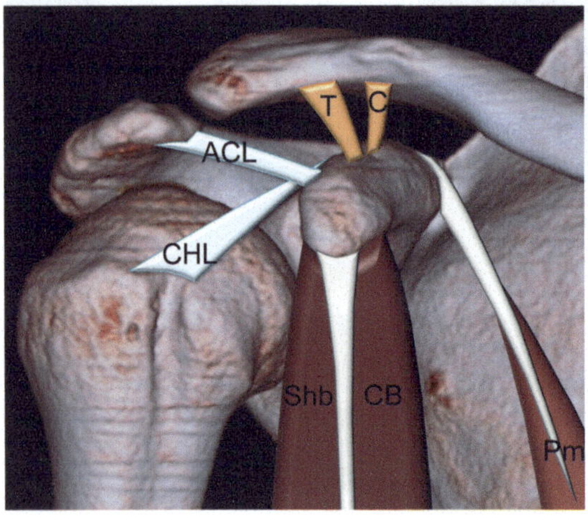

Fig. 3.2 Diagram of tendon and ligament inserts on the coracoid (*ACL* acromiocoracoid ligament, *CHL* coracohumeral ligament, *T* trapezoid ligament, *C* conoid ligament, *Shb* short head of the biceps, *CB* coracobrachial, *Pm* pectoralis minor)

3.3.2 Ultrasound Technique

These ligaments are deep and can be difficult to study. They are also silhouetted by hyperechogenic fat [6]. The positioning of the shoulder is crucial for their study; the retropulsion of the shoulder, hand on the buttock, and the elbow back greatly facilitate their study [7]. However, this position is difficult to achieve on a traumatized shoulder. The ligaments are visualized on the deep side of the deltoid just below the acromial vascular pedicle [8]. The trapezoid ligament is studied on an oblique sagittal oblique cut upward and outward (Fig. 3.3). The conoid ligament is studied on an oblique sagittal cut upward and inward (Fig. 3.4). The probe is initially placed in the axial plane, and its lateral edge is then turned toward the clavicle to obtain the longitudinal section of the trapezoid ligament, about 1 cm inside the acromioclavicular joint. The probe is then slightly translated and oblique within 20–30° to study the conoid ligament.

3.3.3 Pathology

3.3.3.1 Acromioclavicular Sprain

These ligaments can be lesioned in cases of acromioclavicular sprain. Their study makes it possible to differentiate grades 2 and 3 of the

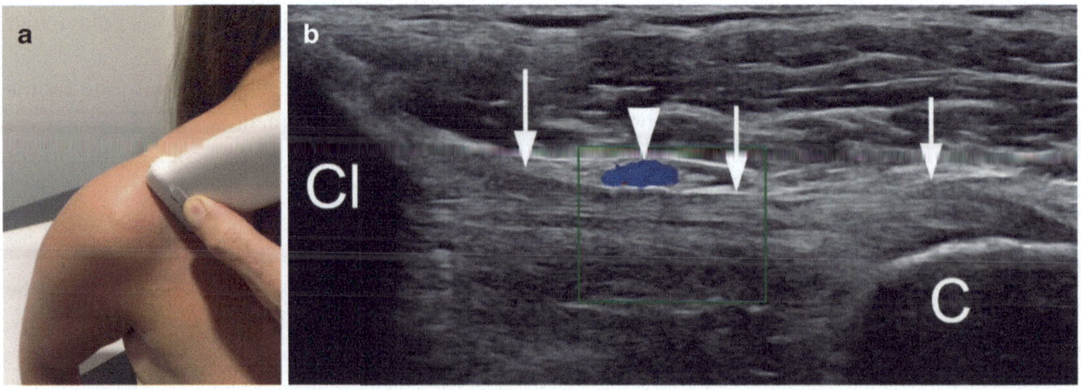

Fig. 3.3 (**a**) Position of the probe for the study of the trapezoid ligament and (**b**) corresponding ultrasound image showing the trapezoid ligament (arrows) under the acromial vascular pedicle (arrowhead) (*Cl* clavicle, *C* coracoid)

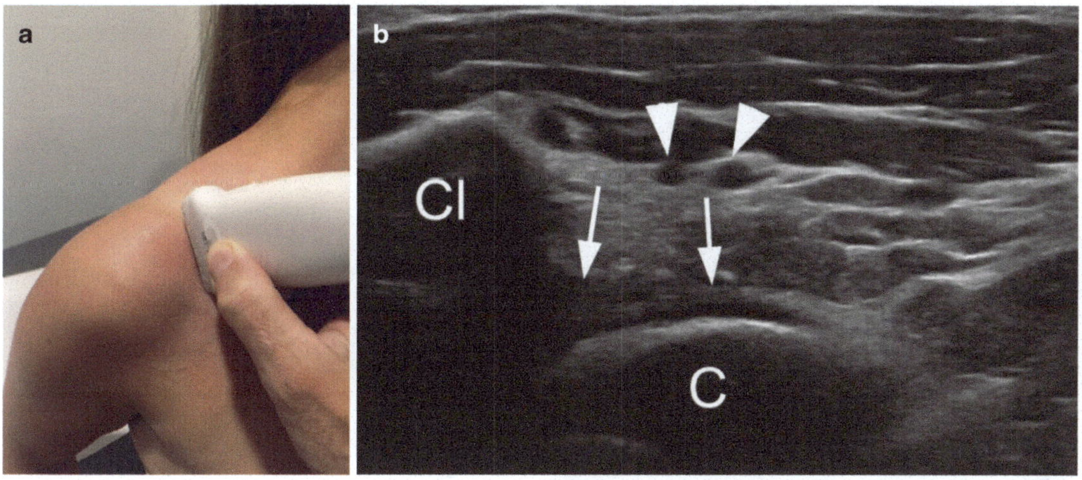

Fig. 3.4 (**a**) Position of the probe for the study of the conoid ligament and (**b**) correlating ultrasound image showing the conoid ligament (arrows) under the acromial vascular pedicle (arrowheads) (*Cl* clavicle, *C* coracoid)

Rockwood classification [9], a differentiation which is not reliable in radiography [10]. Ultrasound semiology is not specific; these ligaments can be elongated, ruptured (Fig. 3.5), or avulsed at their clavicular insertion as well as coracoid [11]. Even if these ligaments are not directly visualized, the increase in the coracoclavicular space on a comparative sagittal section should suggest their rupture [6].

3.4 Coracoid and Glenohumeral Joint

3.4.1 Anatomy

The coracoid serves as an anchor for the coracohumeral ligament (CHL). The CHL helps to strengthen the capsule of the interval of the rotators of which it is the keystone. It participates in the glenohumeral stability limiting the posterior-inferior translation of the humeral head [12]. Jost et al. [13] identified different functions for each anatomical component, with the medial part controlling the lower translation of the humeral head and the lateral part controlling the lateral rotation. LCH contributes to the stability of the long biceps tendon. It has the particularity of being histologically a capsular attachment and functionally a ligament [14]. This ligament is trapezoidal in shape; it inserts on the upper side of the coracoid. Its fibers can be separated into two quotas [13]. The medial band will merge with the superior glenohumeral ligament to support the medial and inferior slope of the intraarticular horizontal portion of the long biceps before inserting onto the lesser tubercle by merging with the upper fibers of the subscapularis. A number of anatomical variants are known for the interpretation of the pathology of the interval. The coracohumeral ligament would correspond to a remnant of the tendon of the pectoralis minor which initially passed in bridge over the coracoid to fit directly into the humeral head. In about 2–11% of the population, the pectoralis minor retains this vestigial insertion, which is responsible for a thickened appearance of the CHL [15, 16]. This ligament may also be absent.

3.4.2 Ultrasound Technique

The arm is placed in external rotation and discreet retropulsion. The proximal insertion of the medial bundle of the CHL is visible on the oblique sagittal section of the acromiocoracoid ligament, just below the coracoid insertion of this ligament (Fig. 3.6) [17].

Then it is sufficient to tilt the probe horizontally to lengthen the ligament body [18]. Once the main axis is identified, it can be studied and

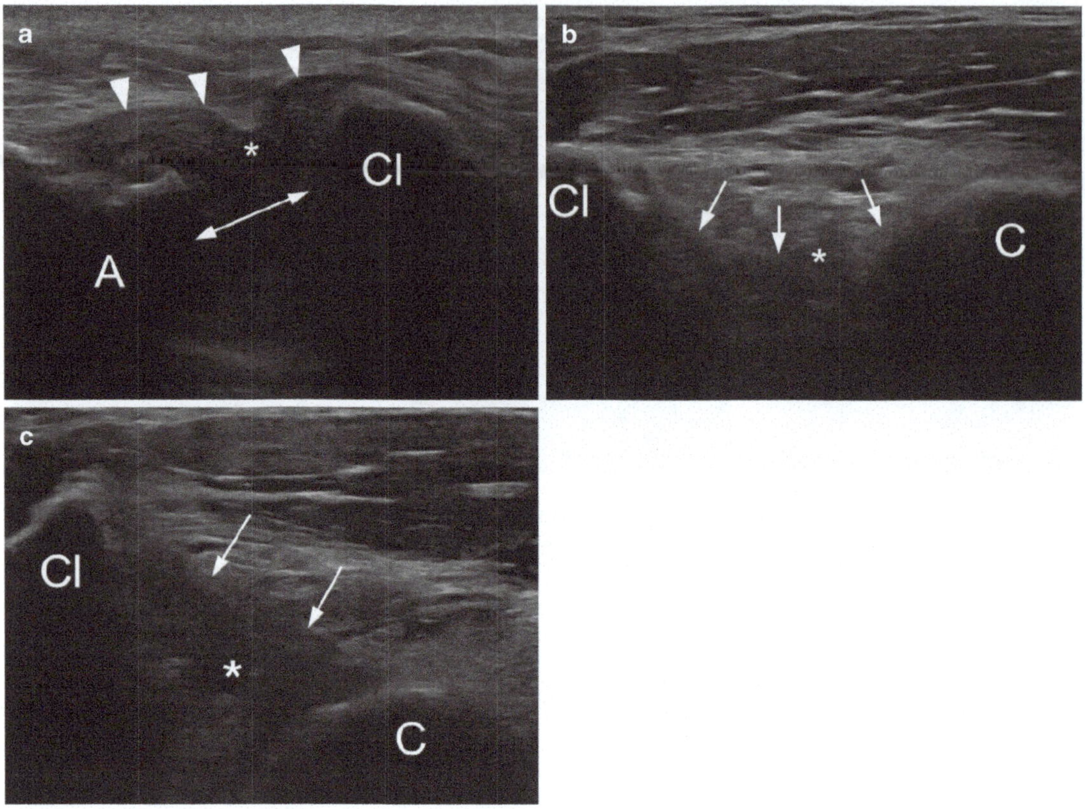

Fig. 3.5 Rockwood classification grade 3 sprain with (**a**) complete rupture (asterisk) of the acromioclavicular upper capsule (arrow heads) with spontaneous upper subluxation of the clavicle (double arrow), (**b**) partial rupture (asterisk) of the trapezoid ligament (arrowheads), which appears hypoechogenic and very relaxed, and (**c**) partial rupture (asterisk) of the conoid ligament, which is very thickened and hypoechogenic (*Cl* clavicle, *Ac* acromion, *C* coracoid)

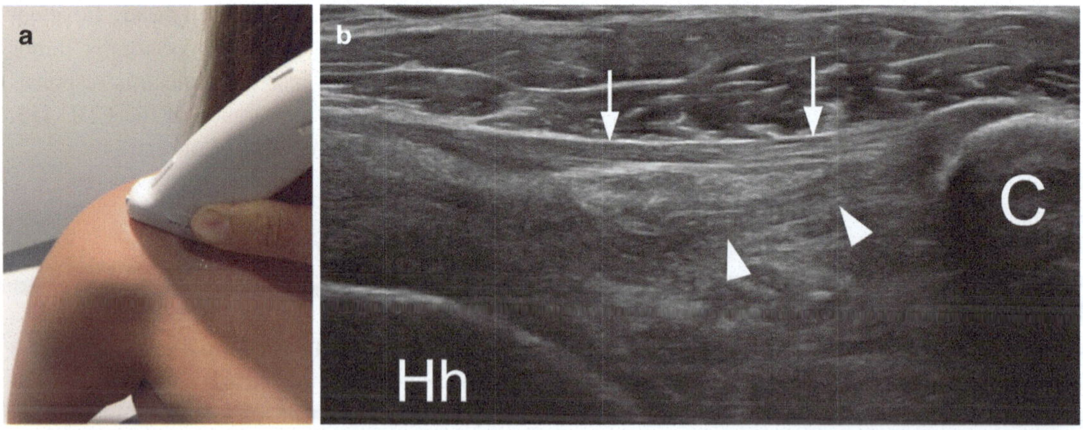

Fig. 3.6 (**a**) Position of the probe for study of the coracohumeral ligament and (**b**) corresponding ultrasound image showing the coracoid insertion and proximal segment of the CHL (arrowhead) under the acromiocoracoid ligament (arrows) (*C* coracoid, *Hh* humeral head)

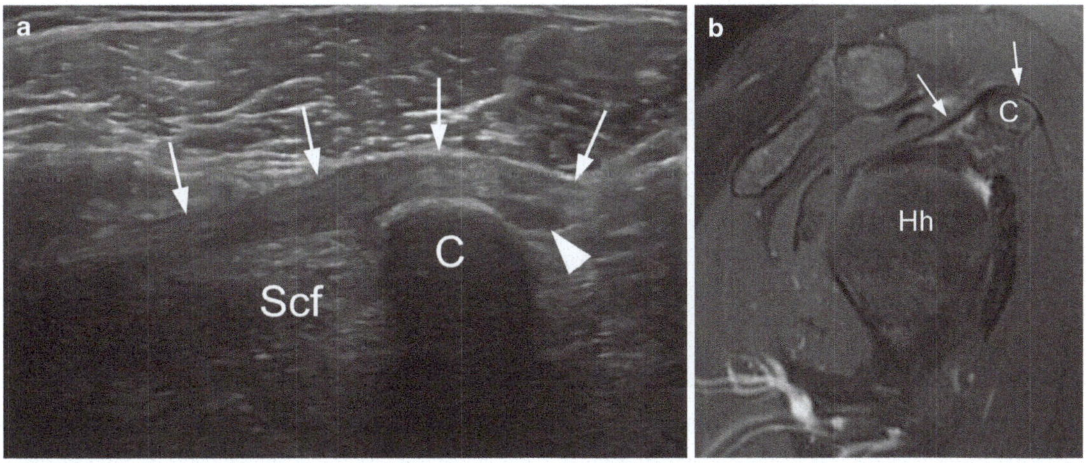

Fig. 3.7 (a) Axial section on the coracoid showing an anatomical variant of the pectoralis minor (arrows) which extends outside the place and place of the coracohumeral ligament, with a thin bursa (arrowhead) in the area of contact with the coracoid (C) and (b) MRI section sagittal in T2 weighting with saturation of the corresponding fat signal (*Scf* subcoracoid fat, *Hh* humeral head)

measured in a cross section. In the normal state, this ligament is thin and difficult to visualize. To differentiate a vestigial insertion of the pectoralis minor (Fig. 3.7) from a pathological thickening, for example, in the case of retractile capsulitis, the dynamic study in an oblique axial section on the coracoid in the internal-external rotation of the arm is indispensable and will show a slippage of the tendon on the upper edge of the coracoid in case of anatomical variant.

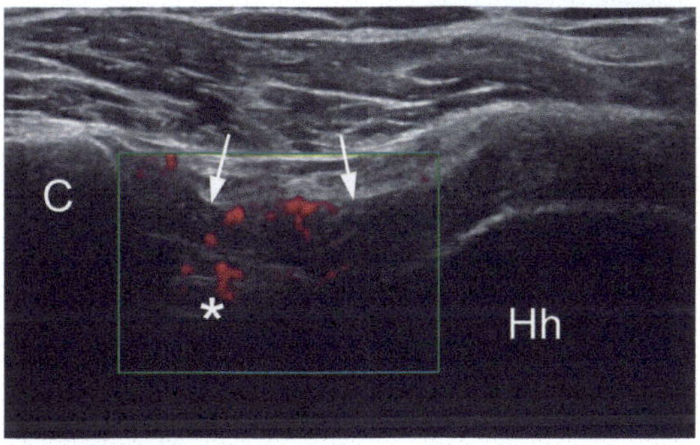

Fig. 3.8 Longitudinal section of a very thickened and hypoechogenic CHL (arrows) vascularized in energy Doppler with adjacent subcoracoid fat hyperemia (*C* coracoid, *Hh* humeral head)

3.4.3 Pathology

3.4.3.1 Retractile Adhesive Capsulitis

A hypoechogenic thickening of CHL (Fig. 3.8) which appears too clearly visible [18], compared to the contralateral side [19], is a very good argument in favor of retractile adhesive capsulitis. However, an insertional variant of the pectoralis minor should not be confused with a thickening of the CHL by performing dynamic maneuvers of rotation of the arm [18]. Hyperechogenic infiltration of subcoracoid fat with hyperemia (Fig. 3.8) and periarticular hyperechogenic infiltration may also be suggestive.

3.4.3.2 Traumatic Injury

LCH and interval may be lesioned in anterior glenohumeral dislocation, but there appear to be isolated traumatic lesions without dislocation with elongation or rupture of one or more components of the interval (Fig. 3.8). In our experience, the anamnesis often found trauma with lowering and forced external rotation of the arm (Fig. 3.9).

3.5 Coracoid and Subscapular Tendon/Subcoracoid Bursa

3.5.1 Anatomy

The underside of the coracoid is smooth and devoid of tendon or ligamentous insertion unlike the other faces. Under the coracoid runs the ten-

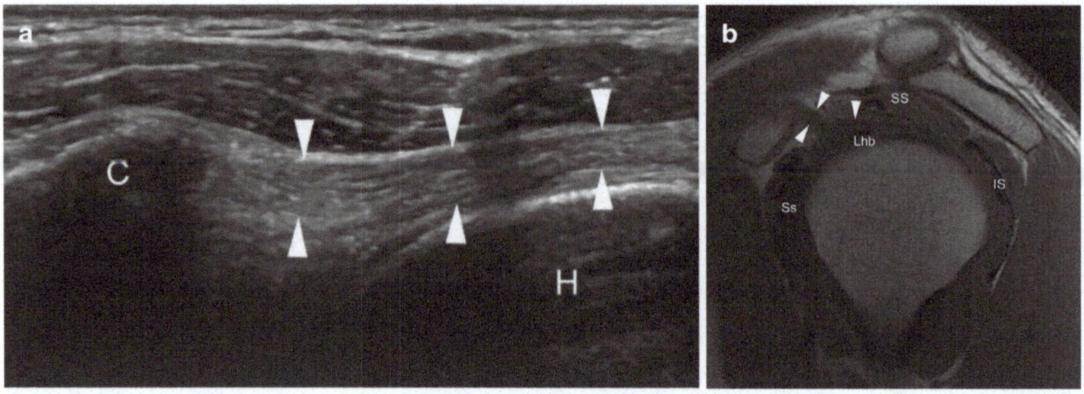

Fig. 3.9 (**a**) Longitudinal section of a thickening sequalae of CHL which is hyperechoic and fibrous. (**b**) Sagittal section MRI in T1 weighting corresponding with T1 isosignal thickening of CHL (arrows) (*Ss* subscapularis, *Lhb* long head biceps, *SS* supraspinatus, *IS* infraspinatus, *H* humerus)

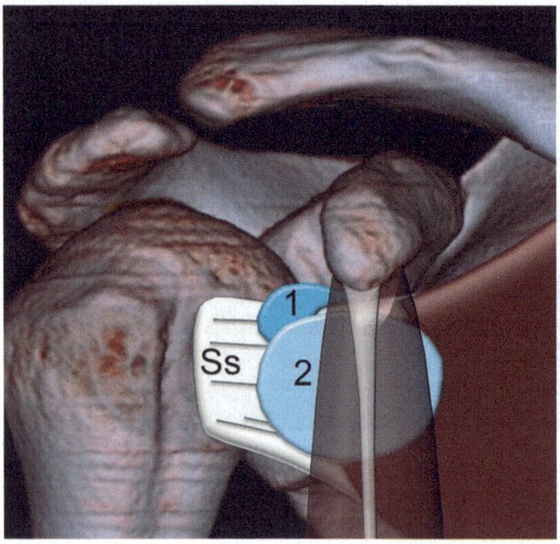

Fig. 3.10 Diagram of subcoracoid space with subcoracoid/subscapular recess. (1) bordering the upper slope of the subscapularis tendon (Ss) and the subcoracoid bursa overlying the tendon (2)

don of the subscapularis. The superficial face of the subscapularis tendon is covered by a synovial bursa, the subcoracoid bursa, the function of which is to reduce friction between the tendon and the coracoid (Fig. 3.10). Some consider it the anterior segment of the subacromiodeltoid bursa with which it can communicate physiologically. However, it never communicates physiologically with the glenohumeral joint [20, 21]. The upper slope of the subscapularis tendon is bordered by the subcoracoidal or subscapular recess, also known as the subscapular bursa (Fig. 3.10). This recess communicates with the glenohumeral joint through an orifice located between the upper and median glenohumeral ligament or between the superior and median glenohumeral ligament. It has very close relations with the subscapularis tendon to which it is fixed by loose connective tissue [22].

3.5.2 Ultrasound Technique

The subcoracoid space is essentially studied on an axial section corresponding to the longitudinal section of the subscapularis. The probe can be shifted inside to also study the medial slope of the space. The coracohumeral space is defined as the smallest distance between the coracoid and the lesser tubercle. It is measured on an axial section centered on the coracoid, with the arm rotating internally. The subscapular recess can be visualized as a water drop-shaped liquid groove in internal rotation at contact with the upper edge of the subscapularis tendon (Fig. 3.11). It completely erases in rotation because the subscapularis then puts itself in tension and compresses the recess. In the normal state, the subcoracoid bursa is not or very difficult to visualize. As with the subacromial impingement, dynamic study is indispensable in order to explore the subcoracoid impingement, with internal and external rotation maneuvers in slight elevation.

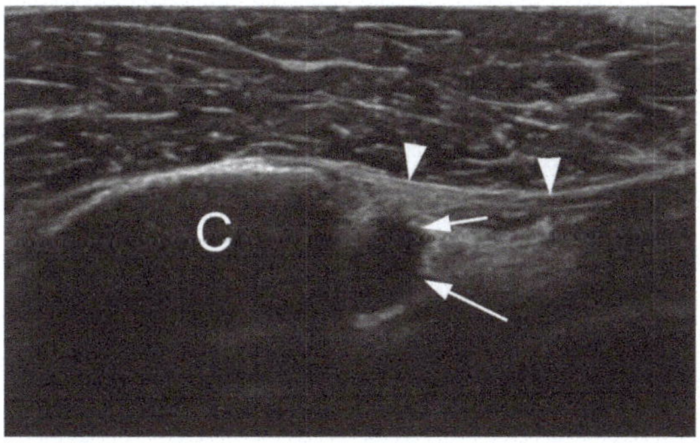

Fig. 3.11 Internally rotating oblique axial section with a rounded liquid image (arrows) below the coracoid (C) and the CHL (arrows) corresponding to the subcoracoidal recess

3.5.3 Pathology

3.5.3.1 Impingement Under the Coracoid

This is a rare but well-known cause of pain in the anterior side of the shoulder [23, 24]. It is the result of compression of the subscapularis tendon, subcoracoid bursa, and anterior capsule between the coracoid process and the lesser tubercle [25, 26]. It can be a result of a long coracoid (Fig. 3.12), posttraumatic stigma, and voluminous calcifications of the upper fascicles of the subscapularis tendon (Fig. 3.13), iatrogenic (surgical equipment) [27] or secondary to a massive

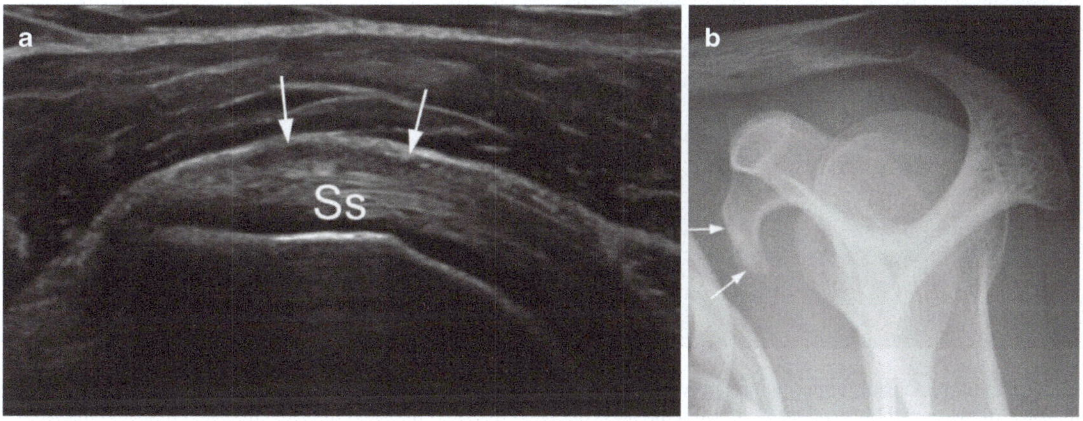

Fig. 3.12 (**a**) Axial/longitudinal section of the subscapularis tendon (Ss) with a discrete hypoechogenic thickening of the subcoracoid bursa (arrows) in a swimmer with anterior scapulalgia with (**b**) coracoid incidence in corresponding false profile showing a long coracoid process (arrows) promoting impingement

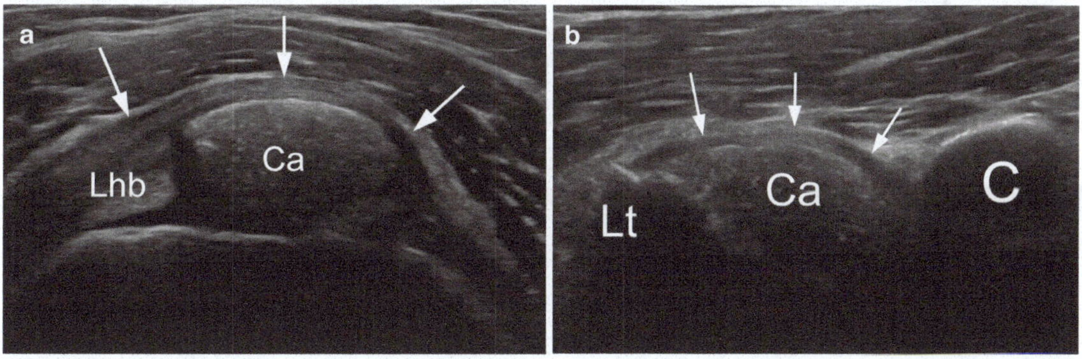

Fig. 3.13 (**a**) Axial/longitudinal section in external rotation of the subscapularis tendon which is the seat of a voluminous calcification (**Ca**) and (**b**) longitudinal section in internal rotation with calcification which stops on the coracoid (C), responsible for a subcoracoid bursitis (arrows) (*Lt* Lesser tubercule)

rupture of the superior cuff with ascent of the humeral head [28].

Repeated coracoid pressure on the surface of the tendon would create an elastic tensile stress on the deep side of the tendon by a *roller winger effect* described by Burkhart [29], responsible for degenerative lesions at the deep side of the tendon called TUFF (*tensile undersurface fiber failure*). The diagnostic criterion is the decrease in coracohumeral distance [30], although its diagnostic value is discussed in the literature [31, 32]. Coracohumeral distance is decreased in symptomatic patients from the contralateral side and asymptomatic subjects (Fig. 3.14) [32, 33]. The normal value of the coracohumeral distance proposed in ultrasound is 12 mm [32], but more than the absolute value of the coracohumeral distance, it seems appropriate to carry out a bilateral comparative measurement in search of an asymmetrical reduction of the space. Impingement can be referred to as subacromial impingement with subcoracoid bursitis involving varying degrees of hypoechogenic thickening and liquid effusion, impinging dynamic maneuvers in adduction, elevation, and internal rotation [32, 34].

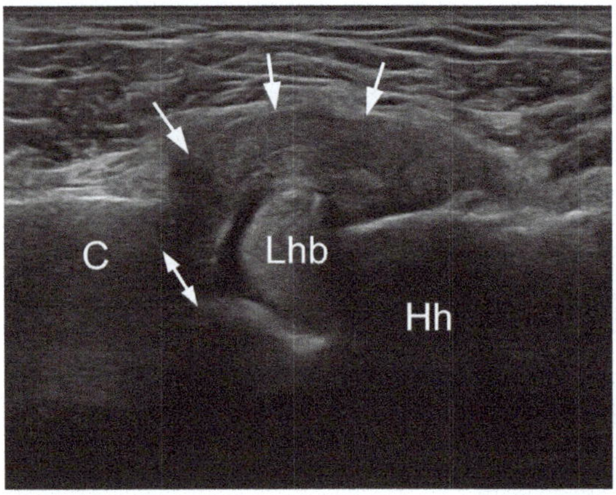

Fig. 3.14 Impingement under coracoid with a sharp decrease in the coracohumeral space (double arrow), the subcoracoid purse outside the coracoid (C), and a long biceps (Lhb) facing the coracoid (*Hh* Humeral head)

3.5.3.2 Effusion/Secondary Osteochondromatosis of Subcoracoid Recess

The subcoracoid bursa can be distended by glenohumeral effusion. It is not always easy to differentiate the subcoracoid bursa from the subscapular/subcoracoid recess. Attention should be paid to studying the relations of the fluid range in front of the subscapularis tendon with the joint cavity and the subscapularis tendon on a sagittal section just outside the coracoid: if the liquid range communicates with the articular cavity above the subscapularis tendon, the image corresponds to the subcoracoid recess, otherwise to the subcoracoid bursa (Fig. 3.15). It is most often associated with effusion of other glenohumeral recesses. This recess can also be the site of secondary osteochondrosis on centered or eccentric

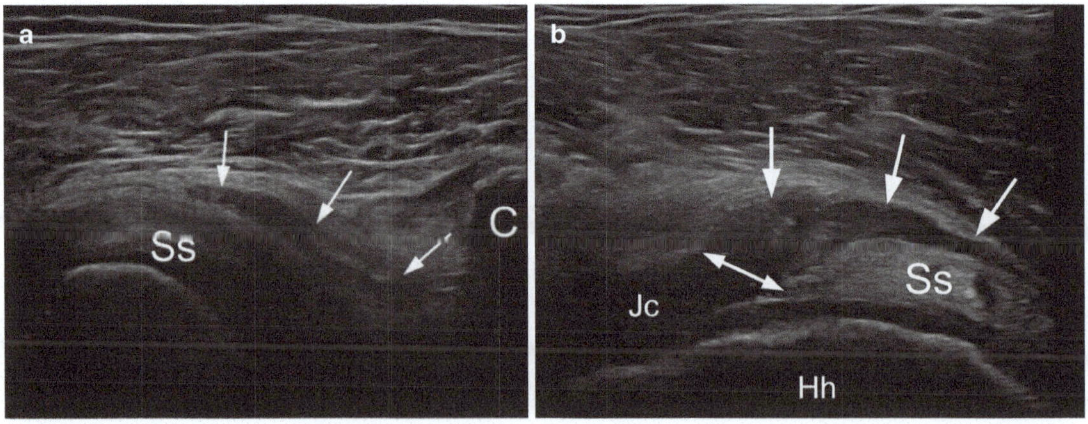

Fig. 3.15 (**a**) Axial section showing an effusion of the subcoracoidal recess (arrows) between the subscapularis tendon (Ss) and the coracoid (C); (**b**) corresponding sagittal section showing the communication (double arrow) between the recess (arrows) and the joint cavity (Jc) at the upper edge of the subscapularis (Ss) and allowing the difference between the bursa and the recess (*Hh* Humeral head)

omarthrosis. They are most often difficult to visualize because they are quite deep and partially masked by the coracoid (Fig. 3.16).

3.6 Traumatic Coracoid

Fractures of the coracoid are rare, accounting for about 1–3% of shoulder fractures [35–37]. It is possible to differentiate between stress fractures that are encountered almost exclusively in rifle shooters [38, 39] and acute traumatic lesions. These acute lesions result from three different mechanisms: direct trauma to the anterior side of the shoulder [35, 37], direct trauma to the humeral head in the event of anterior glenohumeral dislocation, and traction by maximum eccentric contraction of the short head of the biceps and coracobrachialis muscles. Direct trauma is usually responsible for fracture of the base, while traction trauma is responsible for apex avulsion fractures [35, 40, 41]. The avulsions of the upper side of the coracoid correspond to coracoid avulsion of the coracoclavicular ligaments (*see* above). Radiographic diagnosis of coracoid fractures is difficult given the bony overlays, and these fractures are often unknown in radiography [42]. Radiography is nevertheless an obligatory step in case of traumatic shoulder pain, especially to explore the base of the coracoid.

3.6.1 Ultrasound Technique

The coracoid should be systematically explored in the case of a painful posttraumatic shoulder with an oblique sagittal section, "apical oblique" view, in the longitudinal axis of the process [42] by analogy with the apical radiographic incidence [6] as the standard anterior sagittal view only reveals the apex and the distal part of the descending segment (Fig. 3.17a). The "oblique apical" view allows you to explore a larger part of the upper surface of the process and aids in the detection of fractures (Fig. 3.17b).

3.6.2 Pathology

The fracture will be evoked in front of a cortical continuity solution with a per-fractural hematoma (Fig. 3.18a), hyperechogenic edematous infiltration with hyperemia of the soft parts in

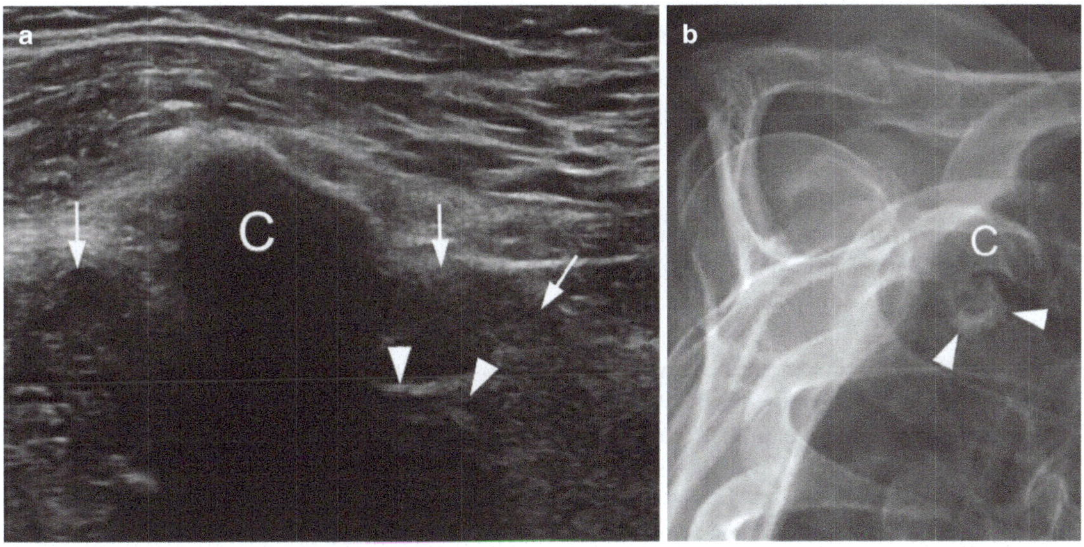

Fig. 3.16 (**a**) Axial section centered on the coracoid with a hypoecho-gene synovial thickening on either side of the coracoid containing a difficultly visualized secondary osteochondroma (arrowhead) and (**b**) corresponding false-profile incidence highlighting the osteochondroma (arrowheads) more easily

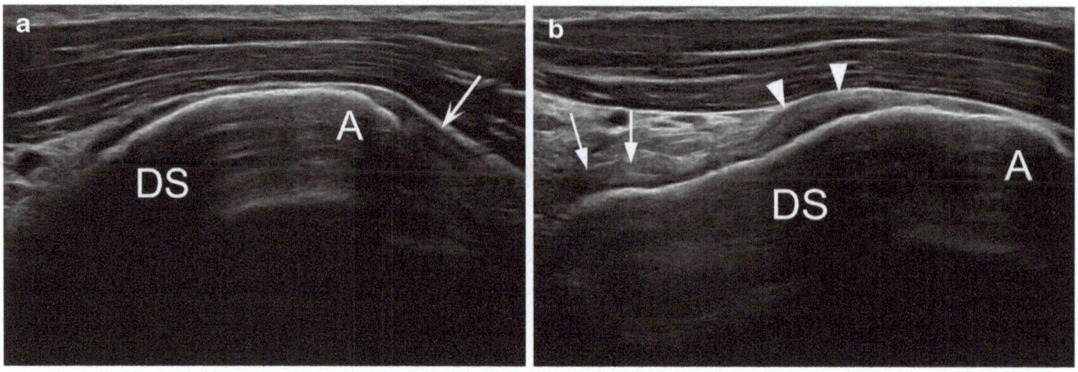

Fig. 3.17 (**a**) Standard sagittal section of the coracoid showing only the apex (A) and the distal part of the descending segment (DS) with the insertion of the short head of the biceps and coracobrachialis (curved arrow). (**b**) The probe is then tilted upwards and inwards to obtain the "apical oblique" view freeing the entire descending segment with the insertions of the pectoralis minor (arrows) and coracoclavicular ligaments (arrows)

contact in case of a recent fracture as opposed to a semi-recent fracture (Fig. 3.19). The traction exerted by the short head of the biceps and coracobrachialis during a thwarted bending of the elbow leads to a lower displacement of the distal fragment, which enhances the effect of the upper cortical release and facilitates detection. Isolated posttraumatic subscapularis bursitis also requires an occult fracture of the coracoid (Fig. 3.18b).

3.7 Coracoid and Tendinous Insertions (Coracobiceps/Coracobrachialis and Pectoralis Minor)

3.7.1 Anatomy

The short head of the biceps and the coracobrachialis insert on the apex of the coracoid. The anteroposterior extension of the coracoid is a lever arm for these muscles with an anterior insertion on the anterior edge of the clavicle. The tendon of the short head of the biceps is inserted on the lateral side of the apex of the coracoid, and the insertion of the coracobrachialis is directly myo-osseous on the medial side of the apex [43] (Fig. 3.19). The two muscles then head down, passing through the back of the pectoralis major. The pectoralis minor tendon is inserted on the medial side of the descending segment (Fig. 3.19).

3.7.2 Ultrasound Technique

The proximal insertion of the short head of the biceps and coracobrachialis is easily accessible by ultrasound. The longitudinal section consists of a strict sagittal section (Figs. 3.20 and 3.21) passing through the apex of the coracoid and the transverse section through a strict axial section. The pectoralis minor tendon is visualized on an oblique sagittal cut at the below and medially (Fig. 3.22).

3.7.3 Pathology

3.7.3.1 Tendinopathy/Enthesopathy

Tendinopathy or ruptures of tendons inserting into the coracoid process are unusual compared to long biceps tendon and cuff tendons [44]. The most common involvement is enthesopathy at the insertion of the short head of the biceps and coracobrachialis with cortical irregularities and/or intratendinous calcifications at the apex. The three muscles taking insertion on the coracoid can nonspecifically be the site of myo-aponeurotic or myotendinous lesions.

3.7.3.2 Traumatic Avulsion

The short head of the biceps and coracobrachialis can avulse the apex of the coracoid in case of large eccentric contraction (Fig. 3.23), as the pec-

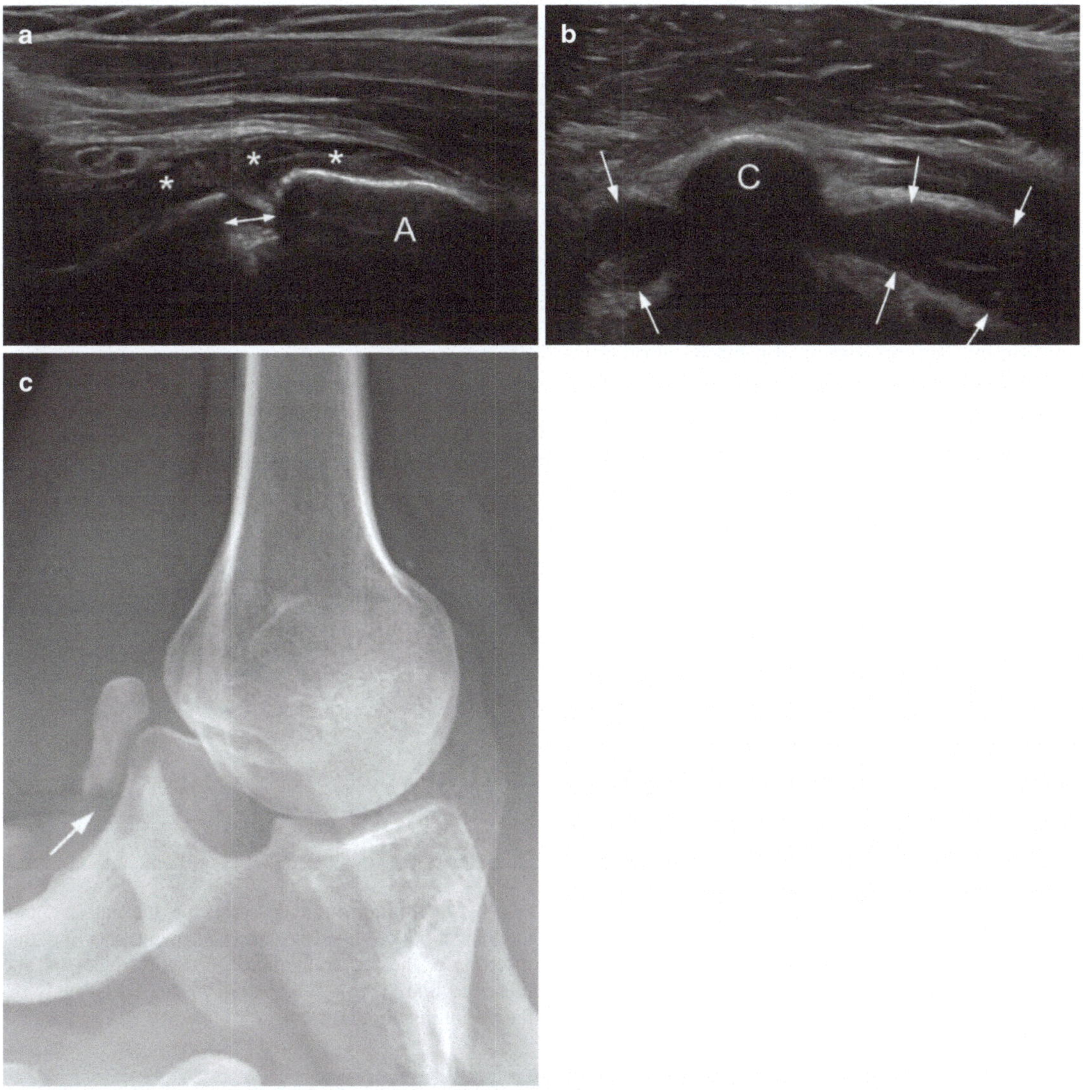

Fig. 3.18 (**a**) Coracoid sagittal section showing a recent fracture of the horizontal segment with widening of the fracture focus (double arrow) and partially fibrous hypoechogenic hematoma (asterisk) and (**b**) axial section on the coracoid distension of the subcoracoid bursa (arrows) on either side of the coracoid (C) associated with the fracture (*A* apex of the coracoid). (**c**) Corresponding Bernageau incidence. This incidence was achieved after ultrasound diagnosis, since the fracture was not visible on the standard effects

toralis minor can avulse the medial slope of the descending segment (Fig. 3.24).

3.7.3.3 Coracobrachialis Accessory

An accessory muscle called accessory coracobrachialis (ACB) can be inserted on the lower side of the coracoid. In the literature, the proximal origin of ACB is described as the lower surface of the coracoid process, with an anterior and inferior oblique path to the subscapularis. It maintains a close relationship with the anterior circumflex humeral artery and musculocutaneous nerve proximally and median nerve and brachial artery distally [45–49]. The ACB is easily visualized in ultrasound, with a typical muscular body appearance, hypoechogenic containing thin internal hyperechogenic linear echoes with fascicular echostructure, sitting in front of the subscapularis tendon and under the subacromiodeltoid bursa and deltoid (Fig. 3.25) [50]. It is separated from the deltoid and the subscapularis by a fine hyperechogenic linear interface. It is important to know this variant so as not to confuse it with subcoracoid bursitis. This anatomical variant may complicate the anterior surgical approach of the shoulder and must therefore be specified in the case of accidental discovery. ACB may be responsible for syndromes of cervicothoracobrachial crossing by compression or impingement on adjacent neurovascular structures. Kopuzc et al. [48] and Flatow et al. [51] reported lesions to the musculocutaneous nerve, median nerve, and lateral trunk of the brachial plexus by this accessory muscular body. When voluminous, the accessory

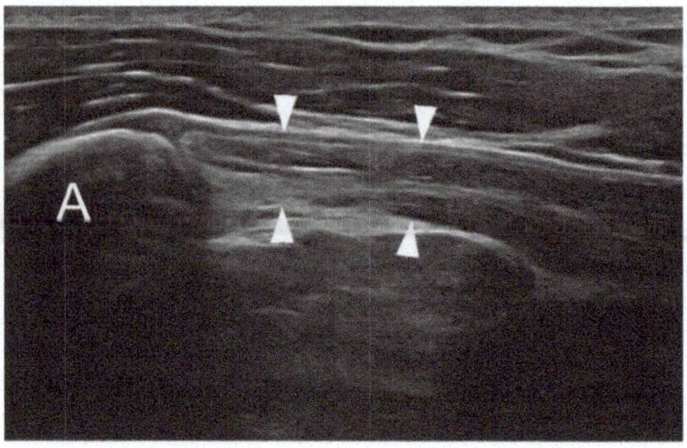

Fig. 3.21 Sagittal section on the medial slope of the apex of the coracoid (A) showing mixed insertion of the coracobrachialis (arrowheads) with a thin anterior fascia and a bone-muscle junction insertion behind

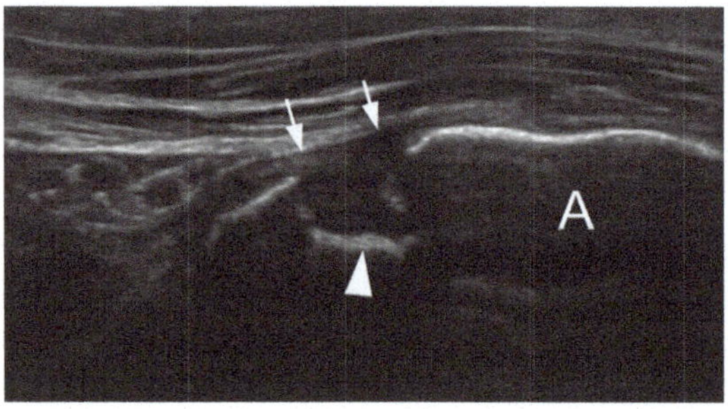

Fig. 3.19 Semi-recent fracture with a fibrous case (arrows) and a rough bone callus (arrowhead) (*A* coracoid apex)

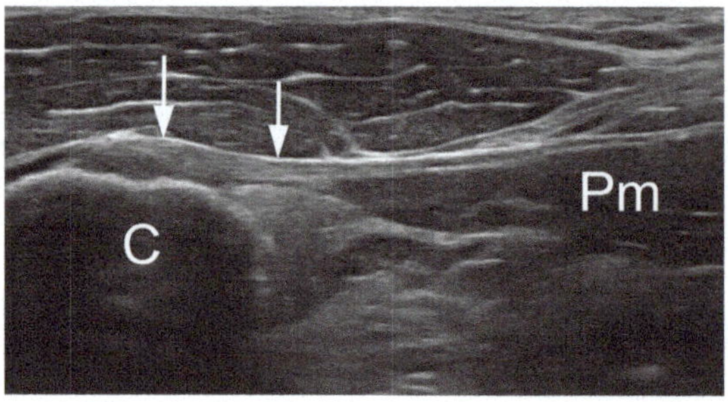

Fig. 3.22 Oblique sagittal section on the anterior and medial slope of the descending segment showing the insertion of the pectoralis minor tendon (arrows) and its muscular body (Pm) (*C* coracoid, *Pm* muscular body of the pectoralis minor)

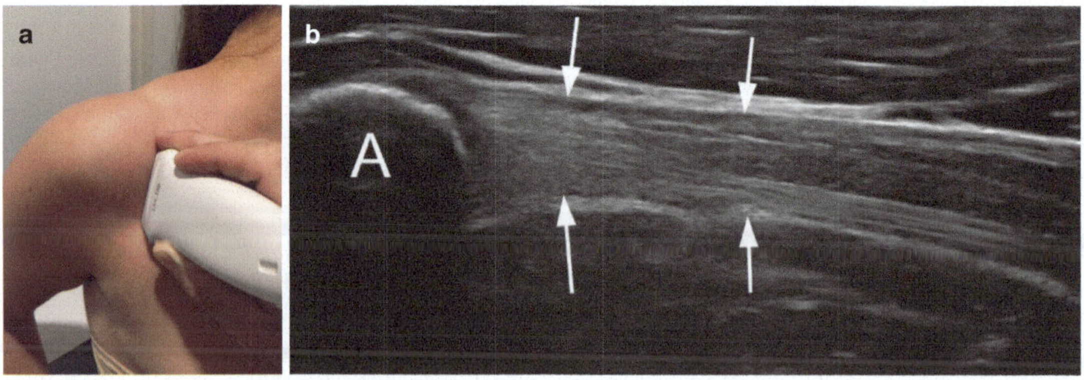

Fig. 3.20 (**a**) Positioning of the probe to study the proximal insertions of the short head of the biceps and coracobrachialis and (**b**) corresponding sagittal section on the lateral side of the apex of the coracoid (A) showing the insertion of the short head of the biceps (arrows)

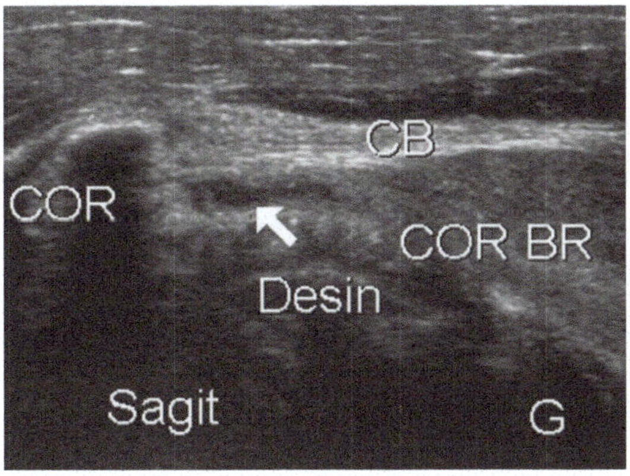

Fig. 3.23 Sagittal section of the coracoidal (arrow) disinsertion of the coracobrachialis (COR BR). (*COR* coracoid, *CB* short head of the biceps)

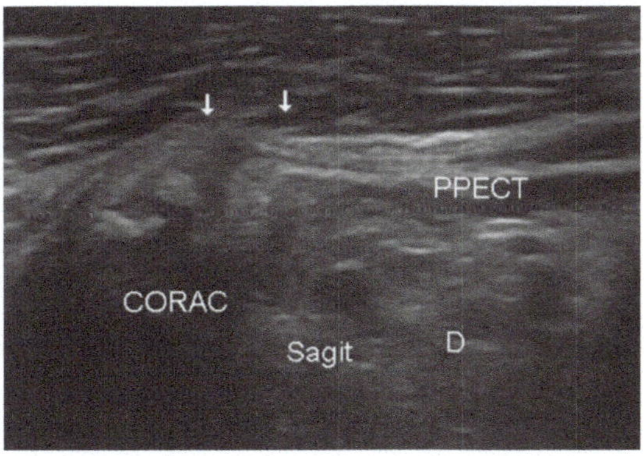

Fig. 3.24 Oblique longitudinal sagittal section of coracoid insertion avulsion (CORAC) of the tendon of the pectoralis minor (PPECT)

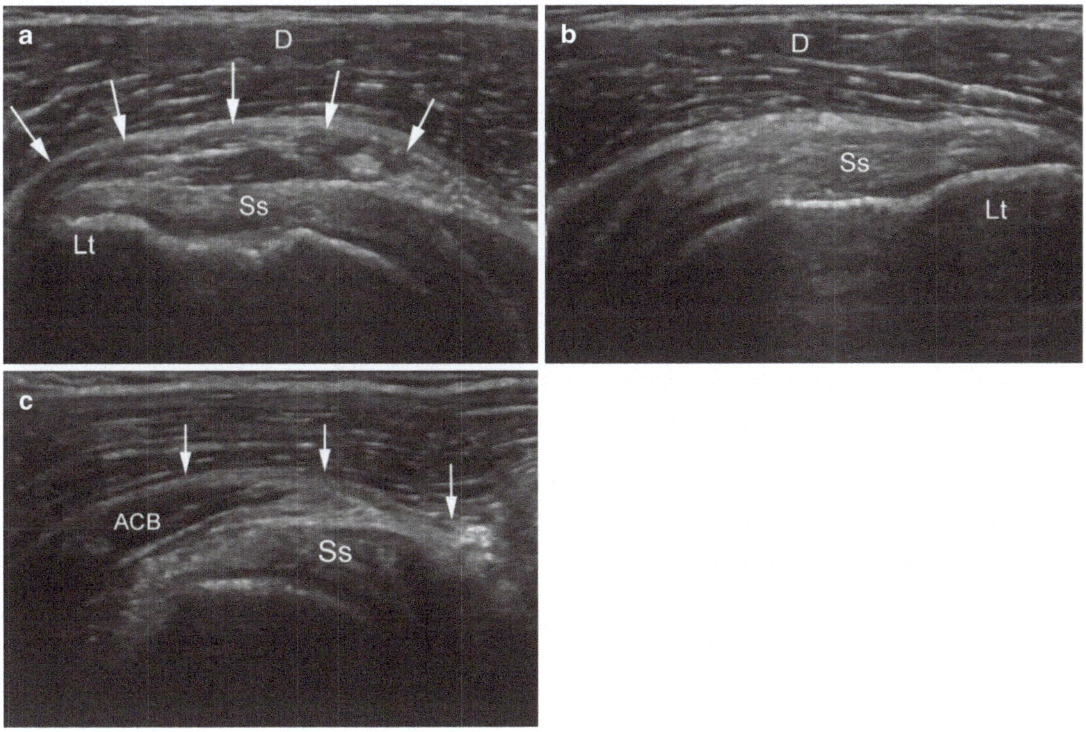

Fig. 3.25 (**a**) Axial ultrasound section of a right shoulder ACB (arrows) anterior to the subscapularis tendon (Ss) and below the deltoid, with a fine hyperechogenic border between these structures (asterisk). (**b**) The comparative ultrasound cut of the left shoulder does not show ACB. (**c**) Corresponding ultrasound sagittal section of the same ACB (arrows) in front of the subscapularis tendon (Ss) and under the deltoid (*C* coracoid, *Lt* lesser tubercule)

coracobrachialis may be responsible for subcoracoid impingement with the coracoid end and proximal segment of the short head of the biceps and coracobrachialis tendons. In dynamic study, the accessory muscular body deforms as it passes under these structures, with a fine subcoracoid bursitis on the surface (Fig. 3.26).

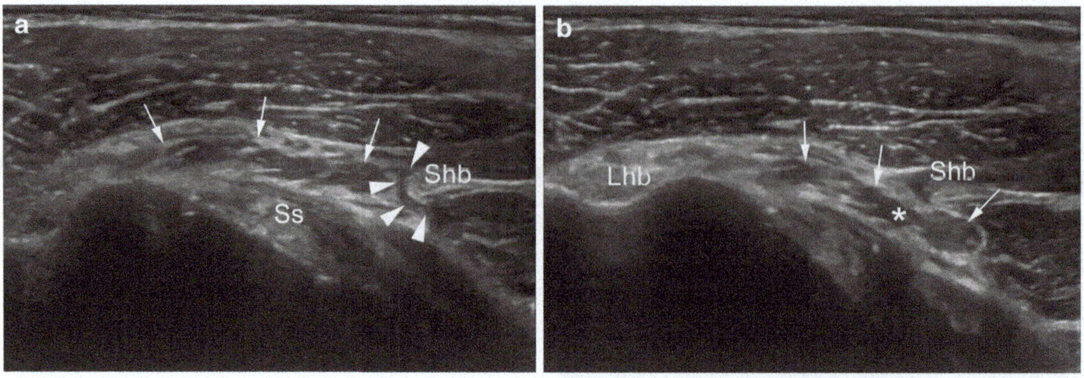

Fig. 3.26 Axial ultrasound section in internal rotation of a right ACB with progressive deformation at the very beginning of internal rotation (**a**) and later internal rotation (**b**) of the muscular body (asterisk) by proximal tendons of short head of the biceps (Shb) and coracobrachialis (Cb) (*Lhb* long head biceps, *Ss* subscapularis)

References

1. Fealy S, Rodeo SA, Dicarlo EF, O'Brien SJ. The developmental anatomy of the neonatal glenohumeral joint. J Shoulder Elbow Surg. 2000;9(3):217–22.
2. Kim SJ, Kim JS, Kim HJ, Yu HW. Bilateral unfused coracoid process: report of a case. J Korean Med Sci. 1998;13(5):563–5.
3. Ferreira Neto AA, Almeida AM, Maiorino R, Zoppi Filho A, Benegas E. An anatomical study of the subcoracoid space. Clinics. 2006;61(5):467–72.
4. Faruch Bilfeld M, Lapegue F, Chiavassa Gandois H, Bayol MA, Bonnevialle N, Sans N. Ultrasound of the coracoclavicular ligaments in the acute phase of an acromioclavicular disjunction: comparison of radiographic, ultrasound and MRI findings. Eur Radiol. 2017;27(2):483–90.
5. Takase K, Yamamoto K. Outcomes and function of conoid ligament on the basis of postoperative radiographic findings of arthroscopic stabilization for the distal clavicle fractures. Conserv Traumatol Surg Res. 2019;105(2):281–6.
6. Bianchi SM, Shoulder C. Ultrasound in musculoskeletal system. Berlin: Springer; 2009. p. 189–332.
7. Peetron P, Bedard JP. Acromioclavicular joint injury: enhanced technique of examination with dynamic maneuver. J Clin Ultrasound. 2007;35(5):262–7.
8. Testut LJ. Treatise of topographic anatomy with medical and surgical applications. Paris: Doin; 1921. p. 756–74.
9. Rockwood CG. Injuries to the acromioclavicular joint. In: Fractures in adults. 2nd ed. Philadephia: Lippincott; 1996. p. 860–910.
10. Bossart PJ, Joyce SM, Manaster BJ, Packer SM. Lack of efficacy of 'weighted' radiographs in diagnosing acute acromioclavicular separation. Ann Emerg Med. 1988;17(1):20–4.
11. Renoux JBG, Zeitoun E, Brasseur JL. Acromio clavicular sprain: ultrasound of coracoclavicular ligaments. In: News in ultrasound of the musculoskeletal system, vol. 6. Montpellier: Medical Sauramps; 2009. p. 23–32.
12. Harryman DT 2nd, Sidles JA, Harris SL, Matsen FA 3rd. The role of the rotator interval capsule in passive motion and stability of the shoulder. J Bone Joint Surg Am. 1992;74(1):53–66.
13. Jost B, Koch PP, Gerber C. Anatomy and functional aspects of the rotator interval. J Shoulder Elbow Surg. 2000;9(4):336–41.
14. Yang HF, Tang KL, Chen W, Dong SW, Jin T, Gong JC, et al. An anatomic and histologic study of the coracohumeral ligament. J Shoulder Elbow Surg. 2009;18(2):305–10.
15. Homsi C, Rodrigues MB, Silva JJ, Stump X, Morvan G. [Anomalous insertion of the pectoralis minor muscle: ultrasound findings]. Radiol J. 2003;84(9):1007–11.
16. Lee SJ, Ha DH, Lee SM. Unusual variation of the rotator interval: insertional abnormality of the pectoralis minor tendon and absence of the coracohumeral ligament. Skeletal Radiol. 2010;39(12):1205–9.
17. Corroller T, Cohen M, Aswad R, Champsaur P. [The rotator interval: hidden lesions?]. Radiol J. 2007;88(11 Pt 1):1669–77.
18. Homsi C, Bordalo-Rodrigues M, da Silva JJ, Stump XM. Ultrasound in adhesive capsulitis of the shoulder. Is assessment of the coracohumeral ligament a valuable diagnostic tool? Skeletal Radiol. 2006;35(9):673–8.
19. Chick NP, Hauger E, Amoretti O. Ultrasound and retractile adhesive capsulitis: focus. In: News in ultrasound of the musculoskeletal system, vol. 7. Montpellier: Sauramps Medical; 2010. p. 199–211.
20. Grainger AJ, Tirman PF, Elliott JM, Kingzett-Taylor A, Steinbach LS, Genant HK. MR anatomy of the subcoracoid bursa and the association of subcora-

coid effusion with tears of the anterior rotator cuff and the rotator interval. AJR Am J Roentgenol. 2000;174(5):1377–80.
21. Rutten MJ, Jager GJ, Blickman JG. From the RSNA refresher courses: US of the rotator cuff: pitfalls, limits, and artifacts. Radiographics. 2006;26(2):589–604.
22. Colas F, Nevoux J, Gagey O. The subscapular and subcoracoid bursae: descriptive and functional anatomy. J Shoulder Elbow Surg. 2004;13(4):454–8.
23. Garofalo R, Conti M, Massazza G, Cesari E, Vinci E, Castagna A. Subcoracoid impingement syndrome: a painful shoulder condition related to different pathologic factors. Musculoskelet Surg. 2011;95(Suppl 1):S25–9.
24. Lappin M, Gallo A, Krzyzek M, Evans K, Chen YT. Sonographic findings in subcoracoid impingement syndrome: a case report and literature review. PM R. 2017;9(2):204–9.
25. Dines DM, Warren RF, Inglis AE, Pavlov H. The coracoid impingement syndrome. J Bone Joint Surg. 1990;72(2):314–6.
26. Osti L, Soldati F, Del Buono A, Massari L. Subcoracoid impingement and subscapularis tendon: is there any truth? Muscles Ligaments Tendons J. 2013;3(2):101–5.
27. Martetschlager F, Rios D, Boykin RE, Giphart JE, Waha A, Millett PJ. Coracoid impingement: current concepts. Knee Surg Sports Traumatol Arthrosc. 2012;20(11):2148–55.
28. Gerber C, Terrier F, Ganz R. The role of the coracoid process in the chronic impingement syndrome. J Bone Joint Surg. 1985;67(5):703–8.
29. Burkhart SS. Fluoroscopic comparison of kinematic patterns in massive rotator cuff tears. Suspension bridge model. Clin Conserv Relat Res. 1992;284:144–52.
30. Lo IK, Burkhart SS. The etiology and assessment of subscapularis tendon tears: a case for subcoracoid impingement, the roller-wringer effect, and TUFF lesions of the subscapularis. Arthroscopy. 2003;19(10):1142–50.
31. Giaroli EL, Major NM, Lemley DE, Lee J. Coracohumeral interval imaging in subcoracoid impingement syndrome on MRI. AJR Am J Roentgenol. 2006;186(1):242–6.
32. Tracy MR, Trella TA, Nazarian LN, Tuohy CJ, Williams GR. Sonography of the coracohumeral interval: a potential technique for diagnosing coracoid impingement. J Ultrasound Med. 2010;29(3):337–41.
33. Friedman RJ, Bonutti PM, Genez B. Cine magnetic resonance imaging of the subcoracoid region. Orthopedics. 1998;21(5):545–8.
34. Drakes S, Thomas S, Kim S, Guerrero L, Lee SW. Ultrasonography of subcoracoid bursal impingement syndromes. PM R. 2015;7(3):329–33.
35. Ogawa K, Yoshida A, Takahashi M, Ui M. Fractures of the coracoid process. J Bone Joint Surg. 1997;79(1):17–9.
36. Haapamaki VV, Kiuru MJ, Koskinen SK. Multidetector CT in shoulder fractures. Emerg Radiol. 2004;11(2):89–94.
37. Jettoo P, Kiewiet G, England S. Base of coracoid process fracture with acromioclavicular dislocation in a child. J Conserv Surg Res. 2010;5:77.
38. Boyer DW Jr. Trapshooter's shoulder: stress fracture of the coracoid process. Case report. J Bone Joint Surg Am. 1975;57(6):862.
39. Sandrock AR. Another sports fatigue fracture. Stress fracture of the coracoid process of the scapula. Radiology. 1975;117(2):274.
40. Eyres KS, Brooks A, Stanley D. Fractures of the coracoid process. J Bone Joint Surg. 1995;77(3):425–8.
41. Rabbani GR, Cooper SM, Escobedo EM. An isolated coracoid fracture. Curr Probl Diagn Radiol. 2012;41(4):120–1.
42. Botchu R, Lee KJ, Bianchi S. Radiographically undetected coracoid fractures diagnosed by sonography. Report of seven cases. Skeletal Radiol. 2012;41(6):693–8.
43. Crichton JC, Funk L. The anatomy of the short head of biceps not a tendon. Int J Shoulder Surg. 2009;3(4):75–9.
44. Bianchi S, Jacob D, Lambert A, Draghi F. Sonography of the coracoid process region. J Ultrasound Med. 2017;36(2):375–88.
45. Wood J. On human muscular variations and their relation to comparative anatomy. J Anat Physiol. 1867;1(1):44–59.
46. Wood J. Variations in human myology observed during the winter session of 1867–1868 at King's college, London. Proc R Soc Lond. 1868;1868(16):483–525.
47. Ogawa K, Takahashi M, Yoshida A. Aberrant muscle anterior to the shoulder joint: its clinical relevance. J Shoulder Elbow Surg. 1999;8(1):46–8.
48. Kopuz C, Icten N, Yildirim M. A rare accessory coracobrachialis muscle: a review of the literature. Surg Radiol Anat. 2003;24(6):406–10.
49. Sugalski MT, Wiater JM, Bigliani LU, Levine WN. Coracobrachialis brevis: anatomic anomaly. J Shoulder Elbow Surg. 2003;12(3):306–7.
50. Bauones S, Morals A. The accessory coracobrachialis muscle: ultrasound and MR features. Skeletal Radiol. 2015;44(9):1273–8.
51. Flatow EL, Bigliani LU, April EW. An anatomic study of the musculocutaneous nerve and its relationship to the coracoid process. Clin Conserv Relat Res. 1989;244:166–71.

Ultrasound of the Acromioclavicular Joint

4

Guillaume Mercy

The conditions of the acromioclavicular joint (AC) including traumatic and degenerative pathologies are some of the most common causes of a painful shoulder. However the involvement of this joint is underestimated, which is nicknamed for this reason "the forgotten articulation" [1].

4.1 Anatomy

The scapula and clavicle form the bony base of the upper chest wall, a V-shaped articulation whose tip is formed by the AC joint (Fig. 4.1).

4.1.1 General

This is a plane joint [2, 3]. The articular surface of the acromion is oval, slightly concave, vertical, almost sagittal, discreetly oriented forward and inward, facing the slightly convex clavicle surface [3, 4].

In half of the cases, the joint is not strictly oriented in the sagittal plane but slightly oblique downwards and inwards, so that the clavicular surface slightly overlaps the acromial surface, up to 50° from the vertical [2, 5].

G. Mercy (✉)
G.H. Pitié-Salpêtrière, Service d'Imageries Spécialisées et des Urgences, Boulevard de l'hôpital, Paris, France
e-mail: guillaume.mercy@aphp.fr

It is elongated in the anteroposterior direction and measures about 19 mm in length and 9 mm in height [6]. The width of the joint space varies from 1 to 3 mm, decreasing with age, reaching down to 0.5 mm after 60 years [1, 4, 7].

4.1.2 Content

The joint contains a capsule, a synovium, a joint cavity, articular cartilages, and an intra-articular disc.

- The disc is discoid or meniscoid in shape ranging from 1 to 4 mm, with its thickness decreasing with age [3, 4, 8–10]. Testut describes up to eight different types of variable development, size, and shape. When complete, it can separate the joint cavity in half or be adherent to the acromion and delimit a single cavity on its clavicular side [3].
- The joint cavity appears only from the age of 23 years [9].
- The cartilage is thicker on the acromial slope [3]. Initially hyaline is gradually transformed into a fibrocartilage from 17 years on the clavicular side and 23 years on the acromial side [3].
- The capsule is thin on the lower side, so that the synovium can easily communicate with the subacromial bursa [11].

T. Apard, J. L. Brasseur (eds.), *Ultrasonography for the Upper Limb Surgeon*,
https://doi.org/10.1007/978-3-030-84234-5_4

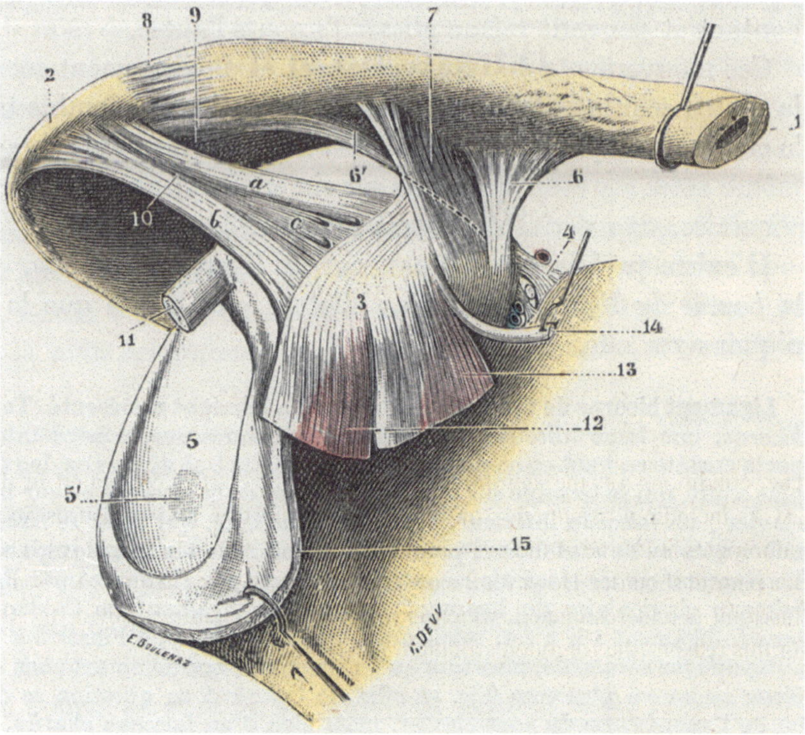

Fig. 4.1 Anatomy of the acromioclavicular joint according to Testut. (1) clavicle; (2) acromion; (3) coracoid process (hidden by 12: short head of the biceps and 13: coracobrachialis); (6) conoid ligament (and 6′ accessory ligament); (7) trapezoid ligament; (8) superior acromioclavicular ligament; (9) inferior acromioclavicular ligament; (10) acromiocoracoid ligament

4.1.3 Ligaments

4.1.3.1 AC Ligaments

The capsule, loose, is strengthened by joint ligaments. Conventionally there are four: superior, inferior, anterior, and posterior [12].

In reality only two are present, one of which is constant [3, 13]:

- The *posterosuperior (or "superior") ligament* is constant, wide, slightly oblique from the anterior edge of the acromion to the posterior edge of the clavicle, "wrapping" around the distal clavicle [8, 14]. Its insertions are in continuity with the periosteum [15], at about 3 mm on the acromial side and 4 mm on the clavicular side [16].
- The *anteroinferior (or "inferior") ligament* is inconstant, thin, and variable in width and orientation [13]. It merges laterally with the acromial insertion of the acromiocoracoid ligament [8]. When present it often does not cover the lower edge of the AC joint, which is therefore usually devoid of ligaments [13].

4.1.3.2 Coracoclavicular Ligaments (CC)

Two other extra-articular ligaments stabilize the AC joint, the coracoclavicular ligaments [2–4, 13, 15, 17–20].

- The *anterolateral or trapezoid CC ligament*: it inserts on the lateral edge of the base of the coracoid, about 2 cm from the tip of the coracoid. It forms a quadrilateral sagittal shaft broadly flared upwards and oriented upwards and outwards to the lower edge of the distal 1/3 of the collarbone. It is inserted on an extended bone ridge from the conoid tubercle of the clavicle medially, up to 1 cm of the articular edge of the clavicle laterally. Its length is very variable, about 15 mm [20].
- The *posteromedial CC ligament or conoid*: it inserts on the medial edge of the base of the coracoid inside the previous one with which it mixes. Then it flares slightly into a cone and turns upwards and slightly backwards to the junction of the medial and lateral third of the clavicle. It is inserted about 4 cm from the joint edge, on an area narrower than the

trapezoid ligament, centered by a small conoid tubercle located on the posterior edge of the clavicle. Its length is variable, in the order of 10 mm [20].

The posterior edge of the trapezoid ligament can merge with the lateral edge of the conoid ligament or leave a gap filled with a serous bursa [3, 4].

4.1.3.3 Variants

- Sometimes a third additional CC ligament starts from the coracoid insertion of the conoid ligament and moves up and out to insert behind the trapezoid ligament [3, 18].
- An additional ligament can line the lower edge of the AC joint and would be a remaining insertion of the subclavian muscle on the acromion [3].
- In some populations (Asia, Africa), the CC space is replaced by a plane neo-articulation [2, 3].

4.1.4 Muscles

The stability of the joint is ensured by these different ligaments but also by the deltoid and trapezius muscles, which have both clavicular and spinoacromial insertions.

On the clavicle, the deltoid is inserted on the anterior side of the lateral third, and the trapezius is inserted on the posterior side [3].

The superficial fascia of the deltoid muscle and trapezius muscle join above the clavicle and extend over the AC joint in the form of a deltotrapezoid fascia [2, 3, 8, 15].

It is commonly referred to as the muscular and conjunctive "deltotrapezial cap," covering the AC joint.

4.1.5 Vascularization and Innervation

The AC joint is irrigated by the suprascapular (subclavian branch) and thoraco-acromial (axillary branch) arteries.

Innervation is provided by the suprascapular and lateral pectoral nerves [21].

4.2 Biomechanics

4.2.1 Function

The clavicle and scapula serve as the original muscular and ligamentous suspension apparatus of the arm. The clavicle is the only bone that brings together the axial skeleton and the upper limb.

Participation of the AC joint in shoulder mobility is low. Indeed, this is largely ensured by scapulothoracic and glenohumeral mobility. The clavicle follows the movements of the scapula, in a synchronism of the scapular and clavicular movements [22–24]. Thus, for Rockwood, when the clavicle rotates 45° in the sternoclavicular, only 5–8° occur in the AC joint [23]. In addition, even after arthrodesis of these two bones, shoulder movements remain possible [25].

4.2.2 Movements

Three types of joint movements are described by Worcester [26]:

- An *anterior and posterior slide* of the scapula on the clavicle with internal or external rotation around a vertical axis, bringing the branches of the acromioclavicular "V" closer to or away from each other, like a compass (accompanies the internal and external rotations of the scapula in the axial plane).
- A *superior rotational movement,* around the AC joint axis, like a hinge, during abduction of the scapula to the clavicle (accompanies the superior rotation of the scapula).
- An *axial rotational movement* around the axis of the clavicle (accompanies the anterior or posterior inclination of the scapula).
- The range of movements is restricted. In complete abduction of the shoulder, the scapula has a movement around the clavicle of the

order of 8° internal rotation, 11° upper rotation, and 19° posterior axial rotation [27].

- However, the amplitude of the upper rotation of the joint during abduction of the shoulder is poorly known: between 5° and 30° according to the authors [2, 12, 23, 27–31].
- *In the next chapters, the movement of the AC joint will be referred to as a displacement of the clavicle relative to the acromion for convenience.*

4.2.3 Stability

4.2.3.1 Ligament Resistance

In vitro tests show that the capsule and AC ligaments are the most resistant, followed by the conoid ligament and then the trapezoid ligament [15].

4.2.3.2 Capsule and Ligaments AC

Capsule and AC ligaments exhibit three times more stability in the anteroposterior plane than in the superior-inferior plane [4, 32].

- In the anteroposterior plane (horizontally), they constitute the primary stabilizer, limiting the posterior clavicular movement largely due to the superior AC ligament [13, 14].
- In the superior-inferior plane (vertically), for displacements of small amplitude, the capsule and superior AC ligament contribute half to joint stabilization, in combination with CC ligaments [14, 15, 33].
- In the axial plane, the superior AC ligament restricts the posterior rotation around the clavicular axis, thanks to its orientation with slight "winding" around the clavicle [13, 14].
- Finally, the capsule and AC ligaments restrict distraction forces (rare) [14, 22].

4.2.3.3 CC Ligamentous Complex

Different ligaments strain differently depending on the direction of movement.

- Vertically, CC ligaments are the primary stabilizer. During weak movements, they absorb about half of the stresses in combination with the capsule and the superior AC ligament. During larger amplitude movements, they take care of 2/3 of the stresses, especially via the conoid ligament [14].
- Horizontally, after section of the capsule and of the AC ligaments, tensions increase in CC ligaments [28]. During posterior stress on the clavicle, the trapezoid ligament undergoes greater tensions than the conoid and vice versa during anterior stress [28, 33].
- In compression, the trapezoid ligament absorbs 3/4 of the stress [14].

In general, experimentally, the conoid ligament undergoes greater tension during anterosuperior loading of the clavicle; the trapezoid ligament undergoes more tension during posterior loading of the clavicle [34].

4.2.3.4 Trapezius and Deltoid Muscles

- Due to its insertion and orientation, the deltoid directly restricts the upper and posterior movements of the clavicle when the ligaments are ruptured [2].
- The trapezius, extended from the axial skeleton to the edge of the acromion, contributes to AC stability by its wide fascial attachment to the upper collarbone [2, 23].

4.2.3.5 Summary

In the experience of Urist [35]:

- Isolated section of coracoclavicular ligaments does not lead to laxity.
- The section of the superior AC ligament with resection of the capsule allows subluxation of the articulation. In case of additional detachment of the deltoid and trapezius, it is possible to displace the clavicle upwards.
- In case of section of the superior AC ligament, with detachment of the deltoid and trapezius muscles, and section of the trapezoid ligament, dislocation of the collarbone upwards but especially backwards is possible.
- In case of section of the superior AC ligament, with detachment of the deltoid and trapezius muscles, and section of the conoid ligament,

the dislocation of the collarbone upwards is major.

In summary, a lesion of acromiocoracoid ligaments is not sufficient to cause laxity but must be combined with a lesion of the capsule and CC ligaments. Lesion of the conoid ligament and/or deltotrapezial fascia aggravates superior displacement. Lesion of the trapezoid ligament aggravates posterior displacement [22].

4.3 Normal Ultrasound

4.3.1 Normal Ultrasound

The reference section plane is frontal, on the upper side of the shoulder stump [36]. Other sagittal sections (disc, CC ligaments, muscle fascia, ultrasound-guided joint infiltration) and axial sections (posterior displacement) may be useful in addition.

4.3.1.1 AC Joint (Anterior Frontal and Sagittal Sections) (Figs. 4.2 and 4.3)

The upper edge of the clavicle and acromion has regular borders. These borders are highly variable in morphology: protruding, planar, or concave [37]. In addition, the joint is slightly more open anteriorly [38].

The joint space, visible as a hypoechoic gap, can be measured at the superficial joint opening. It should be compared to the normal side due to large individual variations [37–39] (average 3 mm, normal <6 mm) [37, 40].

The acromial and clavicular joint edges are normally aligned vertically and horizontally, but in practice slight shifts are frequent and justify the comparison to the normal side [38, 41].

The joint capsule is usually convex but should not bulge more than 3 mm thick, from the tangent to the upper edges of the joint [37, 40].

An articular effusion may be incidentally visible [42].

Disk analysis is possible, although hampered by artifacts [39]. The superficial part of the articular fibrocartilage is constantly visible [37]. It forms a hypoechoic structure under the AC ligament, ovoid in the sagittal plane.

4.3.1.2 Superior AC Ligament (Frontal Section) (Fig. 4.2)

The superior AC ligament is superficial, therefore easily visible on the same frontal section, in the form of hyperechoic thickening of the upper capsule.

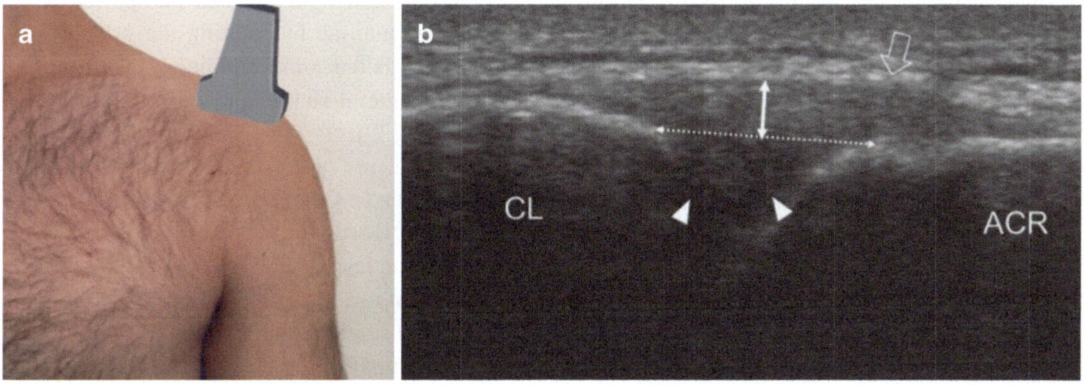

Fig. 4.2 Frontal section on AC joint and superior AC ligament. (**a**) Positioning of the probe. (**b**) Corresponding ultrasound image. The capsule appears thick as it is reinforced on its upper and posterior side by the hyperechoic superior AC ligament, located on the surface of the hypoechoic fibrocartilage (arrowheads). A thin superficial hyperechoic band corresponds to the muscular fascia (hollow arrow). On a comparative section, the width of the surface joint space (double dotted arrow) and the upper capsular thickness (double solid arrow) can be measured. *Cl* clavicle, *Acr* acromion

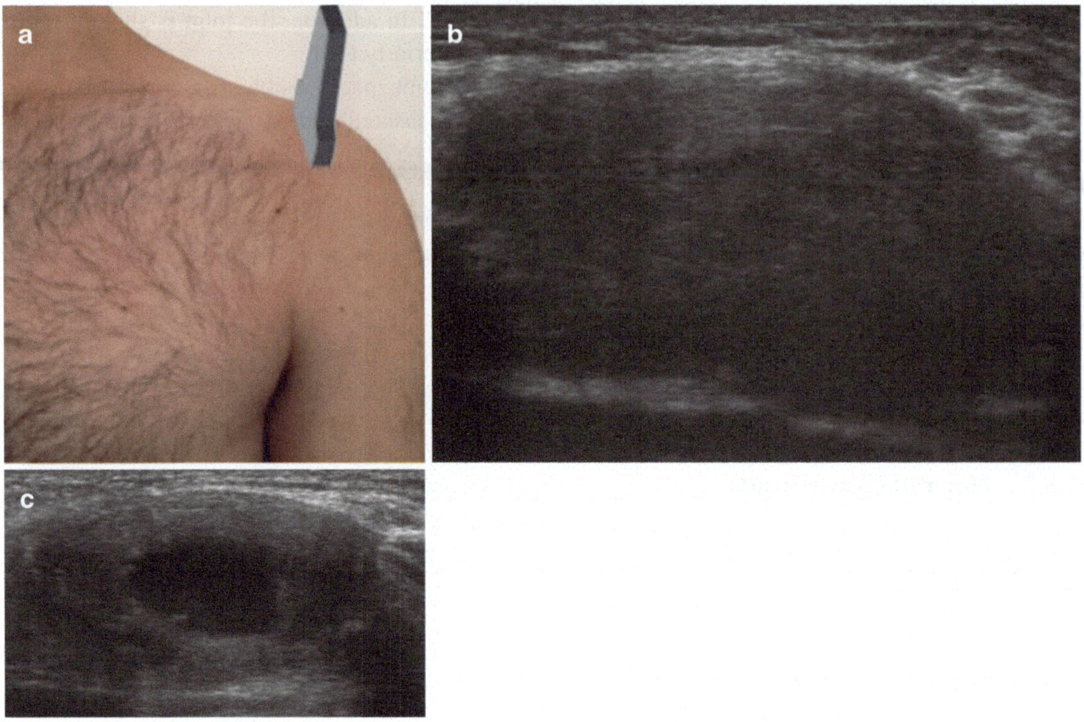

Fig. 4.3 Sagittal section on the AC joint: articular fibrocartilage. (**a**) Position of the probe. (**b** and **c**) Corresponding images in two asymptomatic subjects (**b**: male 33 years; **c**: female 27 years). Fibrocartilage is visible, elliptical in shape, discoid in one case, meniscoid in the other. Note the presence of some anechogenic effusion at the center without clinical translation

4.3.1.3 CC Ligaments (Anterior Sagittal Sections) (Fig. 4.4)

Visualization of CC ligaments is difficult in ultrasound but possible for trained operators. The trapezoid ligament unlike the conoid ligament is constantly accessible. They are located deep under the anterior deltoid muscle. The passage of the lateral acromial artery, branch of the thoraco-acromial artery, superficially to the ligaments, is an excellent landmark [43].

CC ligaments appear on a more or less oblique sagittal section as elongated structures, often hypoechoic because of the anisotropic artifact due to their obliquity [39], which helps to locate them in adjacent fat:

- The conoid ligament, is vertically oriented band, from the base of the coracoid to the clavicle [39]. Its clavicular insertion may not be visible on the posterior edge of the clavicle.
- The trapezoid ligament can be spotted from the previous one by rotating the probe laterally [43]. Is has a more oblique, lateral orientation, a flared shape, and inserts next to the AC joint [39].

4.3.1.4 Muscle Cap (Upper Sagittal Sections) (Fig. 4.5)

In a traumatic lesion, it is indispensable to study the condition of the deltotrapezial muscular cap. On a sagittal section medial to the joint, the muscular attachment of the deltoid muscle is located on the anterior side of the clavicle while that of the trapezius is located on the posterior side [44]. Between the two, the deltopectoral fascia forms a hyperechoic line in continuity with the superficial fascia of the two muscles, which merges laterally with the superior AC ligament [44].

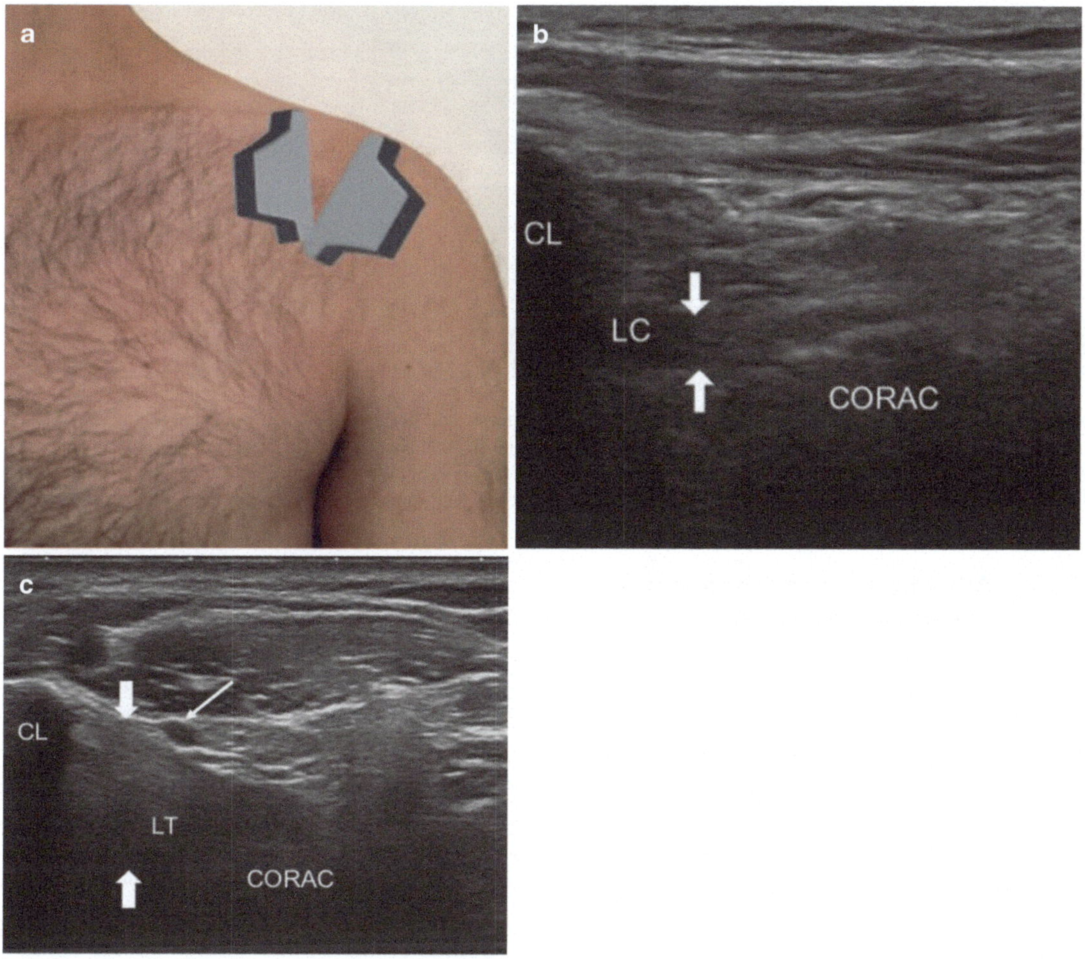

Fig. 4.4 Anterior sagittal sections on the coracoclavicular ligaments. (**a**) Probe positioning: strictly sagittal for the conoid ligament, slightly oblique laterally for the trapezoid ligament. (**b**) Anterior sagittal cut. Conoid ligament (between the two thick arrows). It forms a vertical rectilinear strip, slightly widening upwards. Its proximal part is partially masked by the clavicle, on the posterior edge of which it inserts. (**c**) Oblique anterior sagittal cut, more lateral. Trapezoid ligament (between the two thick arrows). It has a more oblique path, a thicker and more flared appearance than the conoid. The passage of the lateral acromial artery (arrow) into the area of the ligament is a useful landmark. *CL* clavicle, *corac* coracoid, *LC* conoid ligament, *LT* trapezoid ligament

4.3.1.5 Joint Mobility (Dynamic Maneuvers, Frontal Sections)

The analysis is always done by comparison to the normal side.

Joint space is evaluated on a frontal section in search of vertical (frontal plane) or horizontal (axial plane) joint displacement (*see* above).

Some authors also measure the coracoclavicular distance on a sagittal section that reflects the upper clavicular displacement, between the base of the coracoid and the lower edge of the clavicle [39, 45].

Finally, a dynamic "cross arm" maneuver is performed, encompassing an antepulsion and adduction of the shoulder, until the ipsilateral hand reaches the contralateral shoulder [38, 46]; in the normal state, the joint space narrows slightly, and the offset of the bony margins of the articulation changes little relative to the normal side (<1 mm) [38, 46].

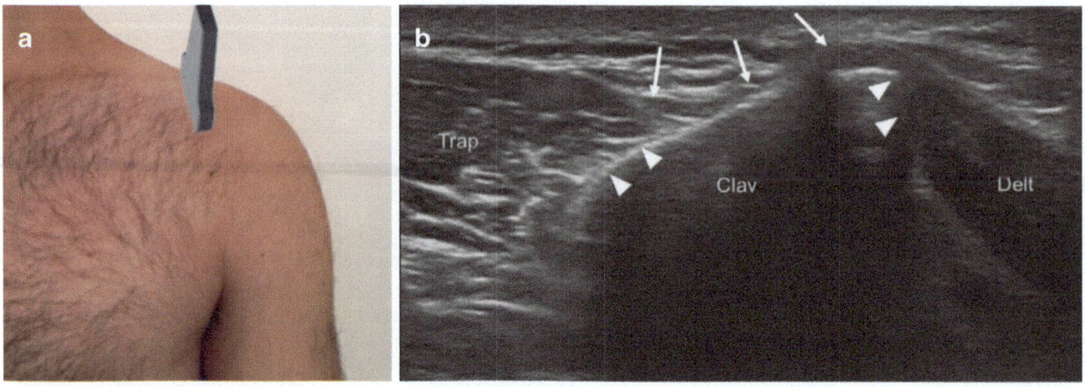

Fig. 4.5 Upper sagittal section on the deltotrapezial cap above the clavicle. (**a**) Position of the probe. (**b**) Corresponding ultrasound image. The trapezius and deltoid have direct myo-osseous insertions (arrowheads) on the anterior and posterior edges of the clavicle, respectively. A superficial fascia (arrows) brings them together and adheres to the superficial side of the clavicle and superior AC ligament. *Trap* trapezius, *Delt* deltoid, *Clav* clavicle

4.3.2 Advantages and Disadvantages of Ultrasound vs MRI

4.3.2.1 Interest of Ultrasound [39, 43, 47]

- Accessible and inexpensive.
- AC joint superficial, thus easily accessible.
- No movement artifacts unlike MRI, especially in acute painful phases.
- Dynamic study.
- Analysis in the plane of the ligaments, unlike most MRI protocols [48, 49].
- Analysis as reliable as MRI to detect capsulo-synovial swelling [39, 40].
- Reliable measurements of joint space and joint swelling (vs. gold standard: MRI or anatomical studies) [50, 51].
- Performed in the sitting position, therefore no reduction of AC movements, especially horizontal, unlike MRI performed in the supine position.
- Guidance for intraarticular infiltration: simple to carry out, controlling on a sagittal section the displacement of the needle, which is introduced anterosuperiorly where the joint space is wider. Studies showed a correct, intra-articular injection in 95–98% of cases, compared with 40–70% without guidance [52–55].

4.3.2.2 Disadvantages of Ultrasound

- No access to the lower edge of the joint.
- Study of the joint disc limited and not as good as in MRI [39]. However, of little clinical interest, due to the frequency of changes with age and the absence of symptomatic correlation.
- More difficult and less reliable analysis of CC ligaments [39, 43, 48, 49]. In our experience, the proximal portion and the clavicular insertion of the conoid ligament are often inaccessible on ultrasound.
- No appreciation of bone edema (arthropathies in inflammatory flare, distal osteolysis of the clavicle, acromial bone, etc.).

4.4 Pathology

4.4.1 Traumatic: AC Sprain

4.4.1.1 Epidemiology and Mechanism

AC sprain is a frequent pathology, the incidence of which is 9 per 1000 per year. It affects athletes in 90% of cases and accounts for 30–50% of shoulder injuries [56].

Two main mechanisms:

- A direct mechanism, by far the most common, by direct contact on the stump of the shoulder, the arm in adduction [4, 25, 57]. It concerns contact or falls sports (two-wheeled, skiing, horse-riding, judo, rugby, American football, hockey, etc.); in rugby they concern one-third of shoulder trauma.
- An indirect mechanism, rare: fall with landing on outstretched hands.

4.4.1.2 Lesion

Direct Mechanism

The direct application of force to the anterosuperior side of the shoulder, in contact with the acromion, induces a rotation of the scapula on itself (tilt) resulting in a l'everage effect on the clavicle, the fulcrum being first the coracoid and, then if the trauma continues, the first rib [58].

The initial lesion corresponds to an elongation without rupture of the AC capsuloligamentous structures [59].

Then the rupture of the capsule usually occurs at the clavicular insertion of the superior AC ligament, above the junction with the fibrocartilage, which remains attached to the acromion. It may be associated with a detachment of the capsule and periosteum at the lower edge of the clavicle [59].

Subsequently, the coracoclavicular ligaments and deltotrapezial fascia rupture, in a lateral to medial direction. In the most severe lesions, the deltoid is torn from the clavicular edge, and the trapezius tears between the fibers inserted on the clavicle and those inserted on the scapular spine [59]. Deltoid is more often lesioned than trapezius [58].

The fall of the scapula downwards, more or less completely disconnected from the clavicle, gives the impression of an ascent of the clavicle (vertical instability). Instability can also be horizontal, corresponding most often to a posterior displacement of the clavicle relative to the acromion.

Indirect Mechanism

Much more rarely, the force is applied from below, the humerus pushing on the acromion. The scapula rotates around the axis of the AC joint itself [58]. This mechanism can explain the anteroinferior displacement of the clavicle in the exceptional Rockwood grade VI [57].

4.4.1.3 Tossy Classification

Tossy [60] proposed a classification in three stages:

- **Grade I**: stretching or partial rupture of AC ligament. Normal X-ray
- **Grade II:** complete rupture of AC ligament and stretching without rupture of CC ligaments. X-ray showing vertical AC subluxation
- **Grade III:** complete rupture of AC ligament and CC ligaments. X-ray showing a vertical AC dislocation ("piano key" image), with an increase in coracoclavicular distance

This classification was virtually abandoned in favor of the Rockwood classification as it considered only ligamentous displacements, excluding those caused by the muscular cap lesions, and neglected posterior displacements. Thus, in a series of about 100 patients, 20% of Tossy II (medical treatment) were reclassified in grade IV in the Rockwood classification and therefore operated [44].

4.4.1.4 Rockwood Classification (Fig. 4.6)

It takes that of Tossy by subdividing grade 3. It is based on a supposed correlation between anatomical lesions and clavicular displacement, in reality very imperfect [43, 44, 61–63].

The clavicular displacement is evaluated by standard X-ray, which involves the production of a front AC view (Zanca type) and an axillary profile (*see* below) [64, 65].

Grade I

Lesions: stretching or partial rupture of AC ligament X-ray normal.

Grade II

Lesions: complete rupture of AC ligament and stretching without rupture of CC ligaments.

X-ray: vertical AC subluxation: slight joint diastasis, elevation of the clavicle relative to the contralateral side with an increase in CC space <25% relative to the contralateral side.

Grade III:

Lesions: complete rupture of AC ligament and CC ligaments.

X-ray: vertical AC dislocation (piano key), with increased CC distance between 25 and 100%.

Grade IV:

Lesions: same as grade 3, and trapezius and deltoid muscles are detached from the distal end of the clavicle. The clavicle is incarcerated in the trapezius posteriorly.

Radiography: increase in CC space <100%. In profile, the clavicle is displaced posteriorly over more than 100% of the joint width.

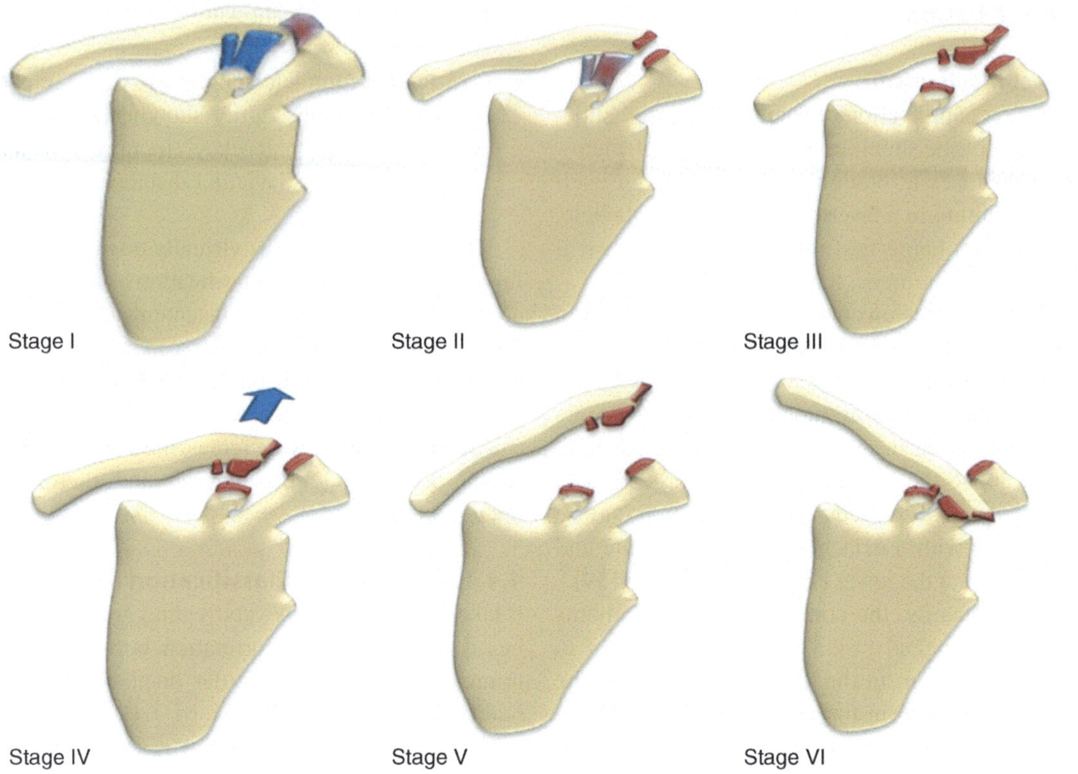

Fig. 4.6 Rockwood classification [61, 62] in six stages

Grade V:

Lesions: same as grade 3, and trapezius and deltoid muscles are detached from the distal end of the clavicle.

X-ray: massive vertical AC dislocation, with increased coracoclavicular distance >100%.

Grade VI (rare):

Lesions: same as grade 3; however, CC ligaments may be intact; trapezius and deltoid muscles may be lesioned or intact.

X-ray: the clavicle is moved forward and down under the acromion (decrease in coracoclavicular distance) or even under the coracoid (subcoracoid dislocation).

Variant: For the bilateral and comparative measurement of the CC, one can substitute the unilateral assessment of the ascent of the clavicle relative to the height of the acromion: up to half the acromion in grade II, the entire height of the acromion in grade III, beyond the acromion in grade V. However, this method seems less reproducible [66].

4.4.1.5 Associated Lesions

In grade III and above, a fracture of the coracoid can be associated with or substitute for ruptures of CC ligaments.

Sometimes the rupture of CC ligaments is replaced by a detachment of the periosteum at their clavicular insertion [22].

Grade IV should seek an associated dislocation of the sternoclavicular joint (bifocal dislocations or "floating clavicle") [67].

Because grades IV and VI are often high energy, vascular or nerve damage to the brachial plexus and other fractures may be associated [67, 68].

4.4.1.6 Reproducibility and Limitations

Intra-observer and interobserver reproducibility is moderate to excellent according to studies for vertical displacement (on front X-rays) [66, 69–71] much less good for horizontal displacement [69, 70].

Thus, grade IV, which accounted for only 0.8% of cases in the initial Rockwood series, would be underdiagnosed and therefore incorrectly operated in the initial phase.

In addition, proper application of the Rockwood classification requires learning: reproducibility is acceptable for trained surgeons but poor for unskilled or poorly experienced physicians [72].

4.4.1.7 Standard X-Rays

Front X-Rays

The classical frontal incidence does not allow the correct visualization of the joint, due to the superposition of the scapular spine on the AC joint from the front [22]. To clear it, either a clavicular view in posterosuperior incidence [73] or a Zanca view, which is an anteroposterior incidence centered on the AC joint with an ascending radius of 15° [1] (Fig. 4.7).

Anteroposterior radiographs should be bilateral and comparative. It allows to search for:

- A widening of the joint space (pathological >6 mm [7], but requiring a comparison to the normal side). It is not specific to instability and can be noted in other pathologies (erosive arthropathies, distal osteolysis of the clavicle, postoperative after acromioplasty).
- A "clavicle ascent": an increase in CC height relative to the normal side.
- A significant posterior horizontal displacement of the clavicle (grade IV) may be suspected when a moderate ascent is accompanied by a widening of the joint space > 60% [74].
- A fracture of the clavicle or coracoid.

Profile X-Rays

For the profile, the axillary incidence is carried out with the arm abducted at 70–90°, beam oriented by 15° laterally and dorsally [75].It allows:

- Identification of a posterior displacement of the clavicle (Rockwood IV).
- To search for a fracture that has gone unnoticed on the front view. In particular, an AC dislocation without a change in CC space should cause a coracoid fracture to be suspected [4].

Stress X-Rays

Comparative front radiographs with abduction [22] and front stress radiographs (carrying a load of 10 kg on each side) [22] are intended to raise awareness of the increase in CC height. In practice, they only unmask Grade III in a small number of cases (4% [76]).

Problem of Posterior Displacement

There is no current consensus to assess posterior clavicular displacement [41]. Axillary view is used in clinical practice and in most studies.

However, the detection of posterior translation on the axillary view faces several difficulties:

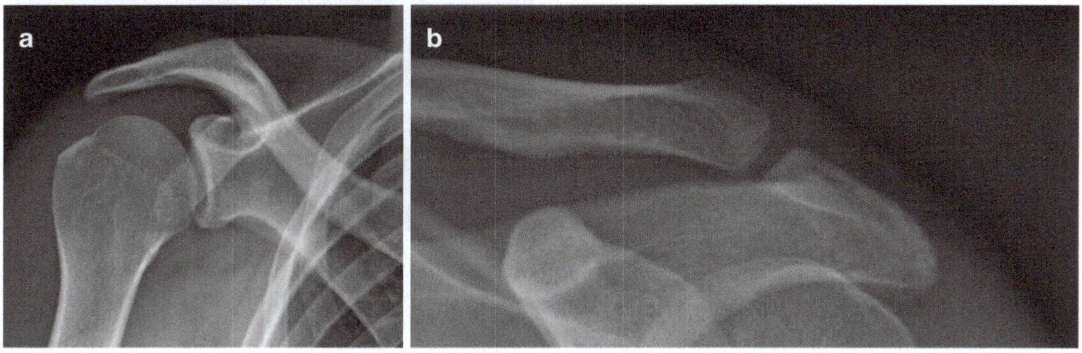

Fig. 4.7 Front X-rays. (**a**) Front shoulder snapshot. The AC joint space is projected onto the spine of the scapula. (**b**) A snapshot centered on the AC joint with a slightly ascending radius (Zanca) allows to visualize the joint space

- Difficulty of moving the shoulder to make the view in the acute phase due to pain.
- Variation of posterior clavicular translation according to radius inclination [75].
- Physiological shift between acromion and clavicle edges in 40% of subjects, with 20% of cases a posterior clavicle translation >2 mm [41] exposing the risk of false positives. The threshold of >100% posterior displacement of the clavicle relative to the acromion retained in grade IV (incarcerated) generally corresponds to the most severe clavicular displacements. In grade III with horizontal instability, therefore less displaced, some retain a posterior clavicular translation >10–12 mm relative to the acromion [77].
- Poor reproducibility of measurements due to curved shape of acromion and clavicle [69].
- The CT scan underestimates horizontal displacements, because it is performed in a supine position (reduction of mobile Grade III lesions).

Authors have therefore attempted to develop "dynamic" X-ray techniques to detect posterior instability in grade III:

- *Tauber* proposed to carry out two axillary radiographs: the usual abduction view as well as an abduction view with 90° anterior antepulsion, allowing the detection of abnormal posterior translational movement of the clavicle [78]. The results are discordant [69, 75].
- The *incidence of Alexander* [22, 77, 79–81]: it corresponds to a view close to the Lamy profile but with maximum adduction (arm crossed against chest, shoulder below the contralateral axillary hollow). The snapshot must be bilateral and comparative. Normally the clavicle and the acromion overlap. In the case of posterior translation, the clavicle is projected above and behind the acromion. Quantitative or semiquantitative measures were proposed [81, 82], which would be repeatable and valid [81]. In addition, this view would be less sensitive to variations in radius angulation of the beam than the axillary image [81].

4.4.1.8 Ultrasound and MRI

Ultrasound allows easy study of the superior AC ligament and rupture of the muscular fascia [44, 50]. In trained hands, it allows a good analysis of CC ligamentous lesions, although less effective than MRI [43, 50]. On the other hand, it allows a better study of displacements and instability (sitting position, contralateral reference, dynamic study).

Joint

Regardless of grade, joint swelling may be observed with or without effusion, as well as Doppler hypervascularization, fibrocartilage lesions [83], and pain under the probe.

Ligaments

The AC ligament can be thickened (grade I) (Fig. 4.8) or broken (grade II) (Fig. 4.9). These are mainly clavicular ligamentous detachments (2/3 of cases) or oblique ruptures starting from the clavicle forward and joining the acromion behind [83]. In high-grade lesions, the ligament is frequently incarcerated in the joint space [83].

CC ligaments can be thickened (grade II) (Fig. 4.10) or broken (grade III) (Figs. 4.11, 4.12, 4.13, and 4.14). CC ligaments are partially visible in ultrasound; however ruptures

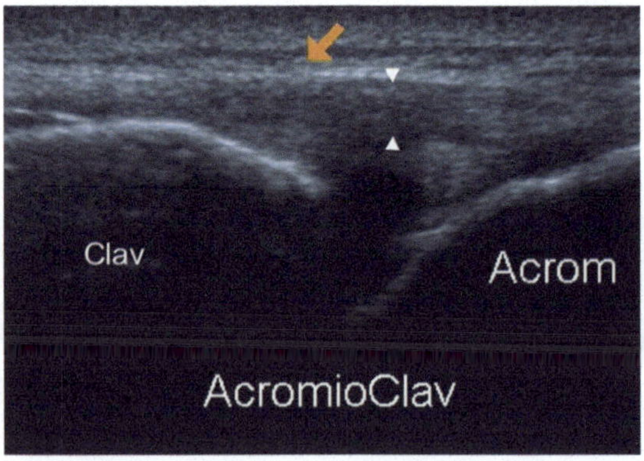

Fig. 4.8 Benign lesion to superior AC ligament during Rockwood I sprain. The superior AC ligament (arrow) is thickened (between arrows) and hypoechoic but continuous

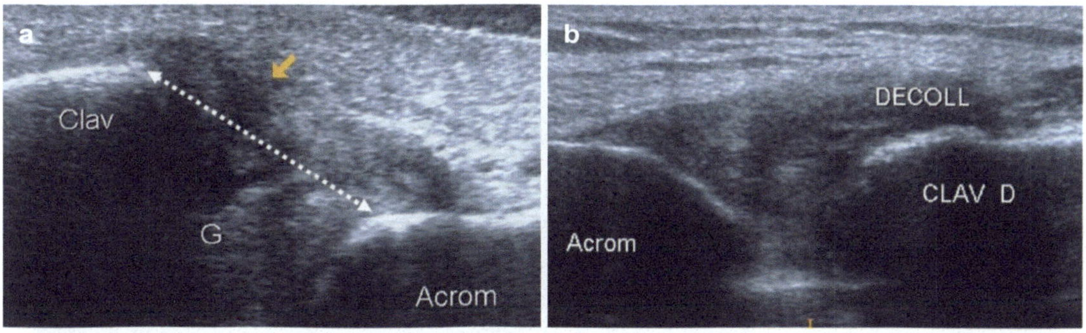

Fig. 4.9 Superieor AC ligament ruptures in Rockwood II sprain. Frontal section. (**a**) Complete detachment of the clavicular side of the superior AC ligament (arrow). Moderate joint diastasis (double dotted arrow) relative to the asymptomatic side (not shown here) and slight upper shift of the clavicle. (**b**) Other patient. Periosteal detachment in continuity with a detachment of the superior AC ligament

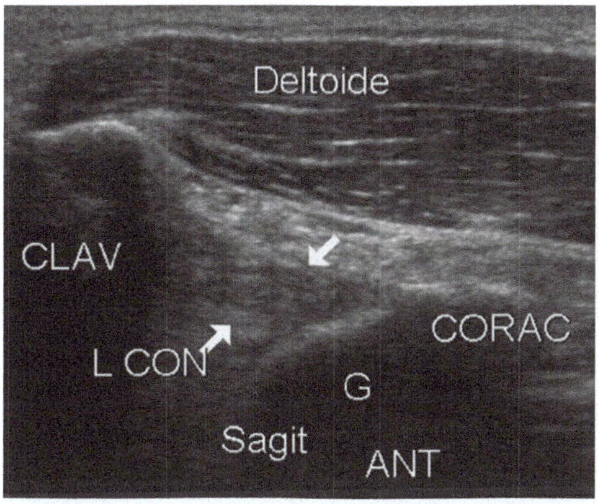

Fig. 4.10 Lesion without rupture of conoid ligament during Rockwood II sprain. Anterior sagittal section. The conoid ligament is thickened, hypoechoic, but well stretched between the base of the coracoid and the posteroinferior side of the clavicle. *L con* conoid ligament, *Clav* clavicle, *Corac* coracoid

are usually located in the ligament body, in areas accessible to ultrasound. In addition, a relaxed appearance of the ligament is an indirect sign of rupture (Fig. 4.11). Only one of the two CC ligaments can be ruptured in grade II [21, 84].

Muscular Cap

Muscle deltotrapezial cap is well analyzed on sagittal sections in ultrasound, in a series of 92 patients [44]:

- Detachment of the fascia without tearing is possible in grade II, occasionally with a tear of only one of the three elements of the muscular cap (fascia tearing, deltoid disinsertion or trapezius disinsertion).
- The rupture of the three elements of the cap is constant in grade V (Figs. 4.13 and 4.14).
- In grades IV as well, yet the disinsertion of the trapezius (within which the clavicle has lodged) may be missing.
- In contrast, lesions vary considerably in grade III: about 50% without significant lesion, 30% intermediate lesions (Fig. 4.15), and 20% with extensive lesions comparable to grade V.

Joint Instability

On a frontal section, the joint may show signs of vertical instability, slight in grade II (often visible only in dynamics), and greater in higher grades:

- In the neutral position, the jont space may be widened relative to the normal side, and there may be a spontaneous superior clavicular shift.
- There may also be an increase in coracoclavicular distance on sagittal sections relative to the normal side [39].
- In dynamic *cross arm* maneuvers, the joint space decreases until direct contact between the two bones, and a joint shift appears (or accentuates), the clavicle rising higher than the acromion [85] (Fig. 4.16).

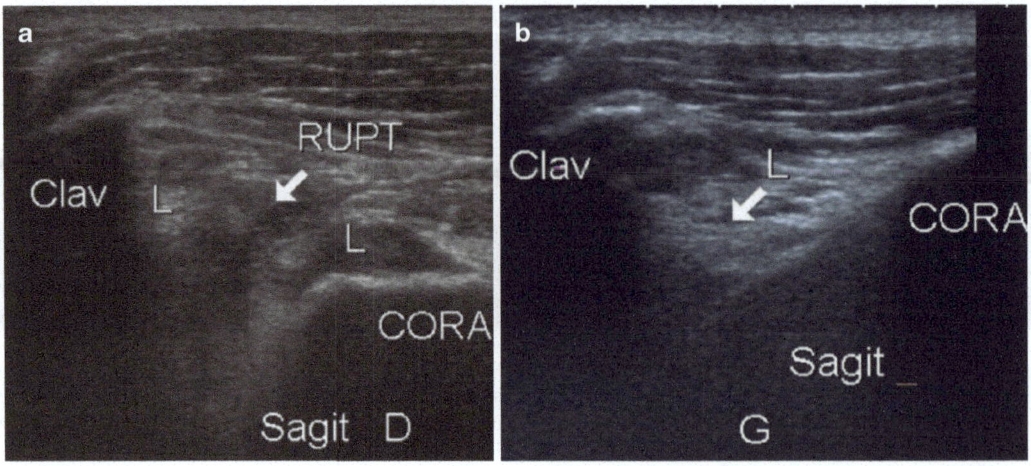

Fig. 4.11 Rupture of the trapezoid ligament in a Rockwood III sprain. Comparative anterior sagittal cut. (**a**) Pathological side. Interruption in the full body of the trapezoid ligament (arrow). *L* proximal and distal ligament stumps, *Clav* clavicle, *Corac* coracoid. (**b**) normal side

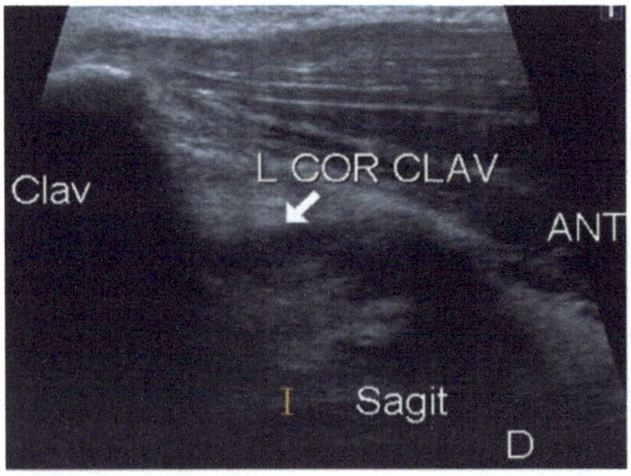

Fig. 4.12 Proximal rupture of conoid ligament during Rockwood III sprain. Anterior sagittal section. The ligament is completely relaxed, taking a curved shape, signifying a rupture (arrow)

In grade IV, ultrasound could objectify posterior clavicular displacement on an anterior axial section, resulting in an increase in the distance between the acromion and the clavicle [39]. The sternoclavicular joint should also be analyzed in these grade IV for bipolar dislocation.

4.4.1.9 Sequelae and Chronic Lesions

In case of persistent symptoms, two nosological frameworks should be distinguished, especially if surgery is envisaged: osteoarthritis and instability; hence the importance of dynamic analysis (dynamic X-rays, ultrasound).

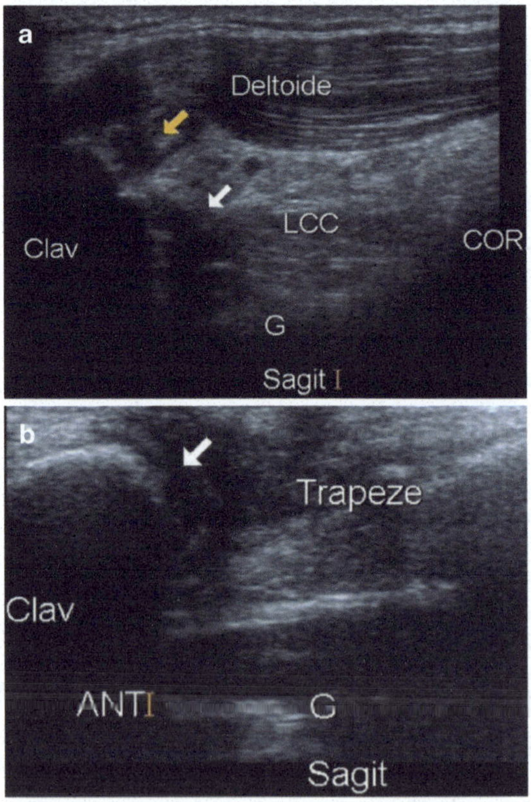

Fig. 4.13 Sprain Rockwood V. (**a**) Anterior sagittal section. Proximal rupture of conoid ligament (white arrow). Rupture of the clavicular insertion of the deltoid muscle (orange arrow). (**b**) Superior sagittal section, same patient. Clavicular detachment of trapezius muscle, with heterogeneous detachment zone (arrow), and heterogeneous retracted muscle. *LCC* coracoclavicular ligament

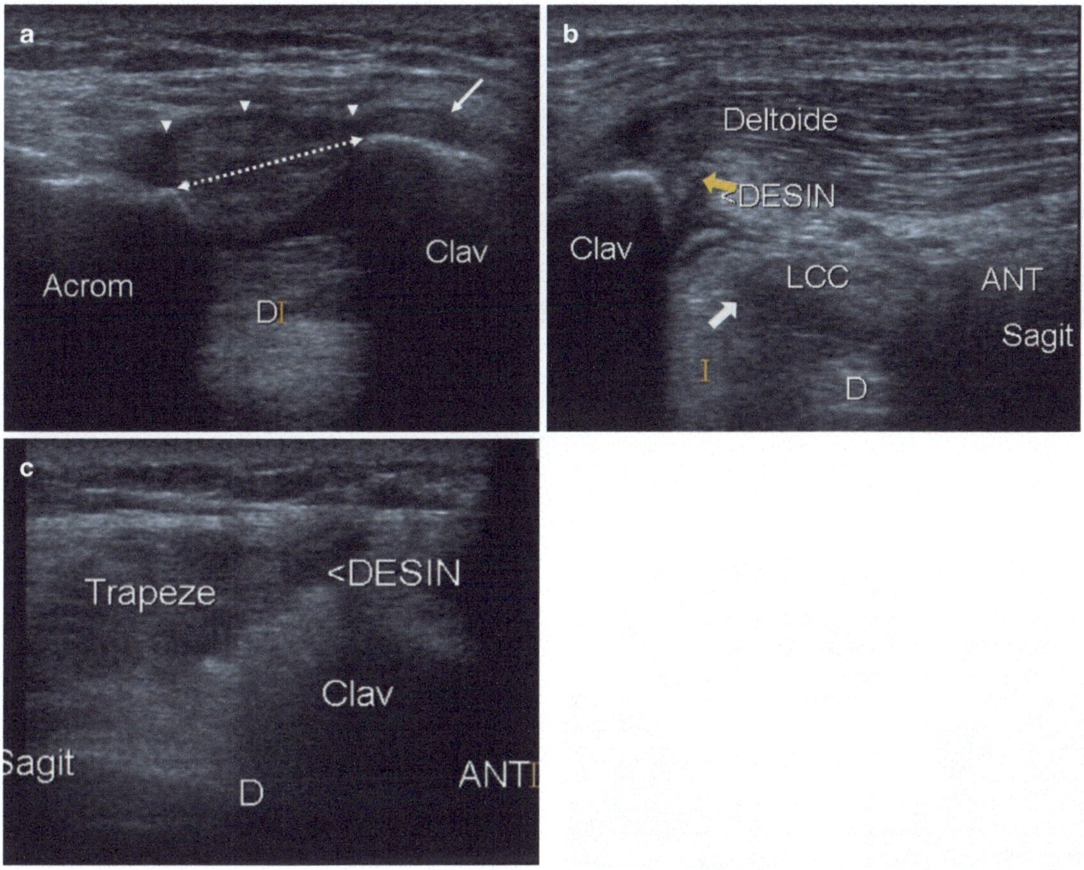

Fig. 4.14 Rockwood V sprain. (**a**) frontal AC section. Detachment of the superior acromioclavicular ligament from the clavicular edge (arrow), with unstretched appearance of the ligament (arrow heads) and articular diastasis (double dotted arrow). (**b**) Anterior sagittal section, same patient. Proximal rupture of the conoid ligament (white arrow) which is otherwise thickened. Lesion of the muscular cap with disinsertion of the clavicular attachment of the deltoid (orange arrow). (**c**) Upper sagittal section, same patient. Disinsertion of the clavicular attachment of the trapezius and retraction thereof

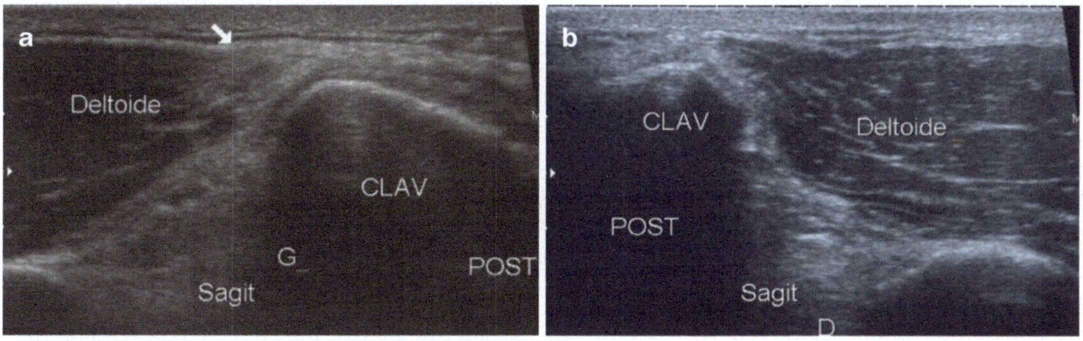

Fig. 4.15 Partial disinsertion of the muscular cap during a Rockwood III sprain. Anterior sagittal section. (**a**) Pathological side: detachment of the deltoid muscle from the clavicle, without rupture of the fascia (arrow). Hyperechoic reactive edema of the muscular parenchyma. (**b**) Normal side

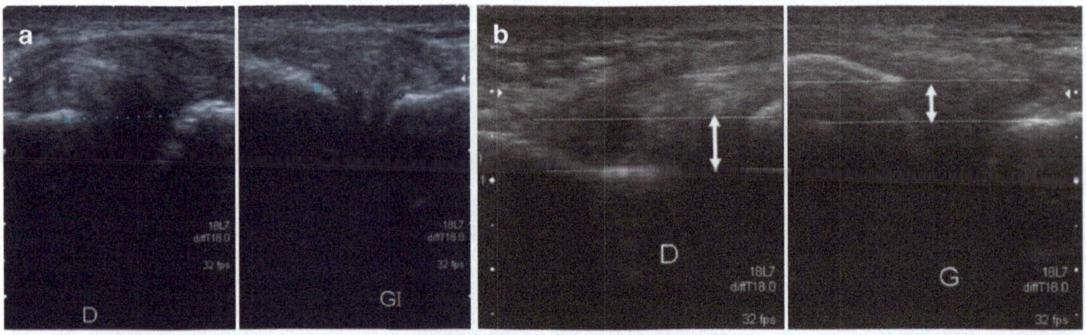

Fig. 4.16 Moderate vertical instability during a Rockwood II sprain of the right shoulder. Bilateral and comparative frontal sections. (**a**) Neutral position. Slight joint diastasis, visible relative to the normal side (dotted segments: 6 mm on the traumatized side versus 4 mm on the left). (**b**) Cross arm maneuver. Upper subluxation of the clavicle during the maneuver with a clavicular shift higher on the traumatized side than on the normal side (double arrows)

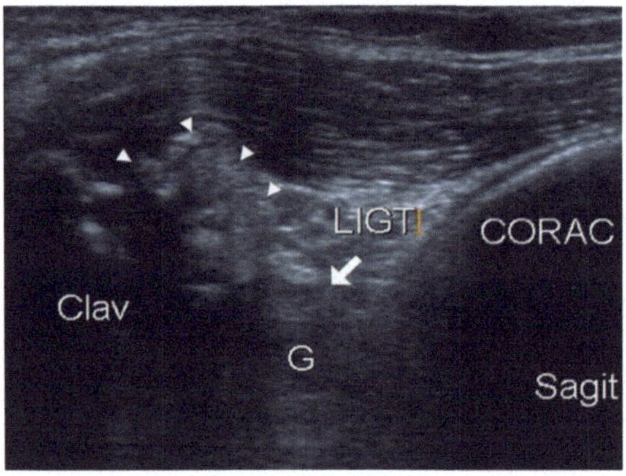

Fig. 4.17 Rockwood III sprain sequelae. Anterior sagittal section. Wide ossifications (arrows heads) of the proximal half of the CC ligament (arrow)

Posttraumatic Osteoarthritis

X-ray and ultrasound: the same presentation as primitive osteoarthritis (see infra), but instead of pinching, some widening of the joint space and vertical AC shift often persist. Ossifications of CC ligaments can be visible in the CC space [48] (Fig. 4.17) or at the insertion of the superior AC ligament (Fig. 4.18).

Chronic Posttraumatic Instability

- Vertical instability, observed in case of a reconstructed ligament rupture or a loss of reduction.
- Persistent horizontal instability after CC surgery without AC stabilization; it causes a posterior abutment of the clavicle on the acromion, progressing toward osteoarthritis [68].
- Radiography and ultrasound: same abnormalities as in acute (*see* above) (Fig. 4.19).

4.4.1.10 Perspectives of Imaging in AC Sprain

Section imaging is not used as a first line in AC sprains. However, it can be useful in targeted cases. There are currently two pitfalls:

- **Detect posterior displacement of the clavicle**: Grade IV not diagnosed in radiography (incarcerated displacement) and grade III with posterior instability of the clavicle, which would have a significant prognostic impact [77].

ISAKOS proposes to subdivide the Rockwood grade III into IIIA (without posterior instability) and IIIB (with posterior instability), based on clinical examination and dynamic X-rays [86].

In practice these dynamic radiographs are rarely performed routinely. MRI and scanner are carried out supine, thus reducing horizontal displacement in grade IIIB.

Ultrasound may have an interest, which remains to be demonstrated, in detecting these posterior instabilities.

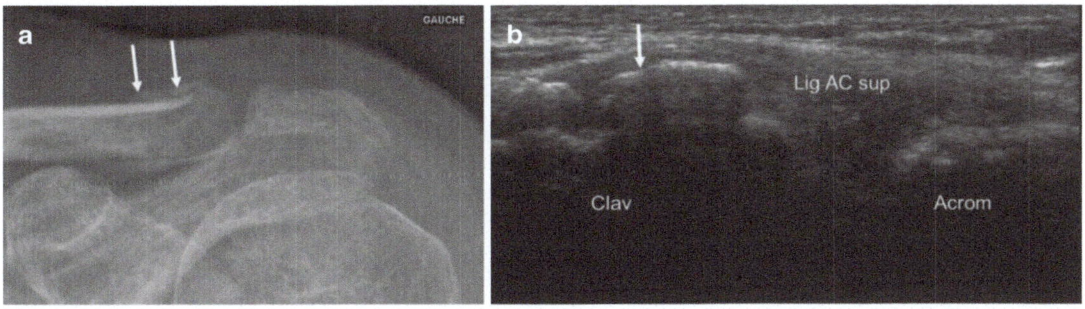

Fig. 4.18 Calcified sequelae of a disinsertion of the superior AC ligament. (**a**) Frontal X-ray. (**b**) Ultrasound, frontal section. Calcifications (arrows) of the clavicular insertion of the superior AC ligament, as well as of the periosteum in continuity

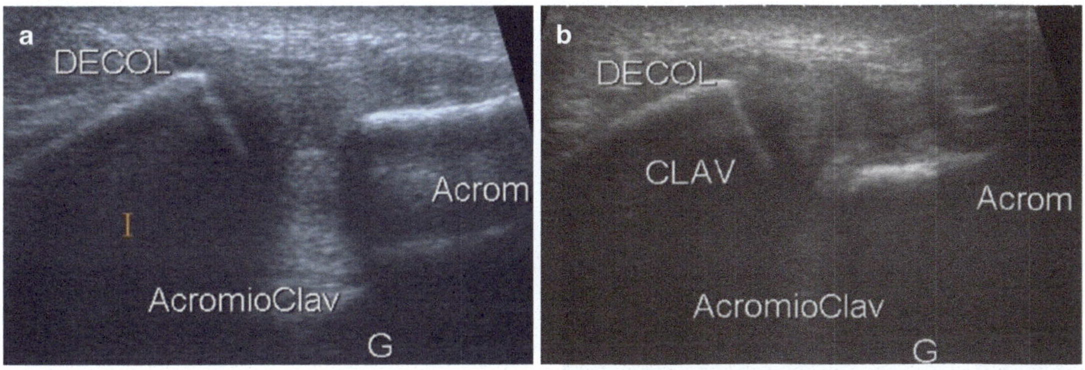

Fig. 4.19 Chronic instability at a distance of Rockwood III sprain in a 25-year-old judoka. Frontal section. (**a**) Neutral position. Spontaneous diastasis and upper shift of the clavicle relative to the acromion. (**b**) Cross arm. Reduction of the diastasis (mobile) and accentuation of the shift of the clavicle upward

- **Determine which grade III is to be operated**, knowing that grade III accounts for 40% of all AC sprains and that surgery at the outset could have better results than later surgery of a chronic instability [87].

In addition to the search for posterior instability, which is difficult to identify, a precise assessment of anatomical lesions could be useful.

The study of CC ligament ruptures has little effect on treatment according to current standards, since grade III is most often treated medically. However, it may be useful in targeted cases where there is a doubt between grade II and grade III when surgery is considered, as X-ray would frequently underestimate the importance of anatomic lesions [43].

Above all, the study of the muscular cap seems decisive to better sort out these grade III lesions. In an ultrasound study with operative control, 20% of grade III had cap lesions identical to grade V [44] and could therefore be candidates for surgery. The long-term utility of ultrasound (and MRI) in this indication remains to be demonstrated.

4.5 Distal Fractures of the Clavicle

Approximately one-quarter of the clavicle fractures are distal [88, 89]. These fractures are more common than acromion fractures and are a differential diagnosis of AC sprains.

They are classified into three types by Neer, depending on the location of the fracture in relation to the clavicular insertions of the CC ligaments [90, 91]:

- Type I: lateral in relation to the CC ligaments.
- Type II: medial relative to the CC ligaments, therefore with displacement of the proximal

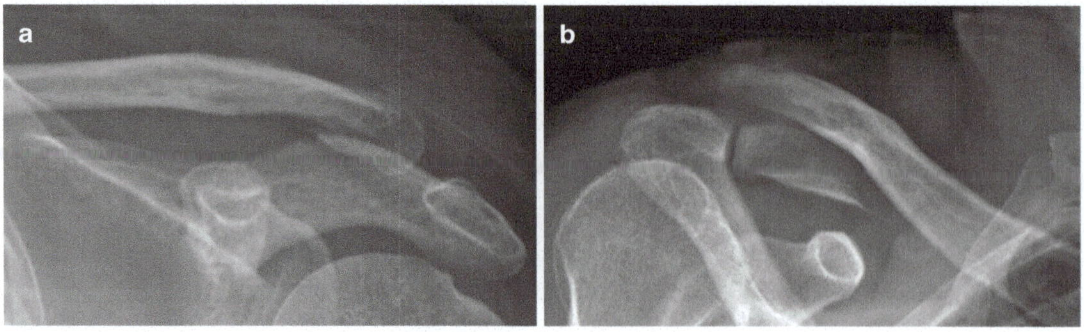

Fig. 4.20 Examples of distal clavicle fractures. (**a**) Neer I fracture. (**b**) Neer II fracture

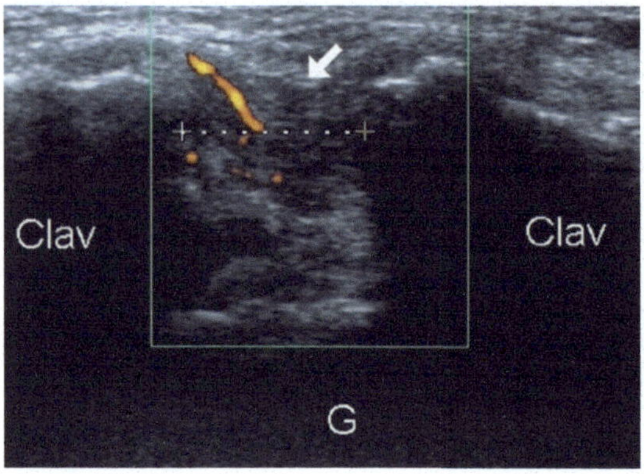

Fig. 4.21 Pseudarthrosis of a Neer II distal clavicle fracture. Frontal section on the clavicle. Wide space separating the two bone fragments (dotted line). Pseudarthrosis was mobile in movements

fragment. In type IIA, both CC ligaments are intact, in IIB the conoid ligament is broken (fracture located between the two CC ligaments).

- Type III: distal joint.

The diagnosis is radiographic (Fig. 4.20). The fracture may however be missed and discovered incidentally during an ultrasound requested for AC sprain. It shows an interruption of the cortical bone of the clavicle (Fig. 4.21). The state of the CC ligaments can also be specified.

4.6 Degenerative AC Arthropathy

Primary AC joint involvement is extremely common. Degenerative arthritis changes are present in 70% before the age of 30 and almost constant after 40 years [92].

Secondary degenerative disorders may be sequalae of lesions that are originally traumatic, microtraumatic, rheumatic, microcrystalline, septic, etc.

4.6.1 Pathophysiology

The incomplete or absent nature of the joint disc and its rapid degeneration are, for some, responsible for the high frequency of degenerative pathology, due to the lack of congruence of articular surfaces [12]. In fact, the disc deteriorates as early as the second decade, fringes, thins, and then perforates until it disappears after 50 years [9, 10]. In contrast, the first lesions of the sternoclavicular articular fibrocartilage appear only after 50 years [9].

Transformations from hyaline articular cartilage to fibrocartilage around the age of 20 may contribute to this rapid joint degeneration [3]. The existence of rotating movements on this near-flat arthrodia and the importance of compression forces associated with the deltoid action may also be involved [2].

Osteoarthritis results in joint remodeling with anteroposterior lengthening of the acromion and rounding of the clavicular surface in mirror, giving a "ball and cup" appearance [93]. Osteophytes developed on the lower slope are implicated in subacromial impingements [12].

4.6.2 Imaging

Standard radiography on classical frontal view can show classical signs: narrowing of the joint space, sclerosis and subchondral geodes, and osteophytes. The Zanca incidence should be preferred, since it allows the clearing of the scapular spine out of the projection of the AC joint (Fig. 4.22).

The scanner is more sensitive but irradiating, not performed in this indication.

Ultrasound (Fig. 4.23) easily highlights osteophytes on the edges of the joint space, narrowing of the space, heterogeneity of the joint disc, sometimes intra-articular osteochondromas. Joint cysts can develop. An effusion has no diagnostic value [40, 42, 94]. Sometimes the joint space is widened in the case of associated instability, erosive remodeling, or osteolysis of the distal clavicle [38].

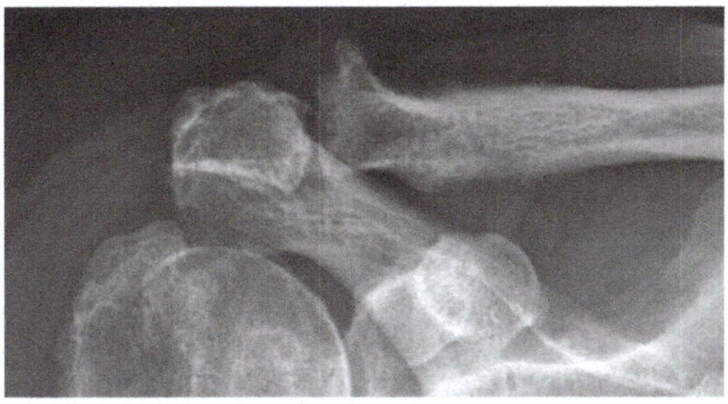

Fig. 4.22 AC Osteoarthritis. Frontal X-ray. Radiograph with ascending radius clears the joint space, allowing to find the cardinal signs of osteoarthritis

Since these abnormalities are very common and often asymptomatic, other signs are necessary to link osteoarthritis to the symptom:

- Swelling with thickening >3 mm of the upper capsular fold.
- Hypervascularization on Doppler.
- Pain during echopalpation or during mobilization in cross arm.

Associated AC instability should also be sought (*see* above).

MRI shows the same abnormalities as ultrasound [95, 96], but also bone edema during relapses, which is correlated with pain; it can be visible on the clavicular side or on both sides of the joint [92, 94, 97].

Anesthetic test: in case of doubt, the acromioclavicular origin of shoulder pain can be confirmed by an anesthetic test with lidocaine 1% or 2% injection guided by ultrasound or radioscopy [12].

4.7 Arthritis

4.7.1 Rheumatic Arthritis

In inflammatory rheumatism (RA), ultrasound may show hypervascularized articular swelling

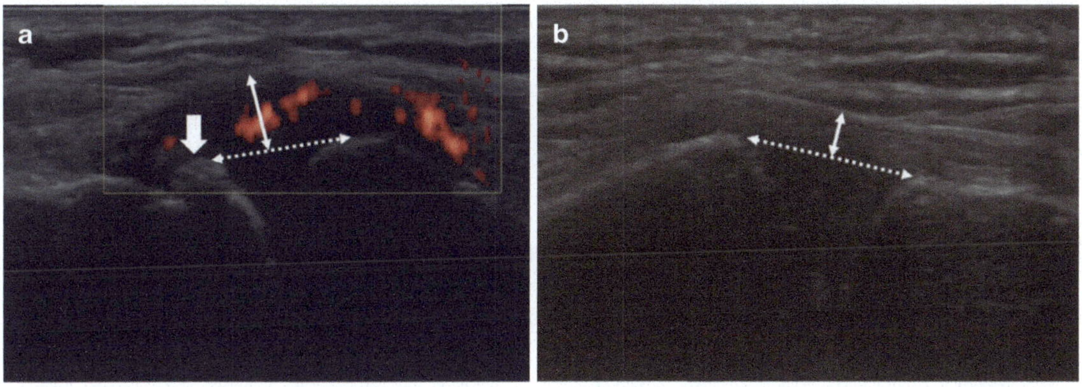

Fig. 4.23 Congestive CA osteoarthritis. 60-year-old woman; sore shoulder on the right. Comparative frontal sections. (**a**) Right side. (**b**) Same patient; left side. Compared to the asymptomatic side, there is a discreet joint pinching (double dotted arrows), marginal osteophytes (wide arrow), and especially a hypervascularized capsular swelling (double arrows) on Doppler

with effusion, with no specificity compared to an osteoarthritis in flare. However, widening of the joint space by bone erosions and static or dynamic signs of joint instability are more common [39].

MRI also allows for the detection of bone edema if performed.

Later, secondary osteoarthritis settles with joint pinching and degenerative changes (*see* above).

4.7.2 Septic Arthritis

Rare due to the low vascularization of the AC joint, it occurs in specific conditions (immunodepression, intravenous drug addiction) or in an iatrogenic setting after puncture, infiltration, or surgery [98].

Ultrasound has no specificity: joint swelling of inflammatory appearance (marked hypervascularization, periarticular and adjacent muscle edema). The absence of effusion makes the diagnosis unlikely [40, 98]. MRI shows the same abnormalities, associated with bone edema. Diagnosis is based on the analysis of the joint puncture.

4.7.3 Microcrystalline Arthritis

AC joint involvement is common in chondrocalcinosis and rare in gout [98]. Imaging is not specific. Diagnosis is based on the analysis of the puncture.

4.8 Joint Cysts

A joint cyst developed on the upper side of the AC joint can be of two types [98–100]:

- "True" joint cyst, due to a capsular valve, as a consequence of joint degradation regardless of its origin (degenerative arthropathy, instability, trauma, infection, metabolic). An ultrasound guided puncture is useful [99].
- "False" cyst after rupture of the rotator cuff (Fig. 4.24) resulting in eccentric omarthrosis and degradation of the lower side of the AC joint. Communication between the glenohumeral, bursal, and acromioclavicular cavities leads to accumulation of fluid in the upper recess of the AC joint, which expands without being encysted. During ultrasound dynamic maneuvers in *cross arm*, the volume of the cyst increases ("geyser sign") [98, 99, 101].

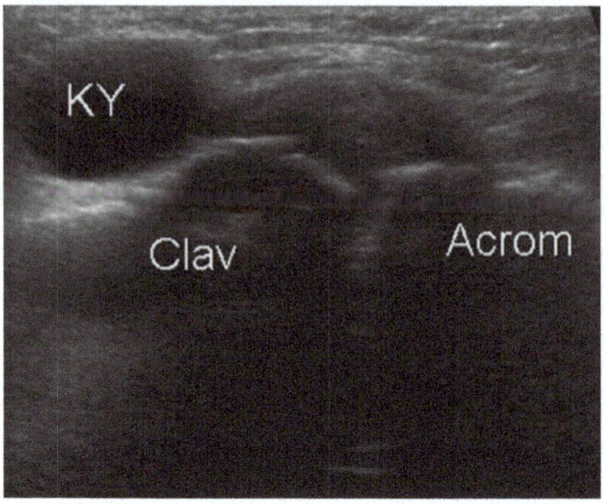

Fig. 4.24 AC joint cyst. Frontal section. The cyst communicates with the joint cavity (arrow). Ultrasound also showed a complete rupture of the rotator cuff with a "geyser sign." *Ky* cyst

4.9 Distal Clavicle Osteolysis (DCO)

It would be the result of compression forces associated with shear movements [2].

The mechanism is poorly known: subchondral microcracks, osteoclastosis, synovial proliferation, and autonomic dysfunction [2, 94].

The causes of an unilateral DCO are either traumatic (6% after AC sprain [102]), or microtraumatic. Infection and bone tumor are differencial diagnoses.

Bilateral DCOs point at a systemic pathology: rheumatoid arthritis, hyperparathyroidism, scleroderma [98].

The X-ray shows widening of the joint space, erosions, and demineralization of the distal clavicle [102].

MRI further shows bone edema (clavicular +/− acromial), joint swelling, and periostitis [94, 102].

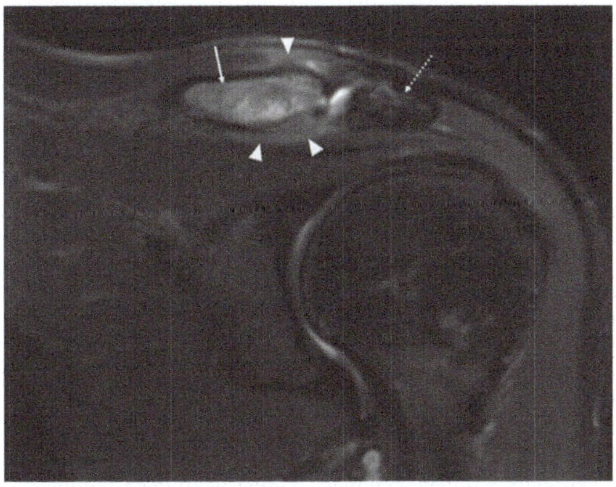

Fig. 4.25 Distal osteolysis of the clavicle. MRI, frontal T2 section with saturation of the fat signal. 38-year-old man; bike fall 6 weeks ago. Bone edema in hypersignal T2 extended on the clavicular side (full arrow), absent on the acromial side (dotted arrow). Moderate periclavicular hypersignal (arrowheads)

The course is generally favorable at 1 year; distal resection of the clavicle may be proposed in case of persistent symptoms [103] (Fig. 4.25).

4.10 Os Acromiale

Os acromiale is an anatomical variant resulting from the non-fusion of a secondary ossification point of the acromion, present in 3–6% of the general population [104].

An os acromiale may be complicated by hypermobility, pain at the junction with acromion, and subacromial impingement in case of an ossified junction [94, 105]. As such, it is a differential diagnosis of AC pain.

The primary ossification nucleus for the coracoid appears at birth. Three or four nuclei of secondary ossification appear after 8–10 years and merge with the rest of the scapula before 25 years [2, 104, 106]. Depending on the non-fusion zone, the positioning of the os acromiale may vary from the tip of the acromion (terminal acromial bone) to the junction with the scapular spine (posterior acromial bone), passing through intermediate forms that are most common (90%) [94, 104].

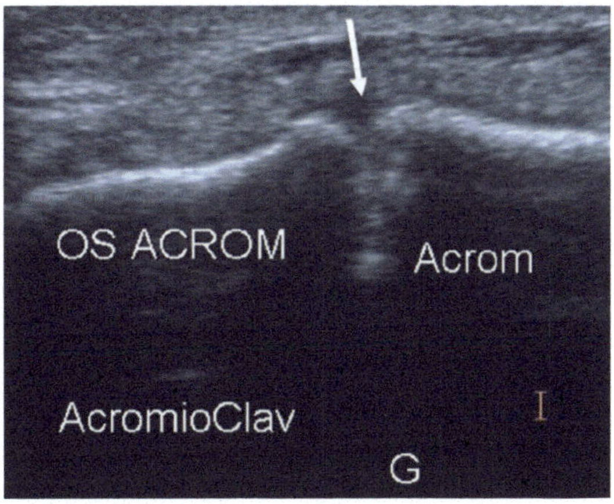

Fig. 4.26 Os acromiale. Oblique frontal section on the acromion. Interruption of the cortex of the acromion, with regular and slightly elevated edges, with pseudo-spacing corresponding to a syndesmotic junction (arrow). *Acrom bone* os acromiale, *Acrom* acromion

The nature of the union between the scapular spine and the acromial bone is variable: synchondrosis, amphiarthrosis, and sometimes true arthrodia [3].

In radiography, the os acromiale is clearly visible on an axillary incidence [12, 94]. However, as this incidence is not usually carried out immediately on the basic radiographic assessment, diagnosis is often performed during ultrasound or MRI.

Ultrasound identifies an os acromiale in 100% of cases [107], provided is is searched for. It shows an interruption of the continuity of the acromion of variable width, between 2 and 8 mm (Fig. 4.26). Bone edges can be flat, pseudo-osteophytic protruding, or blunt [107]. A pathological junction with the acromion is manifested by a local swelling that is vascularized and painful. Ultrasound may look for an abnormal mobilization when performing a slight pressure onto acromion [104].

MRI also allows additional detection of bone edema in case of pain of the junction [94].

4.11 Conclusion

Two acromioclavicular pathologies are particularly common: osteoarthritis and sprains.

Radio-ultrasound pair has a preponderant place in degenerative pathology: detection of an osteoarthritis and confirmation of its symptomatic character.

In traumatic pathology, cross-sectional imaging may have a role in the future to help choose between medical and surgical treatments:

- By helping to detect grade IV (posterior clavicular displacement), to be operated, especially when the radiographic profile is insufficient or not achievable.
- By differenciating several types grade III in operable patients, by analysing posterior instability (grade "IIIB"), ligament workup, and muscle cap.

These issues will need to be further explored in future studies.

References

1. Zanca P. Shoulder bread: involvement of the acromioclavicular joint. (Analysis of 1,000 cases). Am J Roentgenol Radium Ther Nucl Med. 1971;112:493–506.
2. Renfree KJ, Wright TW. Anatomy and biomechanics of the acromioclavicular and sternoclavicular joints. Clin Sports Med. 2003;22:219–37.
3. Testut L, Latarjet A. Traité d' anatomie humaine. 9. éd., rev.corr.et augm. /. Paris: Doin, 1948.
4. Saccomanno MF, De Ieso C, Milano G. Acromioclavicular joint unability: anatomy, biomechanics and evaluation. Joints. 2014;2:87–92.
5. Bucholz RW. Chapter 29: acromioclavicular joint injuries. In: Fractures in adults. Philadelphia: Lippincott Williams & Wilkins; 2001. p. 1210–44.
6. Bosworth BM. Complete acromioclavicular dislocation. N Engl J Med. 1949;241:221–5.
7. Petersson CJ, Redlund-Johnell I. Radiographic joint space in normal acromioclavicular joints. Acta Orthop Scand. 1983;54:431–3.
8. Salter EG, Nasca RJ, Shelley BS. Anatomical observations on the acromioclavicular joint and supporting ligaments. Am J Sports Med. 1987;15:199–206.
9. Depalma AF. Surgical anatomy of acromioclavicular and sternoclavicular joints. Surg Clin North Am. 1963;43:1541–50.
10. Petersson CJ. Degeneration of the acromioclavicular joint. A morphological study. Acta Orthop Scand. 1983;54:434–8.
11. Testut. Traité d'anatomie humaine. 4th ed., revised, corrected and augmented. Paris: O. Doin; 1899.
12. Buttaci CJ, Stitik TP, Yonclas PP, et al. Osteoarthritis of the acromioclavicular joint: a review of anatomy, biomechanics, diagnosis, and treatment. Am J Phys Med Rehabil. 2004;83:791–7.
13. Nakazawa M, Nimura A, Mochizuki T, et al. The orientation and variation of the acromioclavicular ligament: an anatomic study. Am J Sports Med 2016;44:2690–5.
14. Fukuda K, Craig EV, An KN, et al. Biomechanical study of the ligamentous system of the acromioclavicular joint. J Bone Joint Surg Am. 1986;68: 434–40.
15. Renfree KJ, Riley MK, Wheeler D, et al. Ligamentous anatomy of the distal clavicle. J Shoulder Elbow Surg. 2003;12:355–9.
16. Stine IA, Vangsness CT. Analysis of the capsule and ligament insertions about the acromioclavicular joint: a cadaveric study. Arthroscopy. 2009;25:968–74.
17. Rios CG, Arciero RA, Mazzocca AD. Anatomy of the clavicle and coracoid process for reconstruction of the coracoclavicular ligaments. Am J Sports Med. 2007;35:811–7.
18. Harris RI, Vu DH, Sonnabend DH, et al. Anatomic variance of the coracoclavicular ligaments. J Shoulder Elbow Surg. 2001;10:585–8.
19. Xue C, Song L-J, Li X, et al. Coracoclavicular anatomical ligaments reconstruction: a feasibility study. Int J Med Robot Comput Assist Surg MRCAS. 2015;11:181–7.
20. Takase K. The coracoclavicular ligaments: an anatomic study. Surg Radiol Anat. 2010;32:683–8.
21. Rios CG, Mazzocca AD. Acromioclavicular joint problems in athletes and new methods of management. Clin Sports Med. 2008;27:763–88.
22. Jerosch J. Das Akromioklavikulargelenk Orthop. 2000;29:895–908.
23. Rockwood CA, Williams GR, Young DC. Disorders of the acromioclavicular joint. In: The shoulder. Philadelphia: WB Saunders; 1998. p. 483–553.
24. Kennedy JC, Cameron H. Complete dislocation of the acromio-clavicular joint. J Bone Joint Surg Br. 1954;36-B:202–8.
25. Klonz A, Loitz D. The acromioclavicular joint. Unfallsurg. 2005;108:1049–58, quiz 1059.
26. Worcester JN, Green DP. Osteoarthritis of the acromioclavicular joint. Clin Orthop. 1968;58:69–73.
27. Ludewig PM, Phadke V, Braman JP, et al. Motion of the shoulder complex during multiplanar humeral elevation. J Bone Joint Surg Am. 2009;91:378–89.
28. Debski RE, Parsons IM, Woo SL, et al. Effect of capsular injury on acromioclavicular joint mechanics. J Bone Joint Surg Am. 2001;83-A:1344–51.
29. Sahara W, Sugamoto K, Murai M, et al. Three-dimensional clavicular and acromioclavicular rotations during arm abduction using vertically open MRI. J Orthop Res. 2007;25:1243–9.
30. Sahara W, Sugamoto K, Murai M, et al. 3D kinematic analysis of the acromioclavicular joint during arm abduction using vertically open MRI. J Orthop Res. 2006;24:1823–31.

31. Seo Y-J, Yoo Y-S, Noh K-C, et al. Dynamic function of coracoclavicular ligament at different shoulder abduction angles: a study using a 3-dimensional finite element model. Arthroscopy. 2012;28:778–87.
32. Dawson PA, Adamson GJ, Pink MM, et al. Relative contribution of acromioclavicular joint capsule and coracoclavicular ligaments to acromioclavicular stability. J Shoulder Elbow Surg. 2009;18:237–44.
33. Debski RE, Parsons IM, Fenwick J, et al. Ligament mechanics during three degree-of-freedom motion at the acromioclavicular joint. Ann Biomed Eng. 2000;28:612–8.
34. Yoo YS, Tsai AG, Ranawat AS, et al. A biomechanical analysis of the native coracoclavicular ligaments and their influence on a new reconstruction using a coracoid tunnel and free tendon graft. Arthroscopy. 2010;26:1153–61.
35. Urist MR. Complete dislocations of the acromiclavicular joint; the nature of the traumatic lesion and effective methods of treatment with an analysis of forty-one cases. J Bone Joint Surg Am. 1946;28:813–37.
36. Brasseur JL. Ultrasound of the shoulder. Medical and surgical encyclopedia. Musculoskeletal system. 2017;8:30-360-A20.
37. Poncelet E, Demondion X, Lapègue F, et al. Anatomic and biometric study of the acromioclavicular joint by ultrasound. Surg Radiol Anat. 2003;25:439–45.
38. Peetrons P, Bédard JP. Acromioclavicular joint injury: enhanced technique of examination with dynamic maneuver. J Clin Ultrasound. 2007;35:262–7.
39. Heers G, Hedtmann A. Ultrasound diagnosis of the acromioclavicular joint. Orthopade. 2002;31:255–61.
40. Alasaarela E, Tervonen O, Takalo R, et al. Ultrasound evaluation of the acromioclavicular joint. J Rheumatol. 1997;24:1959–63.
41. Barth J, Boutsiadis A, Narbona P, et al. The anterior borders of the clavicle and the acromion are not: always aligned in the intact acromioclavicular joint: a cadaveric study. J Shoulder Elbow Surg. 2017;26:1121–7.
42. Schweitzer ME, Magbalon MJ, Frieman BG, et al. Acromioclavicular joint fluid: determination of clinical significance with MR imaging. Radiology. 1994;192:205–7.
43. Faruch Bilfeld M, Lapègue F, Chiavassa Gandois H, et al. Ultrasound of the coracoclavicular ligaments in the acute phase of an acromioclavicular disjunction: comparison of radiographic, ultrasound and MRI findings. Eur Radiol. 2017;27:483–90.
44. Heers G, Hedtmann A. Correlation of ultrasonographic findings to Tossy's and Rockwood's classification of acromioclavicular joint injuries. Ultrasound Med Biol. 2005;31:725–32.
45. Sluming VA, Scutt ND. The role of imaging in the diagnosis of postural disorders related to low back pain. Sports Med. 1994;18:281–91.
46. Park G-Y, Park JH, Bae JH. Structural changes in the acromioclavicular joint measured by ultrasonography during provocative tests. Clin Anat N Y. 2009;22:580–5.
47. Blankstein A, Ganel A, Givon U, et al. Ultrasonography as a diagnostic modality in acromioclavicular joint pathologies. Isreal Med Assoc J. 2005;7:28–30.
48. Alyas F, Curtis M, Speed C, et al. MR imaging appearances of acromioclavicular joint dislocation. Radiographics. 2008;28:463–79; quiz 619.
49. Antonio GE, Cho JH, Chung CB, et al. Pictorial essay. MR imaging appearance and classification of acromioclavicular joint injury. Am J Roentgenol. 2003;180:1103–10.
50. Heers G, Götz J, Schachner H, et al. Ultrasound evaluation of the acromioclavicular joint. A comparison with magnetic resonance imaging. Sportverletz Sportschaden. 2005;19:177–81.
51. Heers G, Götz J, Schubert T, et al. MR imaging of the intraarticular disk of the acromioclavicular joint: a comparison with anatomical, histological and in-vivo findings. Skeletal Radiol. 2007;36:23–8.
52. Edelson G, Saffuri H, Obid E, et al. Successful injection of the acromioclavicular joint with use of ultrasound: anatomy, technique, and follow-up. J Shoulder Elbow Surg. 2014;23:e243–50.
53. Borbas P, Kraus T, Clement H, et al. The influence of ultrasound guidance in the rate of success of acromioclavicular joint injection: an experimental study on human cadavers. J Shoulder Elbow Surg. 2012;21:1694–7.
54. Peck E, Lai JK, Pawlina W, et al. Accuracy of ultrasound-guided versus palpation-guided acromioclavicular joint injections: a cadaveric study. PM R. 2010;2:817–21.
55. Sabeti-Aschraf M, Lemmerhofer B, Lang S, et al. Ultrasound guidance improves the accuracy of the acromioclavicular joint infiltration: a prospective randomized study. Knee Surg Sports Traumatol Arthrosc. 2011;19:292–5.
56. Pallis M, Cameron KL, Svoboda SJ, et al. Epidemiology of acromioclavicular joint injury in young athletes. Am J Sports Med. 2012;40:2072–7.
57. Bontempo NA, Mazzocca AD. Biomechanics and treatment of acromioclavicular and sternoclavicular joint injuries. Br J Sports Med. 2010;44:361–9.
58. Quigley TB. Injuries to the acromioclavicular and sternoclavicular joints sustained in athletics. Surg Clin North Am. 1963;43:1551–4.
59. Copeland S, Kessel L. Disruption of the acromioclavicular joint: surgical anatomy and biological reconstruction. Injury. 1980;11:208–14.
60. Tossy JD, Mead NC, Sigmond HM. Acromioclavicular separations: useful and practical classification for treatment. Clin Orthop. 1963;28:111–9.
61. Barnes CJ, Higgins LD, Major NM, et al. Magnetic resonance imaging of the coracoclavicular ligaments:

its role in defining pathoanatomy at the acromioclavicular joint. J Surg Orthop Adv. 2004;13:69–75.
62. Nemec U, Oberleitner G, Nemec SF, et al. MRI versus radiography of acromioclavicular joint dislocation. Am J Roentgenol. 2011;197:968–73.
63. Schaefer FK, Schaefer PJ, Brossmann J, et al. Experimental and clinical evaluation of acromioclavicular joint structures with new scan orientations in MRI. Eur Radiol. 2006;16:1488–93.
64. Rockwood CA. Injuries to the acromioclavicular joint. In: Rockwood and Green's fractures in adults. Philadelphia: J. B. Lippincott; 1984. p. 860–910.
65. Rockwood CA, Madsen F. Injuries to the acromioclavicular joint. In: disorders of the shoulder. Philadelphia: Saunders; 1990.
66. Schneider MM, Balke M, Koenen P, et al. Inter and intraobserver reliability of the Rockwood classification in acute acromioclavicular joint dislocations. Knee Surg Sports Traumatol Arthrosc. 2016;24:2192–6.
67. Kim AC, Matcuk G, Patel D, et al. Acromioclavicular joint injuries and reconstructions: a review of expected imaging findings and potential complications. Emerg Radiol. 2012;19:399–413.
68. Mazzocca AD, Arciero RA, Bicos J. Evaluation and treatment of acromioclavicular joint injuries. Am J Sports Med. 2007;35:316–29.
69. Gastaud O, Raynier JL, Duparc F, et al. Reliability of radiographic measurements for acromioclavicular joint separations. Orthop Traumatol Surg Res. 2015;101:S291–5.
70. Cho C-H, Hwang I, Seo J-S, et al. Reliability of the classification and treatment of dislocations of the acromioclavicular joint. J Shoulder Elbow Surg. 2014;23:665–70.
71. Kraeutler MJ, Williams GR, Cohen SB, et al. Inter- and intraobserver reliability of the radiographic diagnosis and treatment of acromioclavicular joint separations. Orthopedics. 2012;35:e1483–7.
72. Pifer M, Ashfaq K, Maerz T, et al. Intra and interdisciplinary agreement in the rating of acromioclavicular joint dislocations. Phys Sportsmed. 2013;41:25–32.
73. Grignon B. Imagerie normale de la ceinture scapulaire, du sternum et des côtes. Encyclopédie Médico-Chirurgicale. Appareil locomoteur. 2013;8:30-370-A10.
74. Vaisman A, Villalón Montenegro IE, Tuca De Diego MJ, et al. A novel radiographic index for the diagnosis of posterior acromioclavicular joint dislocations. Am J Sports Med. 2014;42:112–6.
75. Rahm S, Wieser K, Spross C, et al. Standard axillary radiographs of the shoulder may mimic posterior subluxation of the lateral end of the clavicle. J Orthop Trauma. 2013;27:622–6.
76. Bossart PJ, Joyce SM, Manaster BJ, et al. Lack of efficacy of 'weighted' radiographs in diagnosing acute acromioclavicular separation. Ann Emerg Med. 1988;17:20–4.
77. Wellmann M, da Silva G, Lichtenberg S, et al. Instability pattern of acromioclavicular joint dislocations type Rockwood III: relevance of horizontal instability. Orthopade. 2013;42:271–7.
78. Tauber M, Koller H, Hitzl W, et al. Dynamic radiologic evaluation of horizontal instability in acute acromioclavicular joint dislocations. Am J Sports Med. 2010;38:1188–95.
79. Alexander OM. Dislocation of the acromioclavicular joint. Radiography. 1949;15:260, illust.
80. Waldrop JI, Norwood LA, Alvarez RG. Lateral roentgenographic projections of the acromioclavicular joint. Am J Sports Med. 1981;9:337–41.
81. Zumstein MA, Schiessl P, Ambuehl B, et al. New quantitative radiographic parameters for vertical and horizontal instability in acromioclavicular joint dislocations. Knee Surg Sports Traumatol Arthrosc. 2018;26(1):125–35.
82. Hann C, Kraus N, Minkus M, et al. Combined arthroscopically assisted coraco and acromioclavicular stabilization of acute high-grade acromioclavicular joint separations. Knee Surg Sports Traumatol Arthrosc. 2018;26(1):212–20.
83. Maier D, Jaeger M, Reising K, et al. Injury patterns of the acromioclavicular ligament complex in acute acromioclavicular joint dislocations: a cross-sectional, fundamental study. BMC Musculoskelet Disord. 2016;17:385.
84. Mazzocca AD, Spang JT, Rodriguez RR, et al. Biomechanical and radiographic analysis of partial coracoclavicular ligament injuries. Am J Sports Med. 2008;36:1397–402.
85. Peetrons P, Creteur V, Bacq C. Sonography of ankle ligaments. J Clin Ultrasound. 2004;32: 491–9.
86. Beitzel K, Mazzocca AD, Bak K, et al. ISAKOS upper extremity committee consensus statement on the need for diversification of the Rockwood classification for acromioclavicular joint injuries. Arthroscopy. 2014;30:271–8.
87. Beitzel K, Cote MP, Apostolakos J, et al. Current concepts in the treatment of acromioclavicular joint dislocations. Arthroscopy. 2013;29:387–97.
88. Favard L, Berhouet J, Bacle G. Traumatisme de la ceinture scapulaire. Encyclopédie Médico-Chirurgicale. Appareil locomoteur. 2009;8:14-035-A10.
89. Melenevsky Y, Yablon CM, Ramappa A, et al. Clavicle and acromioclavicular joint injuries: a review of imaging, treatment, and complications. Skeletal Radiol. 2011;40:831–42.
90. Neer CS. Fractures of the distal third of the clavicle. Clin Orthop. 1968;58:43–50.
91. Bouillet B, Moreel P, Descamps S. Prise en charge des fractures récentes de la clavicule. J Traumatol Sport; 26:24–31.
92. Stein BE, Wiater JM, Pfaff HC, et al. Detection of acromioclavicular joint pathology in asymptomatic shoulders with magnetic resonance imaging. J Shoulder Elbow Surg. 2001;10:204–8.

93. Edelson JG. Patterns of degenerative change in the joint acromioclavicular. J Bone Joint Surg Br. 1996;78:242–3.
94. Gordon BH, Chew FS. Isolated acromioclavicular joint pathology in the symptomatic shoulder on magnetic resonance imaging: a pictorial essay. J Comput Assist Tomogr. 2004;28:215–22.
95. Choo HJ, Lee SJ, Kim JH, et al. Can symptomatic acromioclavicular joints be differentiated from asymptomatic acromioclavicular joints on 3-T MR imaging? Eur J Radiol. 2013;82:e184–91.
96. Strobel K, Pfirrmann CWA, Zanetti M, et al. MRI features of the acromioclavicular joint that predict pain relief from intraarticular injection. Am J Roentgenol. 2003;181:755–60.
97. Shubin Stein BE, Ahmad CS, Pfaff CH, et al. A comparison of magnetic resonance imaging findings of the acromioclavicular joint in symptomatic versus asymptomatic patients. J Shoulder Elbow Surg. 2006;15:56–9.
98. Mcdonald S, Hopper MA. Acromioclavicular joint disease. Semin Musculoskelet Radiol. 2015;19:300–6.
99. Chang Chien GC, Best CS, Clay BS, et al. Ultrasonography leads to accurate diagnosis and management of painful acromioclavicular joint cyst. Pain Pract. 2015;15:E72–5.
100. Hiller AD, Miller JD, Zeller JL. Acromioclavicular joint cyst formation. Clin Anat N Y. 2010;23:145–52.
101. Cooper HJ, Milillo R, Klein DA, et al. The MRI geyser sign: acromioclavicular joint cysts in the setting of a chronic rotator cuff tear. Am J Orthop. 2011;40:E118–21.
102. Yu YS, Dardani M, Fischer RA. MR observations of posttraumatic osteolysis of the distal clavicle after traumatic separation of the acromioclavicular joint. J Comput Assist Tomogr. 2000;24:159–64.
103. Nourissat G, Parier J, Radier C. Pathologie chronique acromio-claviculaire. Encyclopédie Médico-Chirurgicale. Appareil locomoteur. 2013: 8: 14-436-A10.
104. Rovesta C, Marongiu MC, Corradini A, et al. Os acromiale: frequency and a review of 726 shoulder MRI. Musculoskelet Surg. 2017;101(3):201–5.
105. Park JG, Lee JK, Phelps CT. Os acromiale associated with rotator cuff impingement: MR imaging of the shoulder. Radiology. 1994;193:255–7.
106. Gumina S, De Santis P, Salvatore M, et al. Relationship between os acromiale and acromioclavicular joint anatomic position. J Shoulder Elbow Surg. 2003;12:6–8.
107. Boehm TD, Kenn W, Matzer M, et al. Ultrasonographic appearance of os acromiale. Ultraschall Med. 2003;24:180–3.

Ultrasound on Shoulder Prosthesis

5

F. Dordain

Ultrasound is used in common practice in the shoulder for the evaluation of rotator cuff pathology.

Its use in shoulder prosthesis is less frequent [1–3].

Yet the exploration of the soft parts on a painful shoulder prosthesis, due to the strong metal presence, cannot be satisfactorily explored other than by an X-ray, because the MRI or the CT scan are highly artifacted.

For the exploration of a painful or deficient shoulder prosthesis, with a normal X-ray, ultrasound is therefore the instrument of choice

It will allow us to explore the rotator cuff and to search for effusions of the subacromial bursa or the glenohumeral joint.

5.1 Ultrasound and Anatomical Shoulder Prosthesis

The anatomical prosthesis, to have optimal function, requires an intact rotator cuff. The appearance of secondary pain on an anatomical prosthesis is quite common.

Once the causes such as infection, a mechanical problem, or an implant loosening are eliminated, the causes due to the soft tissues must be investigated.

F. Dordain (✉)
Private Hospital Saint-Martin, Caen, France

However, these are only rarely sought after.

Ultrasound is an easy, noninvasive, and less expensive examination that will not be disturbed by the presence of the prosthesis that is deeper.

The first cause of pain is a lesion of the rotator cuff.

It can be a lesion of the supraspinatus, either by delamination or even by overstuffing if the prosthetic humeral head is not well positioned or by secondary degenerative rupture.

We will, of course, seek by extension a possible lesion of the infraspinatus.

The other important aspect of the proper functioning of the anatomical prosthesis is the healing of the subscapularis which was tenotomized and reinserted (Fig. 5.1) during the surgical procedure [4].

Numerous studies have shown the importance of healing of the subscapularis to obtain a functional, painless shoulder and to avoid the appearance of an anterior subluxation that promotes the wear of glenoidal polyethylene [5–7].

Ultrasound of the subscapularis on an anatomical prosthesis therefore normally looks like a normal shoulder.

The patient should be seated, elbow to the body, forearm bent at 90°.

Exploration begins with the placement of the probe in a horizontal position, to find the bicipital groove and then, by sweeping, the lesser tubercle and the subscapularis tendon (Figs. 5.2 and 5.3).

T. Apard, J. L. Brasseur (eds.), *Ultrasonography for the Upper Limb Surgeon*,
https://doi.org/10.1007/978-3-030-84234-5_5

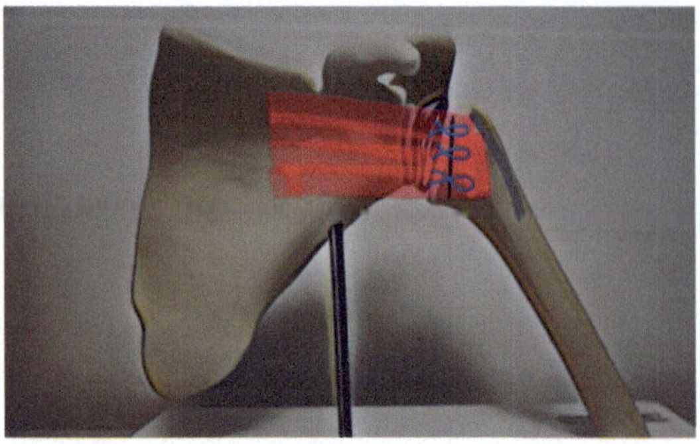

Fig. 5.1 Subscapularis repair in anatomical prosthesis / *Blue* Suture; *Red* SubScapularis; *Grey* Bicipital Groove; *Black* position of ultrasound probe

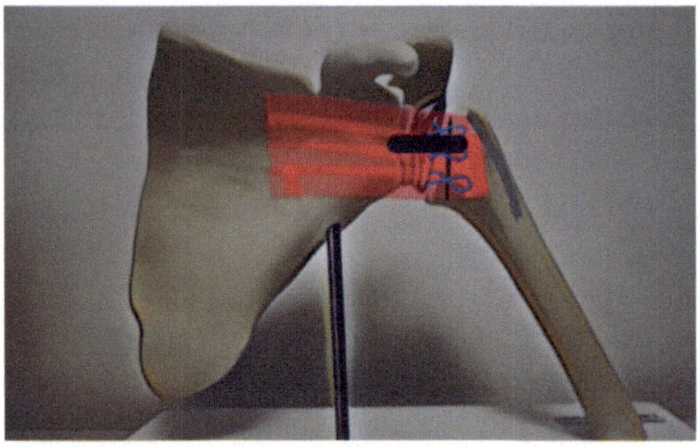

Fig. 5.2 Subscapularis repair in anatomical prosthesis

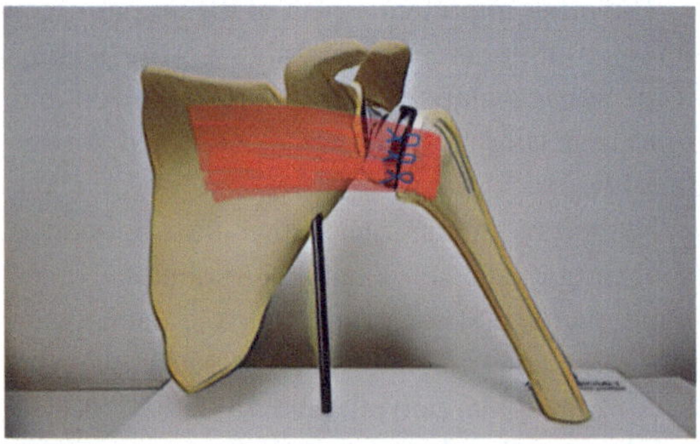

Fig. 5.3 Subscapularis repair in reverse prosthesis

The humeral head will appear much more hyperechogenic than in a normal shoulder due to its metallic composition.

The exploration is then done dynamically by asking the patient to perform external rotational movements.

This allows you to see the subscapularis in length. Suture threads can also be seen, with a structure that is more echogenic than the tendon.

Exploration will look for a possible impingement between the subscapularis and the coracoid or between the humeral head and the coracoid.

An effusion will also be sought, either from the subacromial space, along the long head of the biceps, or intra-articular.

This effusion may be punctured, if necessary, as part of the investigation of an osteoarticular infection.

5.2 Ultrasound and Reverse Prosthesis

Literature is very poor on this subject.

Only a few recent studies have been published, with the search for the healing of the subscapularis tendon to see if this would lead to a better result [8–10].

But there is no description of the ultrasound technique used.

The planes of ultrasound cuts are always the same, according to the standardization of the shoulder.

However, the decrease and the medialization of the center of rotation due to the design of reverse shoulder prosthesis must be taken into account when performing ultrasound.

Here again, an effusion can be sought, either from the subacromial space, along the tendon of the long head of the biceps, or intra-articular.

This effusion may be punctured, if necessary, as part of the investigation of an osteoarticular infection.

For the study of the cuff, very often there is a more or less wide rupture, which has also led to the realization of an inverted prosthesis.

Its study is therefore limited and of modest interest.

The main interest is whether the subscapularis has healed, if it has been reinserted at the end of the procedure.

It is necessary to take into account several elements:

- The tendon will have a more oblique direction inferiorly.
- Its distal insertion will be more medial.

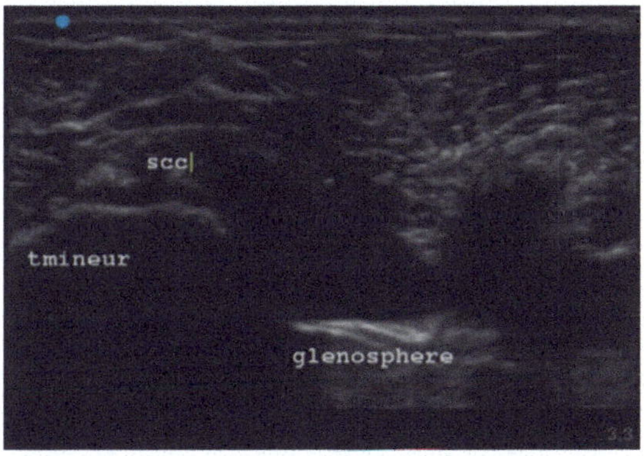

Fig. 5.4 Ultrasound anterior view: superior to inferior. *SSC* SubScapularis; *Tmineur (Tm)* Lesser Tuberosity; *GS* glenosphere

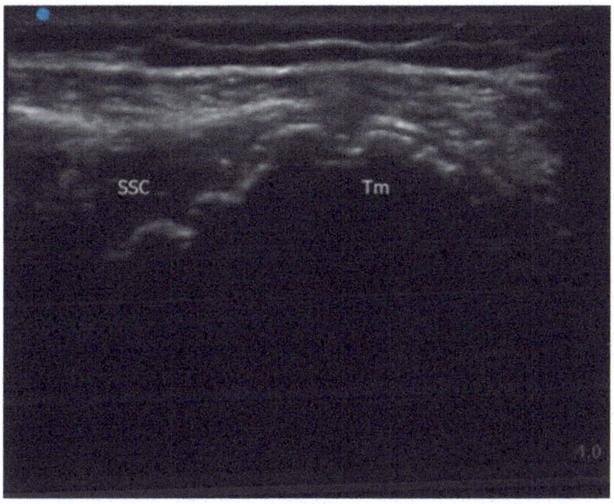

Fig. 5.5 Ultrasound anterior view: superior to inferior. *SSC* SubScapularis; *Tmineur (Tm)* Lesser Tuberosity

- It will be hidden more quickly by the coracoid and coracobiceps.
- In external rotational movements, the humeral epiphysis is guided by the glenoid sphere and has no sliding, rolling motion as on normal anatomy.

Identification of the tendon is therefore difficult, especially when the subject is overweight or obese (Figs. 5.4, 5.5, 5.6, 5.7, 5.8, and 5.9).

The best way to see the joint on an inverted prosthesis remains the posterior cut of the infraspinatus (Figs. 5.10 and 5.11).

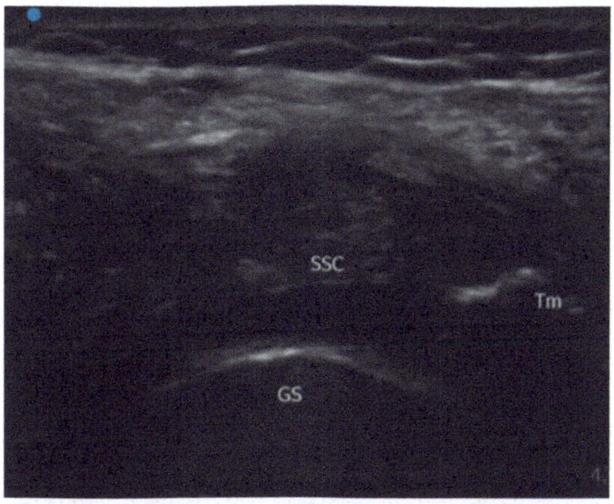

Fig. 5.6 Ultrasound anterior view: superior to inferior. *SSC* SubScapularis; *Tmineur (Tm)* Lesser Tuberosity; *GS* glenosphere

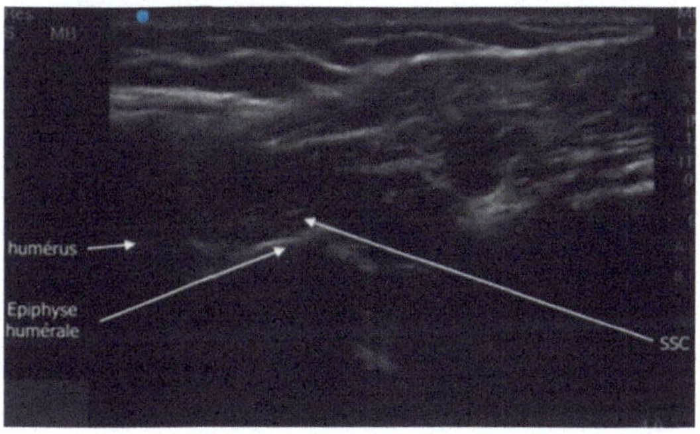

Fig. 5.7 Ultrasound anterior view: superior to inferior. *SSC* SubScapularis

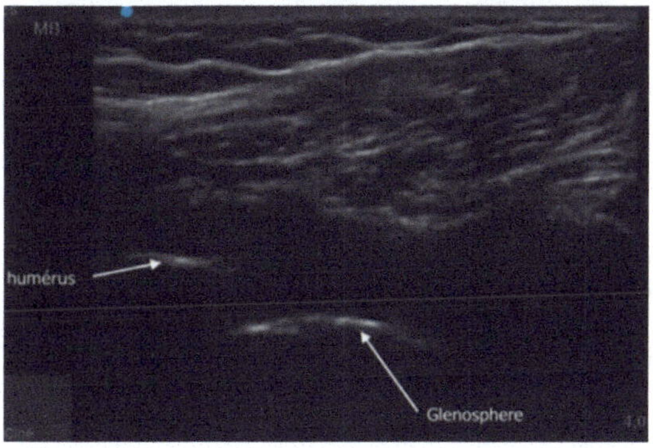

Fig. 5.8 Ultrasound anterior view: superior to inferior

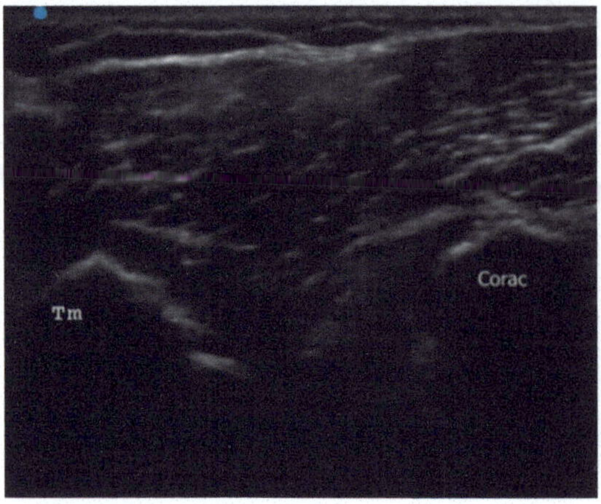

Fig. 5.9 Ultrasound anterior view: superior to inferior. *Tmineur (Tm)* Lesser Tuberosity; *Corac* coracoid

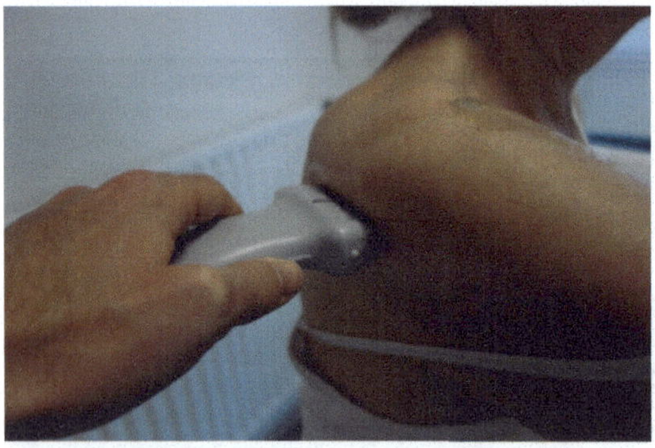

Fig. 5.10 Probe positionning for posterior view: infra spinatus

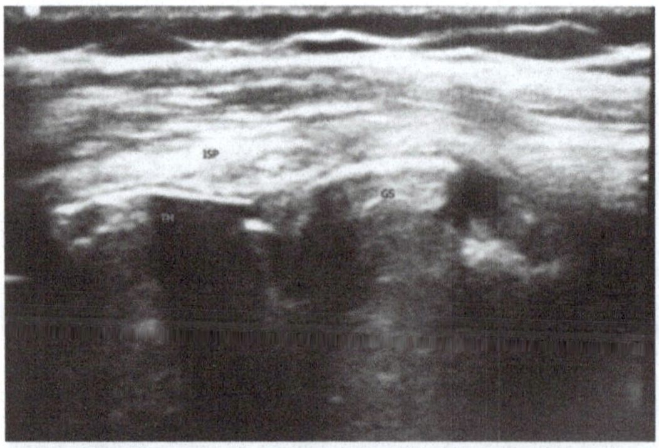

Fig. 5.11 Ultrasound posterior view. *Tmineur (Tm)* Lesser Tuberosity; *ISP* Infra spinatus; *GS* glenosphere

References

1. Westhoff B, Wild A, Werner T, Schneider T, Kahl V, Krauspe R. The value of ultrasound after shoulder arthroplasty. Skeletal Radiol. 2002;31(12):695–701.
2. Chun KA, Cho KH. Postoperative ultrasonography of the musculoskeletal system. Ultrasonography. 2015;34(3):195–205.
3. Parker BJ, Zlatkin MB, Newman JS, Rathur SK. Imaging of shoulder injuries in sports medicine: current protocols and concepts. Clin Sports Med. 2008;27(4):579–606.
4. Miller SL, Hazrati Y, Klepps S, Chiang A, Flatow EL. Loss of subscapularis function after total shoulder replacement: a seldom recognized problem. J Shoulder Elbow Surg. 2003;12(1):29–34.
5. Armstrong AD, Southam JD, Horne AH, Hollenbeak CS, Flemming DJ, Kothari MJ. Subscapularis function after total shoulder arthroplasty: electromyography, ultrasound, and clinical correlation. J Shoulder Elbow Surg. 2016;25(10):1674–80.
6. Armstrong A, Lashgari C, Teefey S, Menendez J, Yamaguchi K, Galatz LM. Ultrasound evaluation and clinical correlation of subscapularis repair after total shoulder arthroplasty. J Shoulder Elbow Surg. 2006;15(5):541–8.
7. Buckley T, Miller R, Nicandri G, Lewis R, Voloshin I. Analysis of subscapularis integrity and function after lesser tuberosity osteotomy versus subscapularis tenotomy in total shoulder arthroplasty using ultrasound and validated clinical outcome measures. J Shoulder Elbow Surg. 2014;23(9):1309–17.
8. Boer FA, van Kampen PM, Huijsmans PE. The influence of subscapularis tendon reattachment on range of motion in reversed shoulder arthroplasty: a clinical study. Musculoskelet Surg. 2016;100(2):121–6.
9. Friedman RJ, Flurin P, Wright TW, Zuckerman JD, Roche CP. Comparison of reverse total shoulder arthroplasty outcomes with and without subscapularis repair. J Shoulder Elbow Surg. 2017;26(4):662–8.
10. Vourazeris JD, Wright TW, Struk AM, King JJ, Farmer KW. Primary reverse total shoulder arthroplasty outcomes in patients with subscapularis re versus tenotomy. J Shoulder Elbow Surg. 2017;26(3):450–7.

Part II

Elbow

Ultrasound of the Lateral Face of the Elbow

6

O. Marès, L. Moscato, P. Kouyoumdjian, N. Cellier, and R. Coulomb

The lateral slope of the elbow is a crossroads with many structures. Ultrasound is a simple and quick examination, which allows an analysis of all the different structures from superficial to deep:

- Subcutaneous structures
- Epicondylar tendons and their main pathology, epicondylitis
- Bone structures: lateral humerus and radial head

6.1 Ultrasound Examination

It must take place in a serene atmosphere where the patient must be comfortably settled, to avoid the need for an unwanted yoga session [1]. For this reason, many authors advise to position the patient in lateral decubitus, which makes it possible to carry out an examination of the external side avoiding bad positioning of the patient (Fig. 6.1). In this position, the patient can follow on the screen machine the entire examination.

The objective of the review is to analyze the various structures mentioned above, which will be the guiding thread of this chapter.

O. Marès (✉) · L. Moscato · P. Kouyoumdjian · N. Cellier · R. Coulomb
Department of Conservative and Traumatological Surgery, Spine Surgery, CHU Carémeau, Nîmes, France

6.2 Superficial Structures: Subcutaneous Tissues, Nerves

6.2.1 Subcutaneous Lesions

The examination should be carried out without pressure because it may crush soft lesions; it allows the visualization of subcutaneous tumors ranging from lipoma to rare glomus tumors [2]. Schwannomas can also be observed.

Tip

To be sure not to perform this examination with too much pressure, you must be able to visualize the superficial veins.

Most of these lesions are found as a well-limited hypoechoic area. Any heterogeneous lesion requires a supplementary assessment (MRI) and a specialized test.

6.2.2 Nerve Lesions

6.2.2.1 Superficial Neuromas

The most pathognomonic sign is pain when the probe is passing the area. A well-defined nodular hypoechoic zone in longitudinal and transverse

T. Apard, J. L. Brasseur (eds.), *Ultrasonography for the Upper Limb Surgeon*,
https://doi.org/10.1007/978-3-030-84234-5_6

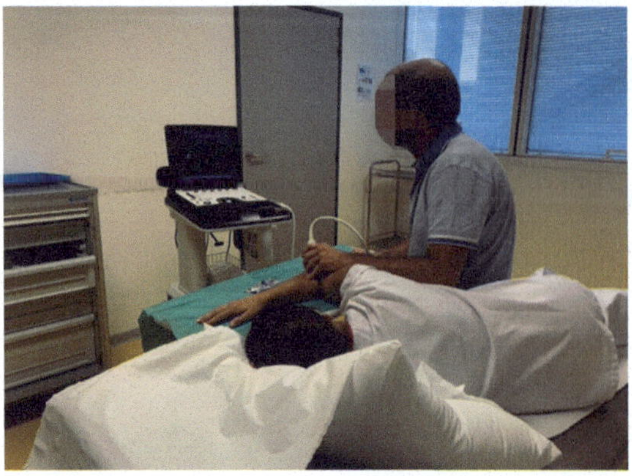

Fig. 6.1 Position for ultrasound: lateral decubitus

section is found on one of the superficial branches of the lateral surface of the elbow: the terminal branch of the lateral cutaneous nerve of the arm or the proximal branch of the lateral cutaneous nerve of the forearm [3]. This hypoechoic zone is in continuity with the nerve in longitudinal section.

6.2.2.2 Radial Nerve

The compression of this branch can be done at five levels [4]:

- At the level of the ECRB extensor carpi radialis brevis
- At the radio capitellum joint
- At the level of Henry's fibers
- At the level of arcade of Frohse, which is the most common
- To the distal edge of the supinator

At the arcade of Frohse, compression is rare but classic, sometimes requiring a surgical procedure. In this case, an appearance of nervous edema is found on ultrasound. The main trunk is located behind the septum separating the brachioradialis from the ECRL extensor carpi radialis longus, in front of the supinator muscle. Its appearance is heterogeneous, with the presence of many vascular formations (Fig. 6.2a and b). The motor branch moves through the two bundles of the supinator, downwards and backwards.

The cross section area is between 4.3 and 14.4 mm^2; beyond that it is necessary to consider a compressive pathology. This is one of the most typical signs of mechanical compression of a nerve branch. But it is always necessary to look for a differential with a contralateral examination in view of interindividual variations.

6.3 Bone Lesions and Entheses Other Than Epicondylitis

6.3.1 Lesions of the Lateral Humerus

Ultrasound has a real interest in the detection of lesions in young children, where it allows to visualize a displacement of the lateral ossification nucleus with either a loss of the external bone alignment and very often associated with a hematoma under the periosteum. But above all it allows, thanks to a cross section, to check the integrity of the growth cartilage which is a major sign of instability, and if it is present it is then lawful to stabilize these fractures [5]. There is a fracture of the intra-articular cartilage with a large hematoma. If this sign is absent, functional treatment is required.

In adults, it allows to visualize cortical tearing or periosteal hematoma linked to direct or indirect trauma, sometimes avoiding misdiagnosis a lesion.

Posterolateral instability is a syndrome that occurs in patients performing throwing sports or may also be present in some cases of epicondylitis. This research is carried out on an oblique section, the probe arranged in the longitudinal direction between lateral epicondyle and radial head. The examiner impels a supination force; the *cut-off* between the distance between the top of the radial head and the humerus is 4 mm. Beyond that, the patient presents almost certain instability [6].

6.3.1.1 Radial Head

Ultrasound has an acute interest in fracture screening, where it allows to visualize occult

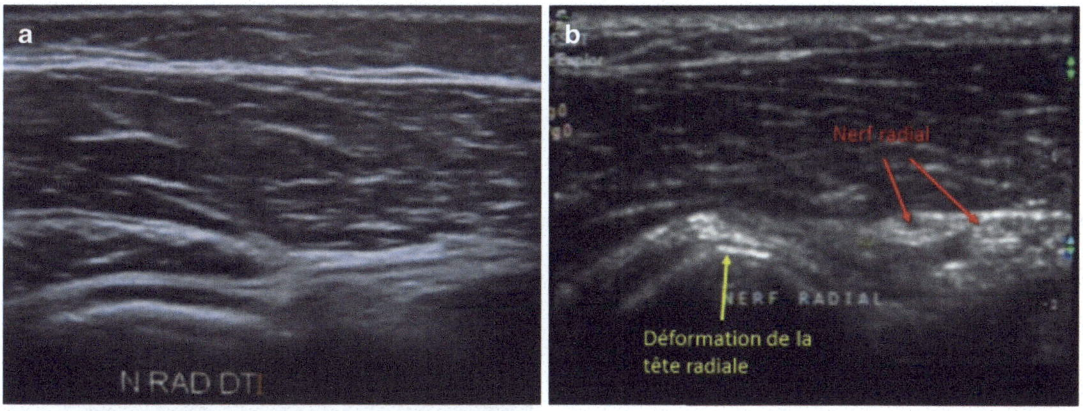

Fig. 6.2 (**a**) Longitudinal section: edema of the deep branch of the radial nerve; too clearly visible. (**b**) Cross section: edema of the deep branch of the radial nerve; too clearly visible

fractures, i.e., with a normal X-ray. The specific sign is a hypoechoic hematic effusion at the neck of the head of the radius with a specificity of 60% and a sensitivity of 83.3% [7]. It also allows you to visualize the classic fractures of Mason type, where effusion is more important and associated with a typical cortical detachment.

It also allows to visualize a kinetic disorder with a jump that can be detected by performing pronosupination movements.

6.3.2 Arthritis Lesions

They are well visualized with effusions and parrot beaks at the side compartment. But ultrasound is of little interest in these lesions compared to conventional examinations. The interest of ultrasound is really in helping to carry out ultrasound-guided procedures.

6.4 Musculo-aponeurotic Lesions

6.4.1 Lateral Epicondylitis

Medial and lateral epicondylitis are frequent pathologies with a significant impact in medico-economic terms [2]. Ultrasound is a first-time analytical examination that provides a wealth of information to best guide therapeutic management. It also makes it possible to carry out percutaneous lengthening tenotomy procedures, paving the way for simplified office practice [8].

6.4.2 The Ultrasound-Guided Review

Its purpose is to analyze the tendino-articular intersection comprising the following structures:

- Humeral radial joint
- Extensor carpal tendons: extensor carpi radialis longus (ECRL) and extensor carpi radialis brevis (ECRB)
- The pronator teres and the branch of the radial nerve

This assessment allows with the Doppler mode to assess the severity of the lesion and also to monitor the progression of inflammation and the effectiveness of the treatments implemented.

The examination takes place with the patient sitting, the elbow slightly bent 30/40° flexion, the arm on the table, and the examiner positions himself on the side of the arm.

The examination begins with the exploration of the skin tissue for subcutaneous lesions and then on cross section, and the patient performs wrist extension movements in order to identify the following three bundles: brachioradialis, extensor carpi radialis brevis, and extensor carpi radialis longus. Their analysis is done in two stages.

6.4.3 Longitudinal Exploration

The first step is a longitudinal exploration in order to identify the humeral radial joint line. It is then unrolled to analyze the radial head and the interval for signs of chondropathy, effusion, and/or rare synovial plicae [9]. This static workup is then supplemented by a dynamic workup that looks for blockage, kinetic disorder, or any other cause that could explain epicondylitis.

The examination then focuses on the enthesis of the tendon, looking for signs of tendinopathy:

- In mode B:
  - The presence of calcifications with their classic shadow cone is analyzed in mode B.
  - Signs of cracking, longitudinal hypoechoic images that may evoke partial disinsertion of the joint tendon. These images associate with images of fibrillar disorganization. It is also possible to observe complete disinsertions (Fig. 6.3). Images of pseudo-menisci can also be found in exceptional ways (Fig. 6.4).
- In Doppler power mode:
  - Signs of hypervascularization, which also allow for a progressive monitoring of the medical treatment (Fig. 6.5).
- These signs are not specific, and they are frequently found on the contralateral side without clinical signs. Moreover the interobserver variability is great [10]. In daily practice, two ultrasound signs are essential for diagnosis: elective pain when passing the probe and hypervascularization in color Doppler.

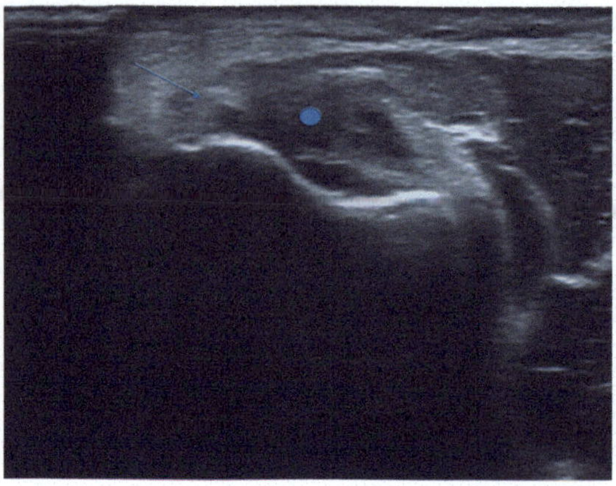

Fig. 6.3 Epicondyle longitudinal section (arrows: calcification; round: disinsertion of the common extensor on the epicondyle)

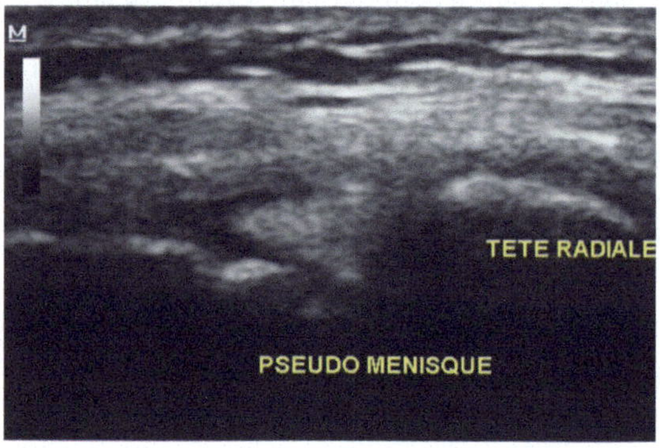

Fig. 6.4 Image of pseudo-meniscus

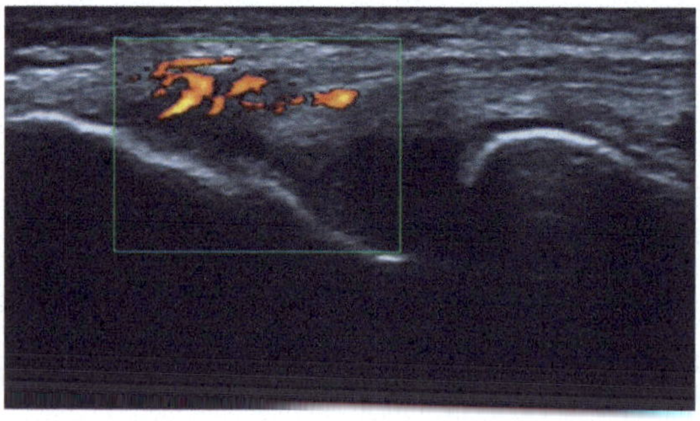

Fig. 6.5 Longitudinal cut power Doppler evidence of active lesions

6.4.4 Cross-Sectional Exploration

The assessment is supplemented by an analysis in the transverse direction which allows to identify three important elements: ECRB and ECRL and the pronator teres (Fig. 6.6).

It is also necessary to make a dynamic assessment to analyze the kinetics of the extensor carpi

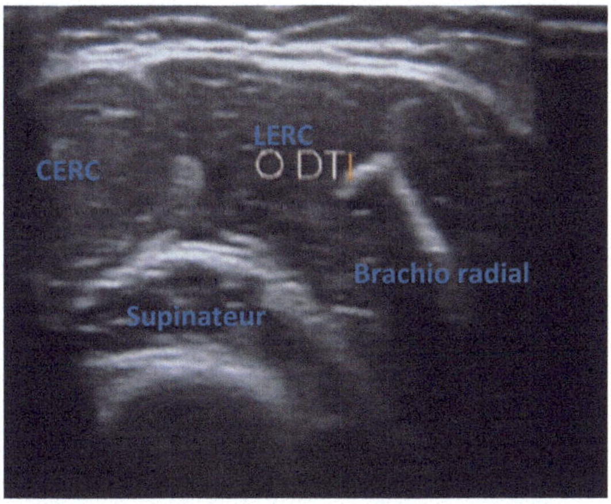

Fig. 6.6 Transverse cross section image locating the various anatomical elements

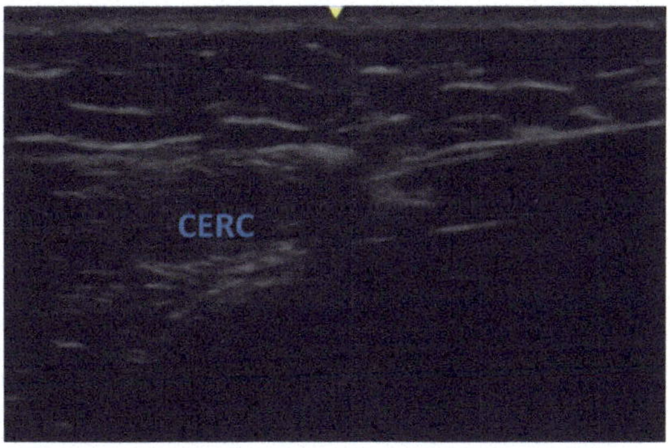

Fig. 6.7 Transverse image during ultrasound-guided section of the joint tendon

muscles vis-à-vis the pronator teres. In pronation, as in supination, the radius and the supinator rotate under the superficial epicondyles up to about 45° on both sides, and the patient is free of pathology.

If the patient is symptomatic, synkinesis movements will be found as early as 30° pronation. The partition between ECRB and ECRL should also be analyzed during active wrist extension. Apart from pathological cases, the septum of the ECRB bulges toward the ECRL, while in pathological cases this fascia works differently. This assessment must be of course comparative and bilateral.

6.4.5 Ultrasound in the Treatment of Epicondylitis

Lateral epicondylitis is the most common condition affecting the elbow and in most cases resolves on its own [11]. However, when orthopedic treatment fails, surgical intervention is necessary for resistant cases.

Ultrasound coupled with effective anesthesia also allows to perform a therapeutic procedures (Fig. 6.7) by achieving a fascia release of the ECRB and at the tendon level by performing a dynamic percutaneous elongation tenotomy [8, 12].

In conclusion, ultrasound makes it possible to make a thorough assessment and eliminate external causes of epicondylitis. In addition, the development of guided ultrasound techniques makes it a new tool in the therapeutic arsenal. The place that remains to be defined is the view of the variable results obtained by the various means of medical and surgical treatment in cases of chronic epicondylitis, as reported in the latest meta-analysis [12].

6.5 Conclusion

Ultrasound is an essential examination in the management of elbow pathologies. It makes it possible to diagnose and eliminate most differential diagnoses. Its use does not eliminate the use of an X-ray during the initial assessment to clear any intra-bone pathology.

In addition, in the case of lateral epicondylitis, the development of ultrasound-guided procedures of tenotomy offers new treatment options.

References

1. Mezian K, Sobotová K, Angerová Y. Sonographic elbow scanning is not yoga exercise. Adv Rheumatol. 2019;59:33. https://doi.org/10.1186/s42358-019-0079-3.
2. Lunn J, Stanton J, Arya A. Glomus tumour of the elbow: an unusual complication of surgery. Shoulder Elbow. 2016;8:197–8. https://doi.org/10.1177/1758573216640190.
3. Chiavaras MM, Jacobson JA, Billone L, Lawton JM, Lawton J. Sonography of the lateral antebrachial cutaneous nerve with magnetic resonance

imaging and anatomic correlation. J Ultrasound Med. 2014;33:1475–83. https://doi.org/10.7863/ultra.33.8.1475.
4. Xiao TG, Cartwright MS. Ultrasound in the evaluation of radial neuropathies at the elbow. Front Neurol. 2019;10:216. https://doi.org/10.3389/fneur.2019.00216.
5. Li X-T, Shen X-T, Wu X, Chen X-L. A novel transverse ultrasonography technique for minimally displaced lateral humeral condyle fractures in children. Orthop Traumatol Surg Res. 2019;105:557–62. https://doi.org/10.1016/j.otsr.2019.02.005.
6. Camp CL, O'Driscoll SW, Wempe MK, Smith J. The sonographic posterolateral rotatory stress test for elbow unability: a cadaveric validation study. PM R. 2017;9:275–82. https://doi.org/10.1016/j.pmrj.2016.06.014.
7. Malahias M-A, Manolopoulos P-P, Kadu V, Shahpari O, Fagkrezos D, Kaseta M-K. Bedside ultrasonography for early diagnosis of occult radial head fractures in emergency room: a CT-comparative diagnostic study. Arch Bone Jt Surg. 2018;6:539–46.
8. Capa-Grasa A, Rojo-Manaute JM, Rodriguez-Maruri G, de Las Heras Sánchez-Heredero J, Smith J, Martín JV. Selective 360° percutaneous extensor carpi radialis brevis tendon release for tennis elbow: an experimental study. J Ultrasound Med. 2012;31:1193–201. https://doi.org/10.7863/jum.2012.31.8.1193.
9. Lee HI, Koh KH, Kim J-P, Jaegal M, Kim Y, Park MJ. Prominent synovial plicae in radiocapitellar joints as a potential cause of lateral elbow pain: clinico-radiologic correlation. J Shoulder Elbow Surg. 2018;27:1349–56. https://doi.org/10.1016/j.jse.2018.04.024.
10. Levin D, Nazarian LN, Miller TT, O'Kane PL, Feld RI, Parker L, McShane JM. Lateral epicondylitis of the elbow: US findings. Radiology. 2005;237:230–4. https://doi.org/10.1148/radiol.2371040784.
11. Bateman M, Littlewood C, Rawson B, Tambe AA. Surgery for tennis elbow: a systematic review. Shoulder Elbow. 2019;11:35–44. https://doi.org/10.1177/1758573217745041.
12. Yoo SH, Cha JG, Lee BR. Ultrasound-guided percutaneous bone drilling for the treatment of lateral epicondylitis. Eur Radiol. 2018;28:390–7. https://doi.org/10.1007/s00330-017-4932-7.

7 Ultrasound of the Median Nerve at the Elbow

G. Candelier

Discussions around ultrasound imaging of the median nerve most often concern carpal tunnel syndrome, where it has become a relevant, well-codified, and reproducible diagnostic tool. At the elbow, the situation is less clear. On the one hand, the pathology of the median nerve is still being systematized, and the differences between anterior interosseous nerve syndrome, pronator syndrome, and lacertus fibrosus syndrome remain a source of discussion. In contrast to what happens at the wrist, where the consequences of nerve compression can be directly analyzed, the pathology of the median nerve at the elbow, except in particular cases, appears as a dynamic pathology for which the measurement of static parameters is faulty.

7.1 Anatomy of the Median Nerve at the Elbow [1–3]

The median nerve runs down the arm into the brachial canal which is bounded by the brachial fascia medially, the anterior brachialis muscle posteriorly, and the biceps on the outside. It is then most often located inside the brachial artery, which it crossed during its journey away from the musculocutaneous nerve. It passes in front of the medial intermuscular septum (Zone I).

At the bend of the elbow the median nerve, which is always in front of the anterior brachialis, lies inside the artery medial to the tendon of the biceps. The latter gives its aponeurotic expansion, the lacertus fibrosus, which will join the superficial fascia of the pronator teres (PT). The biceps tendon marks the separation point from the musculocutaneous nerve that passes outside the biceps tendon (Zone II). At the PT, the humeral artery is divided into several branches, the two main ones being the radial artery that has a lateral and superficial path and the ulnar artery that goes deep. The nerve then passes between the two bundles of the PT (Zone III). The ulnar bundle of the PT covers the ulnar artery. The radial artery passes to the above the ulnar bundle and under the humeral bundle. The anterior interosseous nerve arises from the posterior surface of the median nerve as it passes between the two heads of the PT. The path of the median nerve is then made under the fibrous arch formed by the meeting of the humeroulnar and humeroradial bundles of the superficial flexor muscle (Zone IV) (Fig. 7.1).

These four anatomical zones will serve as the basis for ultrasound analysis of the median nerve. This topographic division corresponds to the

Supplementary Information The online version of this chapter (https://doi.org/10.1007/978-3-030-84234-5_7) contains supplementary material, which is available to authorized users.

G. Candelier (✉)
Hand Surgery Department, Saint Martin Private Hospital, Caen, France

T. Apard, J. L. Brasseur (eds.), *Ultrasonography for the Upper Limb Surgeon*,
https://doi.org/10.1007/978-3-030-84234-5_7

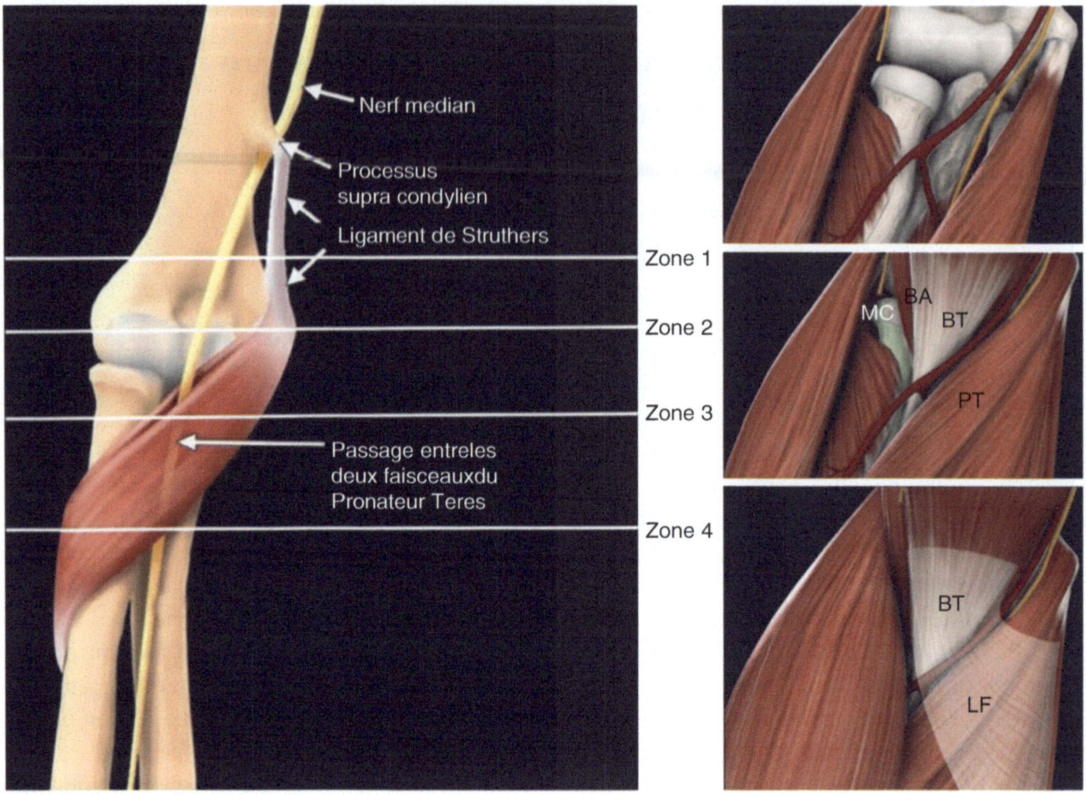

Fig. 7.1 Anatomical relationships of the median nerve from proximal to distal, passage through different zones of possible impingement. *BA* anterior brachialis, *BT* biceps tendon, *PT* pronator teres, *LF* lacertus fibrosus, *MC* musculocutaneous nerve

potential sites of anatomical variations and nerve compression.

7.2 Ultrasound of the Median Nerve at the Elbow

Ultrasound examination of the elbow is performed with the patient sitting in front of the examiner. The forearm is placed on a table with the elbow slightly bent the palm of the hand in complete supination. The examiner will thus be able to perform contraction maneuvers in flexion and pronation.

A linear probe is used with a frequency range from 6 to 12/15 MHz, allowing examination of the surface and deep structures (humeroulnar joint). Color Doppler mode can be used to clarify vascular structures. The examination will be bilateral and comparative. It starts with a cross section called the BAM section (Fig. 7.2).

The displacement of the probe in ascension will allow the analysis of muscle, tendon, vascular, bone, joint structures, and above all the monitoring and analysis of the nerve (Videos 7.1 and 7.2).

- **Zone I:** The probe is placed at the distal part of the arm; the anatomical reference is the medial epicondyle. The anterior brachialis, nerve, artery, and emergence of the tendon sheath of the biceps are visualized (Fig. 7.3).
- **Zone II:** Landmark: humeral trochlea. Exposure of the muscular body of the humeral bundle of the PT, from the distal portion of the anterior brachialis, the nerve is placed inside the PT and outside the artery. On this BAM section, the lacertus fibrosus starting from the

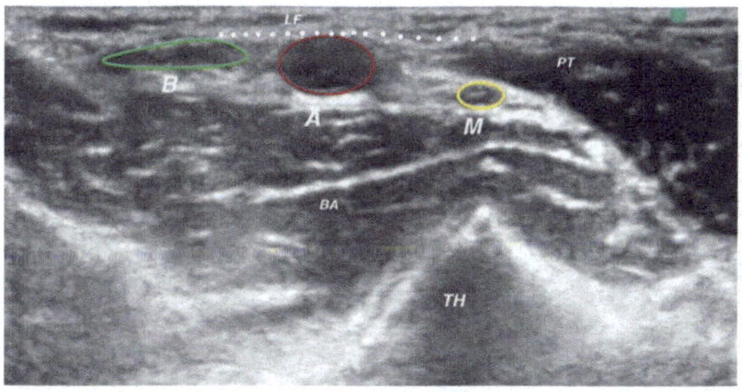

Fig. 7.2 The BAM cut is performed elbow in slight flexion; the probe is placed transversely to the fold of the elbow. The tendon of the biceps (B), the brachial artery (A), and the median nerve (M) are visualized from outside to inside. Its anatomical reference is the humeral trochlea (TH). By moving the probe from top to bottom or from bottom to top, we visualize the path of the nerve that passes between first the pronator (humeral bundle) and the anterior brachialis (BA) and then between the two heads of pronator teres (PT) (Videos 7.1 and 7.2). Lacertus fibrosus (LF) is inserted on the medial edge of the biceps and ends on the superficial fascia of the PT

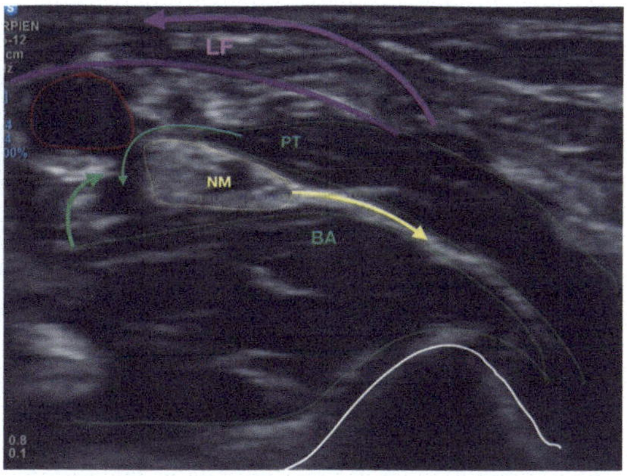

Fig. 7.4 Syndrome of the median nerve canal at the elbow (PMNE) is due to dynamic compression of the median nerve below the PT. This is caused by the traction exerted on its muscular body by lacertus fibrosus (LF), which is put into tension by the contraction of the biceps. This clamp is well highlighted in ultrasound when performing dynamic tests (Video 7.3)

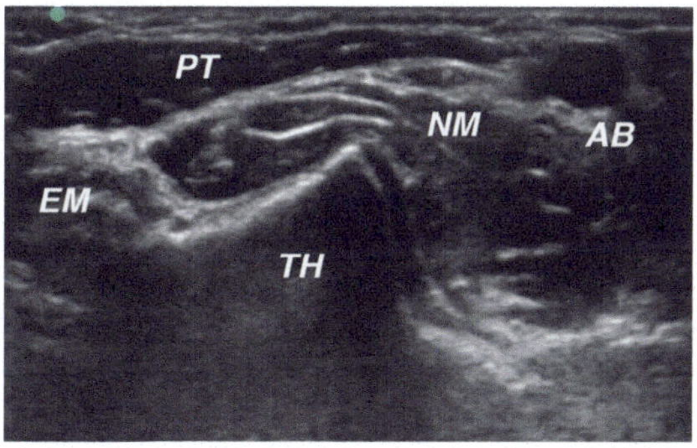

Fig. 7.3 Zone I cross section whose anatomical reference is the medial epicondyle

medial edge of the biceps and covering the artery is the nerve and merging with the superficial fascia of the humeral head of the PT. In dynamics (aggravated flexion of the elbow) the contraction of the biceps causes tension on the lacertus, which compresses and moves laterally the muscular body of the PT. The nerve is then driven under the humeral bundle of the PT (sign of lobster claw) (Fig. 7.4 and Video 7.3). The basilic vein is laid on the surface of the lacertus and is an excellent anatomical landmark.

- **Zone III:** Coronoid process and radial head. The two bundles of the PT are then visualized. We observe the division of the humeral artery. The ulnar artery goes under the ulnar bundle of the PT when the radial artery remains above it. The nerve passes between the two muscle bodies; one can sometimes visualize the emergence of the anterior interosseous nerve to the deep surface of the nerve (Fig. 7.5).
- **Zone IV**: Beyond the coronoid process: the arch of the superficial flexor and the passage of the median nerve and potentially the path of the anterior interosseous nerve to the interosseous membrane are exposed.

Throughout the examination, longitudinal sections are performed as well as oblique sections in the axis of the PT and lacertus fibrosus.

7.3 Anatomical Variants [1, 4, 5]

Numerous variations in anatomical relationships from the median nerve to the elbow have been described.

The median nerve receives a nerve contingent from the musculocutaneous nerve. This anastomosis occurs in the majority of cases just

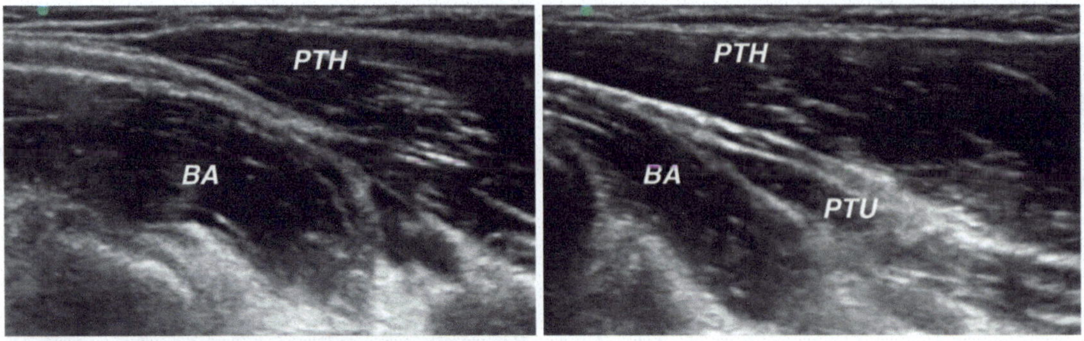

Fig. 7.5 On the longitudinal sections, the passage of the median nerve between the two bundles of the pronator teres muscle (PTH and PTU) is visualized. The passage from a strictly longitudinal section in the forearm axis to a more oblique positioning of the probe from inside to outside and from proximal to distal makes it possible to clear the path of the median nerve better

after the musculocutaneous nerve has passed through the coraco-biceps. In rare cases (13%) this anastomosis of the musculocutaneous nerve to the median nerve occurs at the elbow in Zone I.

Anatomical variations in the muscular bodies of the PT are possible. The deep head is absent in 22% of patients (Zone III).

High insertion of the humeral bundle is most often associated with the existence of a Struthers ligament. This ligament is stretched from the supracondylar process to the medial epicondyle (Fig. 7.6).

This should not be confused with the Struthers arch, which is a very common reinforcement of the medial intermuscular septum and which maintains close anatomical relationships with the ulnar nerve. The Struthers ligament may be responsible for vasculo-nervous compression. It is difficult to see (Zone I) but can be suspected in the presence of a high insertion of the humeral bundle of the PT and the presence of a supracondylar process. One can help by visualizing a damping of the flow from the humeral artery to the elbow during extending supination of the forearm.

The humeral artery may also exhibit anatomical variations. Sometimes the artery can be located inside the nerve, which can change the understanding of the BAM cut. An upper division of the humeral artery is possible and visible from Zone I (Fig. 7.7).

7.4 Pathology [6–10]

Pathologies from the median nerve to the elbow are numerous, be it extrinsic compression of the nerve or intraneural tumor pathologies, for example. Some anatomical problems may cause structural distress of the median nerve as it travels to the elbow.

Ultrasound will thus be very useful in flushing out a compression by a hematoma, a synovial cyst, a tumor of adjacent structures, a pseudoaneurysm of the humeral artery or its branches, a fracture sequelae, a tumor of the median nerve, etc.

Canal syndromes from the median nerve at the elbow are often unrecognized because their clinical semiology is protean and sometimes unspecific. Interosseous nerve syndrome at the stage of paralysis of the long flexor of the thumb and deep flexors of the index finger (and pronator quadratus PQ) is easily diagnosed. Symptomatology of PMNE (proximal median nerve entrapment) can be caused by simple pain in the forearm and lack of grip strength. Sometimes this involvement of the median nerve at the elbow may mimic a carpal tunnel syndrome with which it may otherwise be associated. The very etiology of these canal syndromes at the elbow is discussed. Round-pronator syndrome is a debate. It is now well established that damage to the anterior interosseous nerve is not due to compression below the arch of the superficial flexor but may involve damage to the trunk of the nerve prior to the

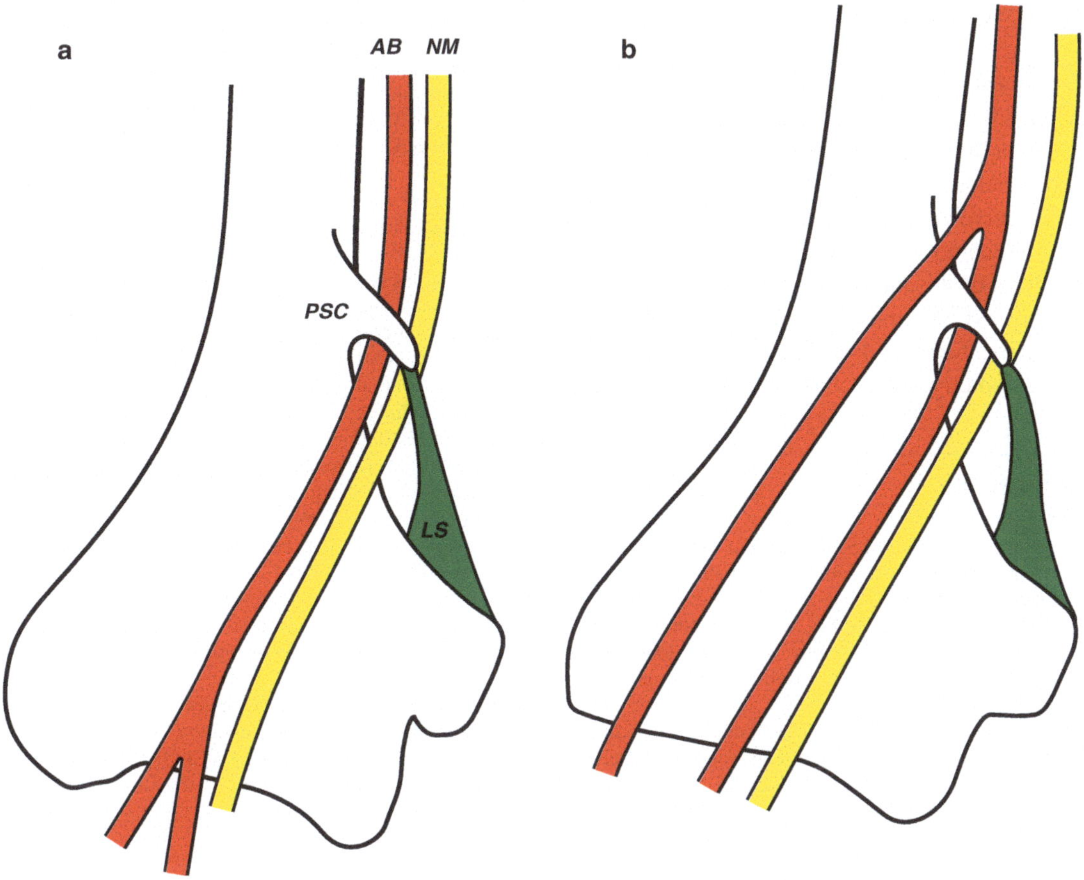

Fig. 7.6 The Struthers ligament is inserted proximal on the supracondylar process and distal on the medial epicondyle. An upper division of the humeral artery (Fig. 7.7) must cause this anomaly to be suspected. Evidence of the supracondylar tubercle (PSC) on transverse sections may help visualize compression on the nerve. (**a**) The median nerve (NM) and the artery move together in the channel formed by the supracondylar process, the Struthers ligament (LS), and the humerus. (**b**) Upper division of the artery

emergence of AION. The diagnosis of PMNE is based on rigorous muscle testing, the search for a sign of Tinel under the lacertus fibrosus, and the positivity of the scratch collapse test which negatively affects the application of cold in the lacertus zone. EMG is most often normal (except for AION paralysis). Ultrasound can explain a dynamic compression of the median nerve under the humeral head of the PT by compression of the latter by pulling the lacertus during the thwarted flexion of the elbow. The section of the lacertus fibrosus, whether in open air or in mini open under ultrasound guidance, allows for the disappearance of symptoms even in the event of paralysis of the AION.

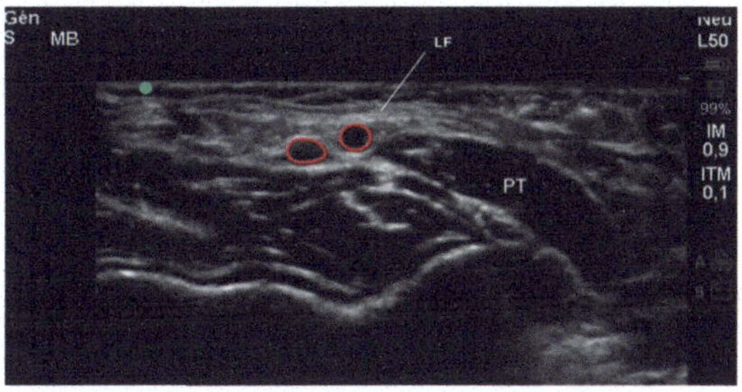

Fig. 7.7 Patient with a clinical picture of paresis of the anterior interosseous nerve. The consultation ultrasound found an upper division of the brachial artery suggesting the possibility of a Struthers ligament. The MRI and X-ray of the humerus did not reveal it. The ultrasound-guided release of lacertus fibrosus was followed by a disappearance of symptomatology. *LF* lacertus fibrosus, *PT* pronator teres, circled with red the upper division of the brachial artery

7.5 Conclusion

The morphological analysis of the median nerve enabled by ultrasound is an essential contribution to the daily routine of a hand surgery consultation. It helps to highlight the structural anomalies of the nerve and its environment. Its contribution to the diagnosis of PMNE and even more in paralysis of the anterior interosseous nerve must be clarified but already seems promising. In the future the functional analysis of muscle bodies by elastometry will probably be of great interest.

References

1. Creator V, Madani A, Sattari A, Bianchi S. Sonography of the pronator teres: normal and pathologic appearances. J Ultrasound Med. 2017;36(12):2585–97.
2. Choi S-J, Ahn JH, Ryu DS, Kang CH, Jung SM, Park MS, et al. Ultrasonography for nerve compression syndromes of the upper extremity. Ultrasonography. 2015;34(4):275–91.
3. De Maeseneer M, Brigido MK, Antic M, Lenchik L, Milants A, Vereecke E, et al. Ultrasound of the elbow with emphasis on detailed assessment of ligaments, tendons, and nerves. Eur J Radiol. 2015;84(4):671–81.
4. Nebot-Cegarra J, Perez-Berruezo J, de la Torre FR. Variations of the pronator teres muscle: predispositional role to median nerve entrapment. Arch Anat Histol Embryol. 1991–1992;74:35–45.
5. Mat Taib CN, Hassan SNA, Esa N, Mohd Moklas MA, San AA. Anatomical variations of median nerve formation, distribution and possible communication with other nerves in preserved human corpses. Folia Morphol. 2017;76(1):38–43.
6. Pham M, Bäumer P, Meinck H-M, Schiefer J, Weiler M, Bendszus M, et al. Anterior interosseous nerve syndrome: fascicular motor lesions of median nerve trunk. Neurology. 2014;18:598–606.
7. Arányi Z, Csillik A, Dévay K, Rosero M, Barsi P, Böhm J, et al. Ultra-sonographic identification of nerve pathology in neuralgic amyotrophy: enlargement, constriction, fascicular entwinement, and twisting. Muscle Nerve. 2015;52:503–11.
8. Burnier M, Sneag D, Nwawka O, Feinberg J, Arányi Z, Lee S, Wolfe S. The lesion of anterior interosseous nerve syndrome is not in the forearm. 2018;6003(6):329–464.
9. Hagert E. Clinical diagnosis and wide-awake surgical treatment of proximal median nerve entrapment at the elbow: a prospective study. Hand (N Y). 2013;8(1):41–6.
10. Candelier G, Apard T, Favennec YE, Treatment of compression of the median nerve at the elbow by echoguided section in WALANT of the lacertus fibrosus. 2017;5206(6):389–509.

Ultrasound of the Ulnar Nerve at the Elbow

8

Jean Louis Brasseur

The lesions of the ulnar nerve at the elbow are the most common nerve damage to the upper limb after that of the carpal tunnel [1].

Thanks to its comparative study, but also its dynamic specificity and in particular the lift technique, ultrasound is at the forefront in the screening and characterization of ulnar nerve damage to the elbow [2–10].

In addition to general and tumor pathologies, two types of lesions are particularly sought after: impingements with numerous conflicting etiologies and abnormal mobility.

8.1 Anatomy and Sonoanatomy

The ulnar nerve has a complex path [2–7, 11]. We find it:

- To the lower third of the arm in the Struthers canal (not to be confused with the ligament of the same name that can compress the median nerve) (Fig. 8.1) [12–14]
- To the posterior and medial surface of the distal humerus where it is plated with a retinaculum (or Osborne ligament) (Fig. 8.2)
- Next to the humeroulnar interval
- To its passage under the arch of the flexor carpi ulnaris (Fig. 8.3) formed by the arched ligament stretched between the two heads of this muscle

It is easily spotted in ultrasound thanks to its "honeycomb" structure in the axial plane (Fig. 8.4) and by the lift technique that sweeps this area in a comparative way. If there is a suspicion of nerve damage, the nerve is placed in the middle of the screen and the probe rotated by 90° to analyze the nerve in its main axis, locate a disparity in caliber, and then measure its surface comparatively (Fig. 8.5). A comparative bending maneuver is systematically performed in search of mobility (anterior translation or compression against the pallet); changes in pressure on the nerve are important during this maneuver [15–20] (Fig. 8.6).

8.2 Pathological Appearances of the Nerve in Ultrasound

Acutely, the pathological nerve [2–5], presents:

- Hypoechogenic swelling in the lesioned area or upstream of the compression zone or friction zone (Fig. 8.7); the measurement of this swelling is controversial; an area greater than 10 mm^2 or a difference of more than 2mm^2

J. L. Brasseur (✉)
Department of Radiology, G.H. Pitié-Salpêtrière, Paris, France
e-mail: jlbrasseur@impf.fr

T. Apard, J. L. Brasseur (eds.), *Ultrasonography for the Upper Limb Surgeon*,
https://doi.org/10.1007/978-3-030-84234-5_8

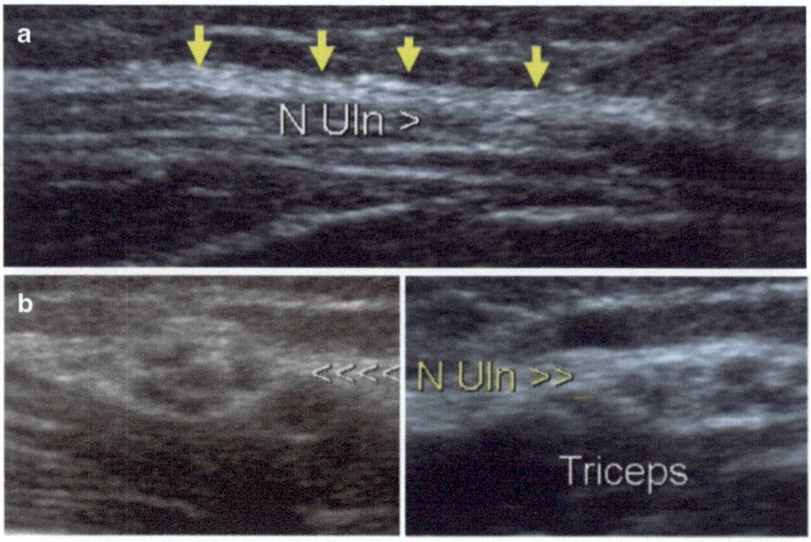

Fig. 8.1 Ulnar nerve in the Struthers canal (arrows) (**a**); comparative axial view of the nerve (**b**) at this level showing the deformation of the left nerve by comparison at the right

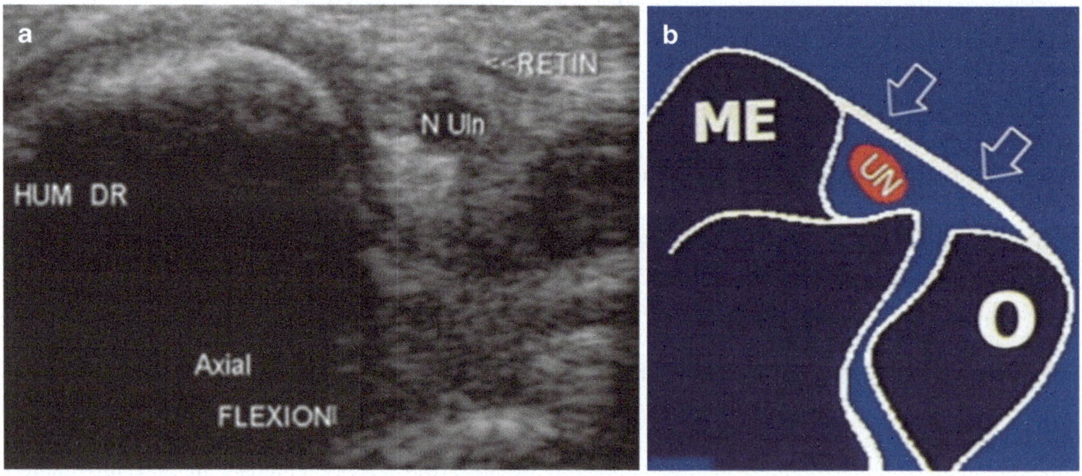

Fig. 8.2 Ulnar nerve held in place at the posterior face of the distal humerus by the retinaculum (or Osborne ligament) slightly deformed here in bending (**a**); corresponding pattern (**b**) (Dr Lhoste)

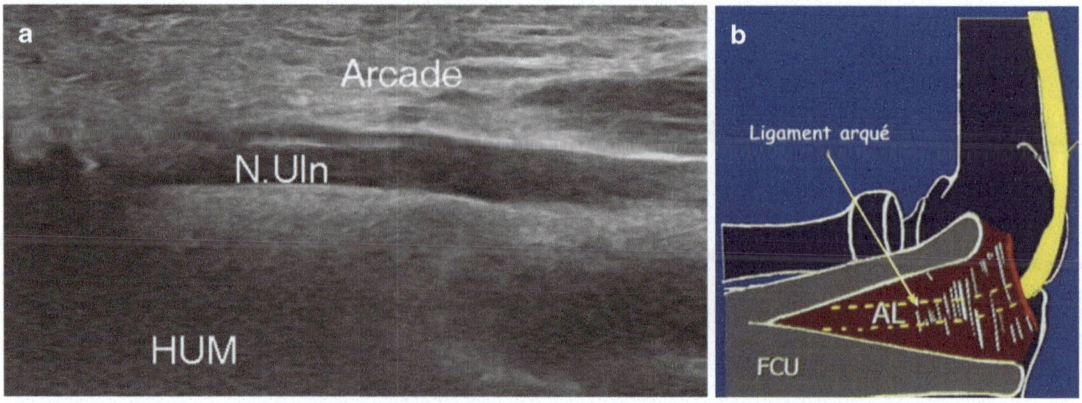

Fig. 8.3 Sagittal section of the ulnar nerve passing under the arch (or arched ligament) of the flexor carpi ulnaris (FCU) (**a**); corresponding diagram (**b**) (Dr. Lhoste)

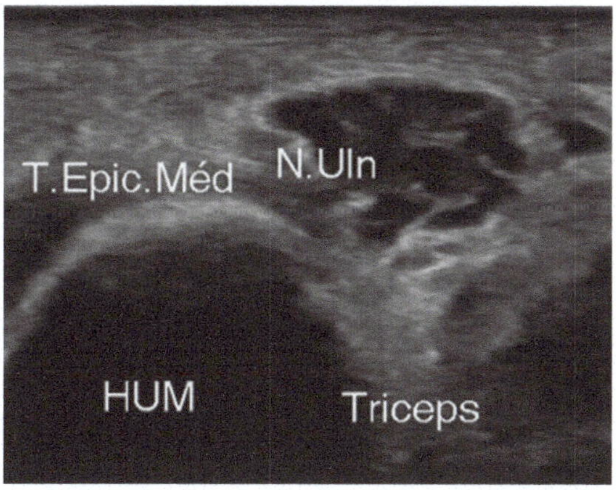

Fig. 8.4 Axial section showing the "honeycomb" structure of the ulnar nerve

between the two sides seems to be the values to be retained to date [21–27].

- A notch and/or a decrease in size at the area of compression (Fig. 8.8).
- A disappearance of the "cable" structure with blurred appearance of the axonal contours (Fig. 8.9).
- Doppler hyperemia (Fig. 8.10).

Elastography could assist in the detection of this nerve lesion [28, 29].

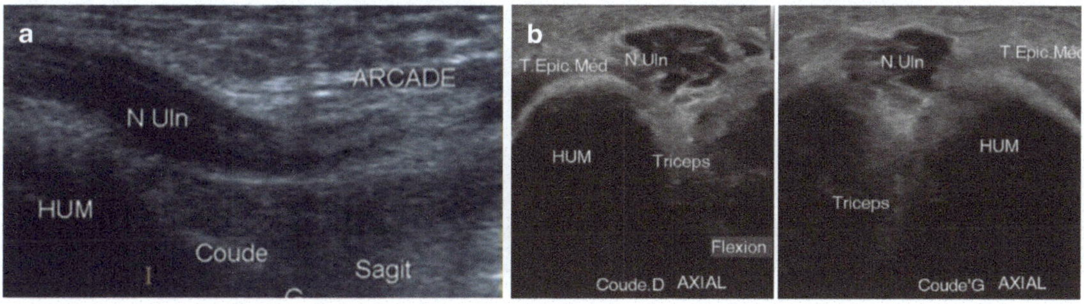

Fig. 8.5 Analysis of the nerve in its main axis showing swelling upstream of the passage under the arch (**a**); comparative measurement of the surface of the nerve on a cut divided into two to allow to take the same marks and be sure to be at the same level (**b**)

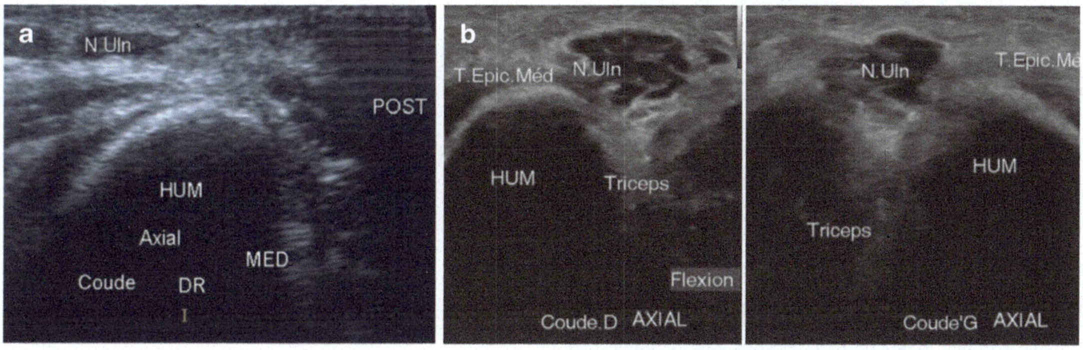

Fig. 8.6 Flexion maneuver showing anterior dislocation of right nerve (**a**) and deformation of the right nerve thickened against the pallet in another patient (**b**)

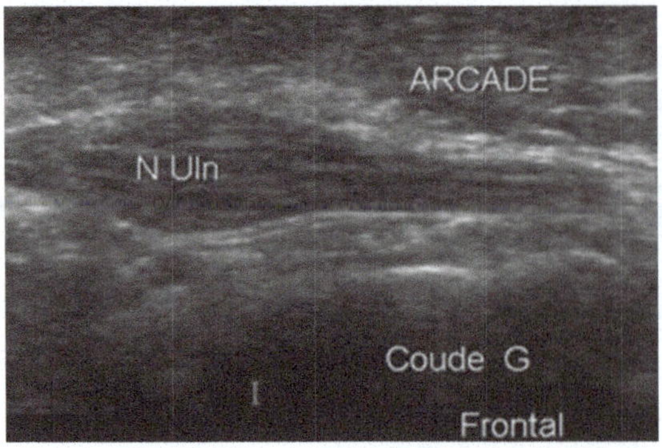

Fig. 8.7 Significant swelling of the ulnar nerve upstream of compression (here by the FUC arch)

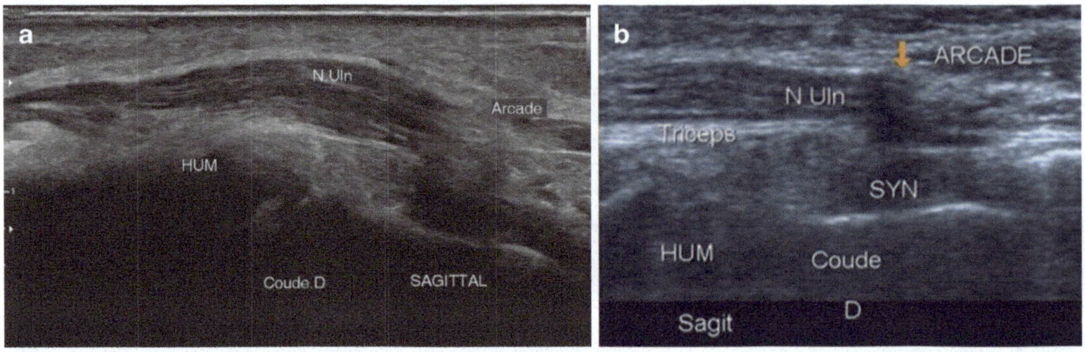

Fig. 8.8 Marked deformation in the area of compression with decreased caliber at this level (and upstream swelling) (**a**); single notch without caliber asymmetry in another patient (**b**)

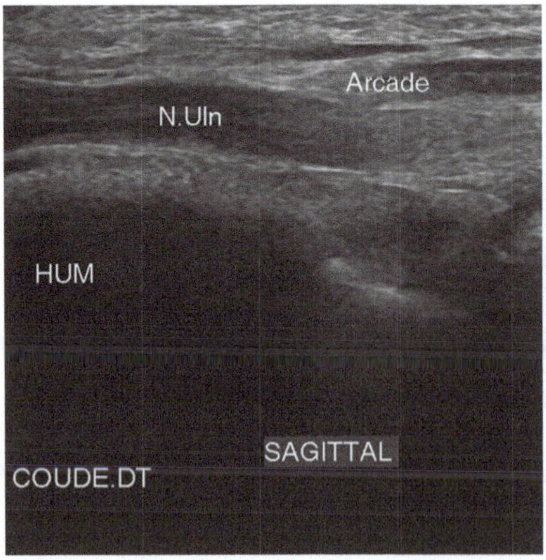

Fig. 8.9 Disappearance of the "cable" structure of the nerve upstream of compression

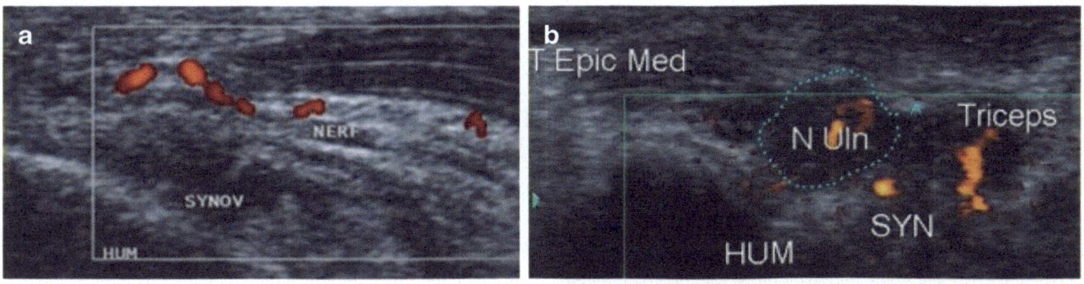

Fig. 8.10 Hyperemia of ulnar nerve in the vicinity of compression caused by hypertrophic synovitis (**a**); pronounced thickening and vascularization of an ulnar nerve in the axial plane in another patient (**b**)

Fig. 8.11 Anterior dislocation of right ulnar nerve during comparative flexion test

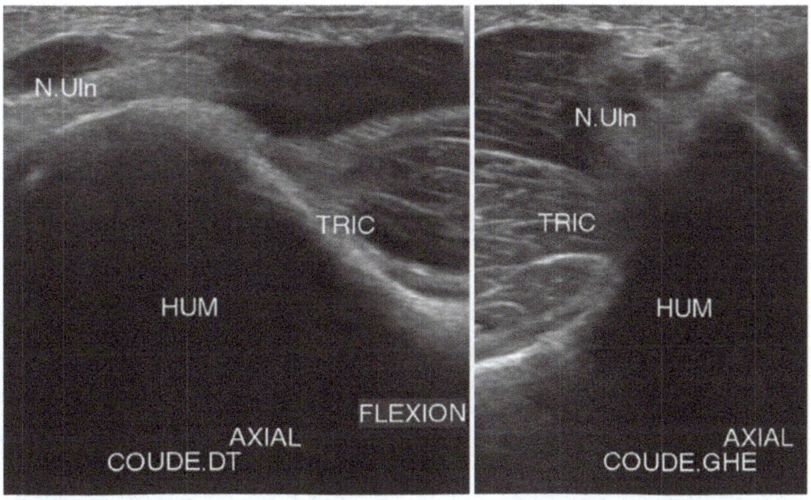

8.3 Etiologies of Ulnar Nerve Damage at the Elbow

8.3.1 Nervous "Irritation" in Case of Abnormal Mobility

The flexion maneuver is the great advantage of ultrasound over other techniques. Comparatively, the anterior displacement of the ulnar nerve is visualized (Fig. 8.11). It then "climbs" the ulnar contour of the humeral pallet causing a repeated "friction" that generates nerve irritation.

Congenital insufficiency or absence of the retinaculum is the cause of this abnormal mobilization; it is common (about 10%), and this abnormal mobilization is often asymptomatic. It is often associated with the anterior translation of an accessory bundle of the triceps muscle that accompanies the nerve in its anterior translation (Fig. 8.12) [30–33].

Sometimes, in case of simple relaxation of the retinaculum, compression of the ulnar nerve against the pallet is observed (Fig. 8.13), which can lead to a symptomatology especially in thin patients who do not have a fatty sheath interposed between the nerve and the cortex.

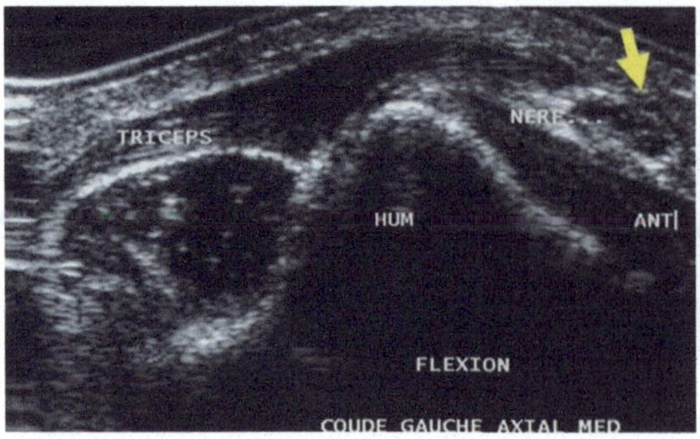

Fig. 8.12 Anterior dislocation of an accessory bundle of the triceps accompanying the anterior translation of the ulnar nerve in flexion

8.3.2 Locations and Etiologies of Nerve Impingement

Etiologies are multiple, and the purpose of ultrasound, in addition to visualizing a nervous anomaly, is the detection of its origin. Here are the main ones.

8.3.2.1 Struthers Arcade [12–14]

This etiology is little known and often seems to be unrecognized. It was well analyzed by Jacob [12]. This arch is clearly visible in some patients, and the deformation of the nerve is then well visualized (Fig. 8.14).

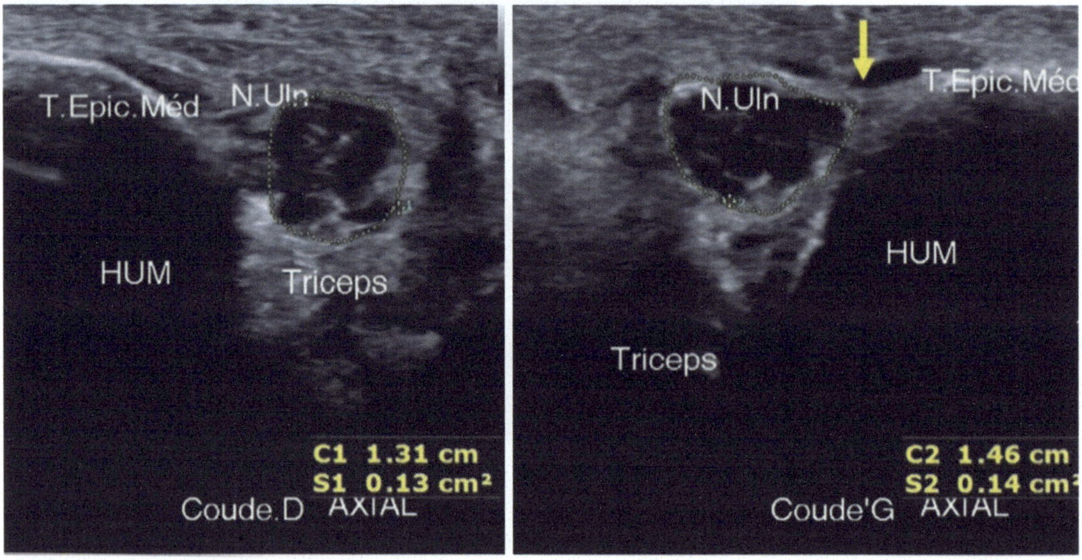

Fig. 8.13 In the flexion maneuver, the left ulnar nerve comes into contact with the humeral cortex, while on the right a fatty hyperechogenic border "protects" the nerve

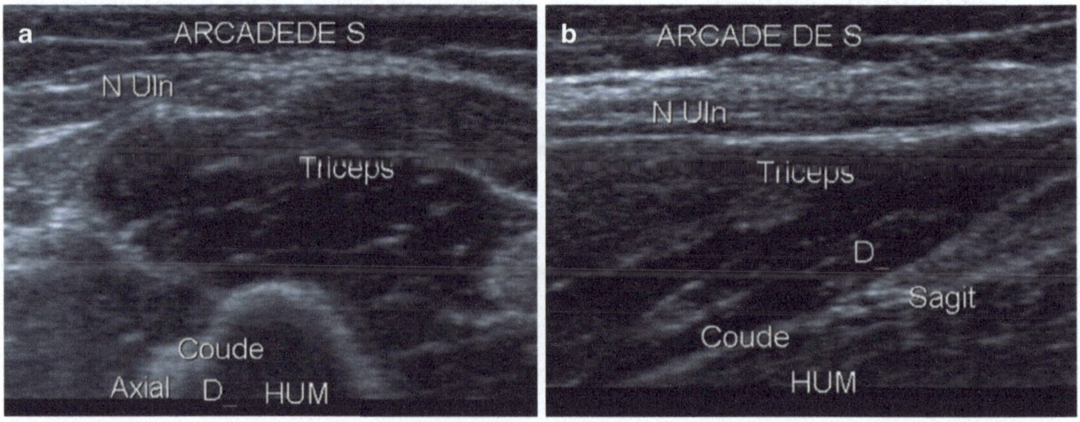

Fig. 8.14 Thickening of the Struthers arch clearly visible in the axial (**a**) and longitudinal (**b**) plane

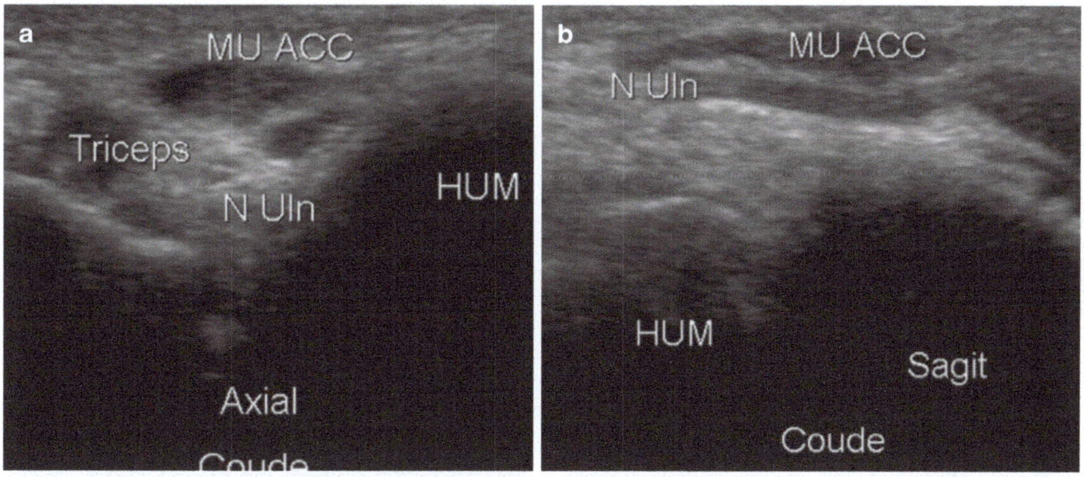

Fig. 8.15 Accessory muscle (epitrochleo-anconeus) compressing the ulnar nerve in the axial (**a**) and longitudinal (**b**) plane

8.3.2.2 Accessory Muscle

It is mainly the ancillary (or epitrochleo-anconeus) anconeus muscle, often bilateral, which can be compressive (Fig. 8.15) [34, 35]. Other muscles have been described, but the mechanism is identical. Accessory bundles of the triceps or abnormal insertions of this muscle were also described.

8.3.2.3 Hypertrophy of the Triceps Muscle

These congenital anomalies must be differentiated from the hypertrophy of the triceps muscle that is encountered in some athletes after intensive training leading to a compression of the nerve limited to the dominant arm.

8.3.2.4 Tumor Formations

These are not nerve tumors but juxta-nerve tumors that can compress the ulnar nerve; these are mainly lipomas and lymph nodes that cause this type of compression (Fig. 8.16).

8.3.2.5 Lesions at Joint Origins

They are multiple and easily detected in ultrasound: a cyst [36, 37] (Fig. 8.17), a synovial swelling, a juxta-articular ossified nodule (Fig. 8.18), but also an osteophytic spicule or even a liquid distension of the ulnar recess may be pathogenic (Fig. 8.19).

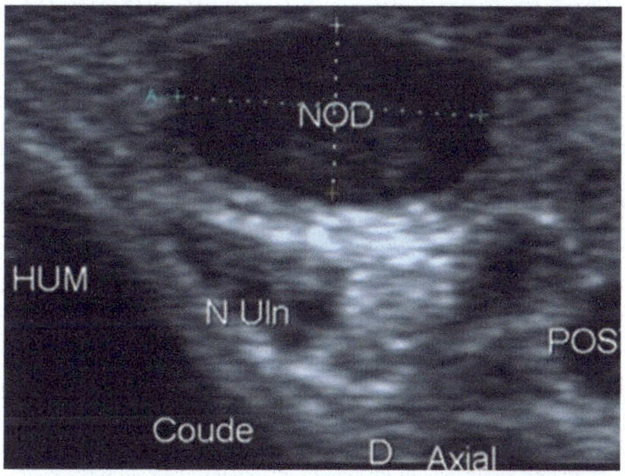

Fig. 8.16 Hypoechogenic nodular formation (here a ganglion, as part of a cat scratch disease) causing compression of the ulnar nerve

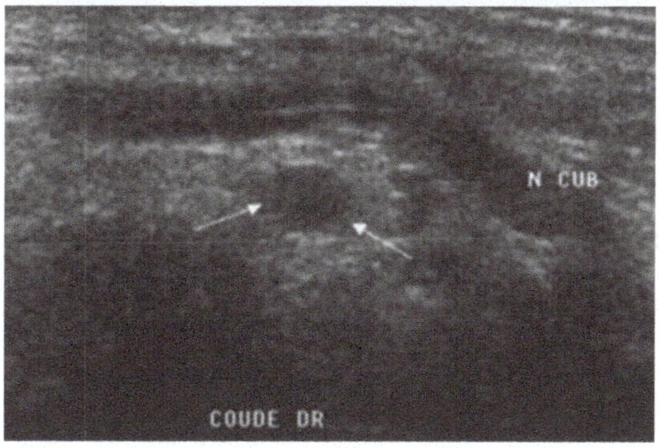

Fig. 8.17 Mucoid cyst deforming the ulnar nerve

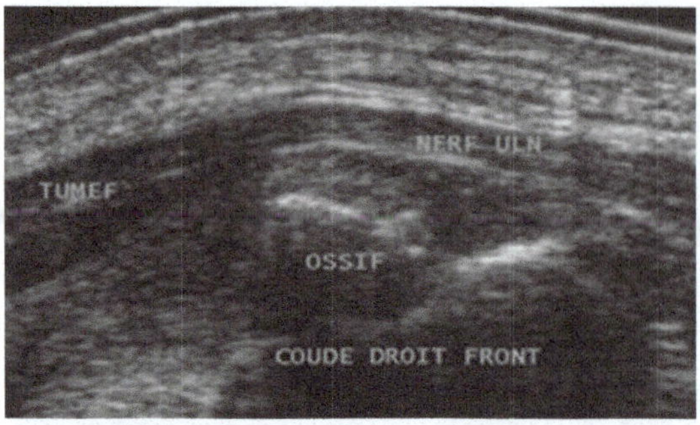

Fig. 8.18 Juxta-articular ossified nodule compressing the ulnar nerve

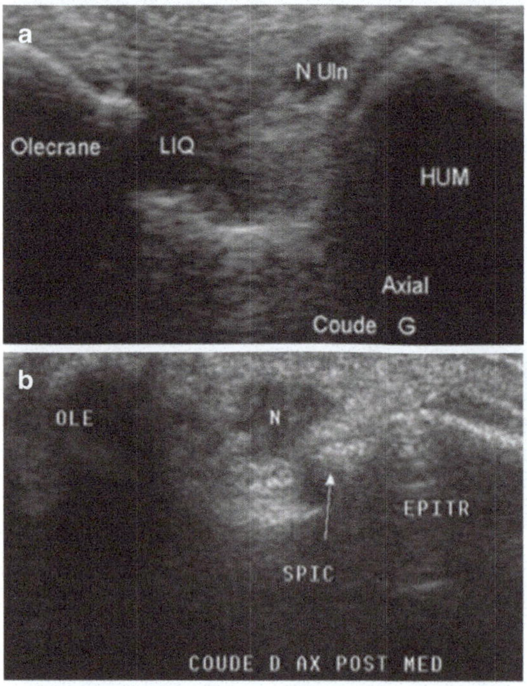

Fig. 8.19 Liquid distension of the joint recess causing impingement with the ulnar nerve (**a**); in another patient, it is an osteophytic spicule that causes the impingement (**b**)

8.3.2.6 Thickening of the Retinaculum

This anatomical element that keeps the nerve in place is sometimes thickened (due to chronic traction phenomena?) compressing the nerve with each flexion (Fig. 8.20).

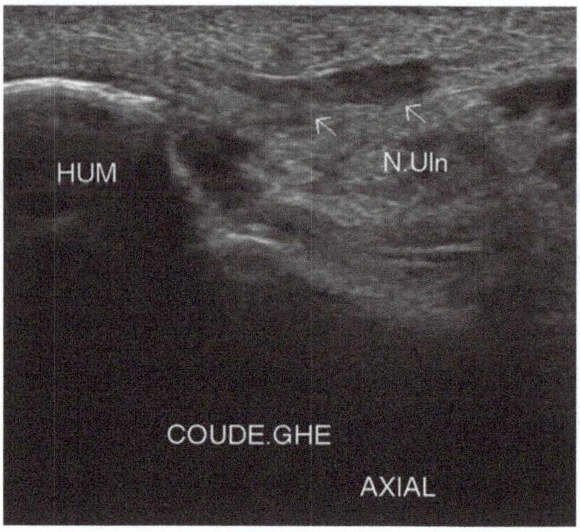

Fig. 8.20 Marked thickening of the retinaculum compressing the nerve in its retro-humeral path

8.3.3 Nerve Irritation in Case of Neighboring Lesion

The ulnar nerve, the insertion of the medial epicondyle, and the medial collateral ligament (LCM) (especially its transverse bundle) are three very close structures, and the involvement of one of them can affect the others. Thus, swelling of the transverse bundle of the LCM can lead to a hematic and fibrous neighboring reaction reaching the adjacent nerve (Fig. 8.21).

8.3.4 Direct Trauma

In addition to posttraumatic shocks and lacerations, it should always be borne in mind that a simple prolonged compression of the elbow on a hard plane can cause pain (Fig. 8.22), the origin of which is sometimes unknown. Scars, especially postoperative ones, can also cause compression or even traction.

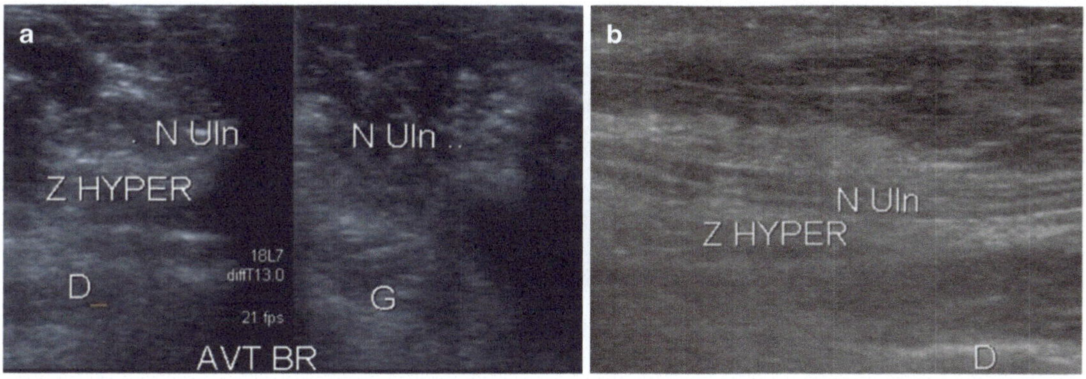

Fig. 8.21 Sequelae of medial collateral ligament lesion causing a right hyperechogenic cicatricial (Z HYPER) fibrous patch in conflict with ulnar nerve as shown by comparison on the opposite side in the axial plane (**a**); the conflicting hyperechoic zone is indeed found in the longitudinal plane (**b**)

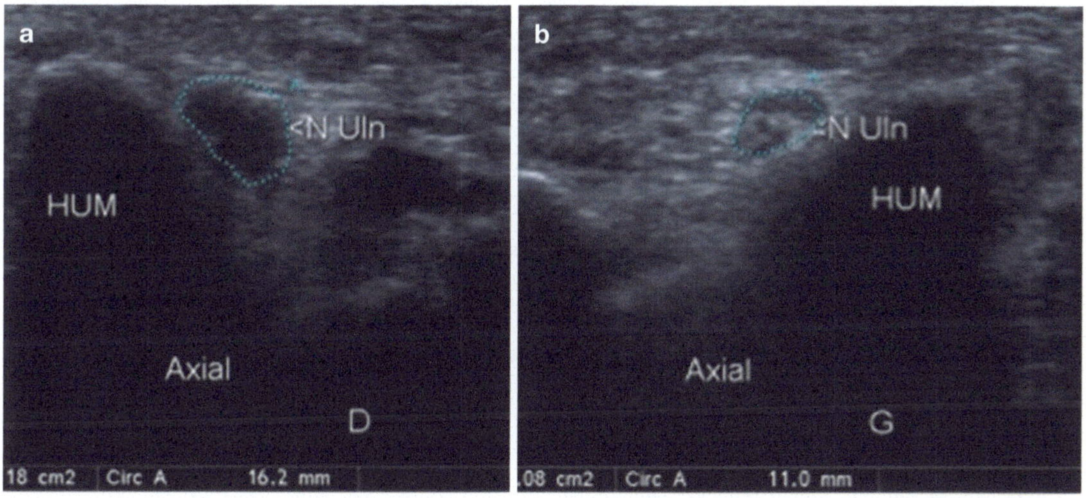

Fig. 8.22 After prolonged pressure on a hard plane, there is a hypoechogenic swelling of the right nerve (**a**) clearly visible by comparison on the opposite side (**b**)

8.3.5 Other Lesions of Ulnar Nerve

Nerves may be subject to tumor damage (mainly schwannomas and neuromas) (Fig. 8.23) but also thickened in a diffuse way mainly in the case of leprosy, which is a growing pathology in our country [38, 39] (Fig. 8.24).

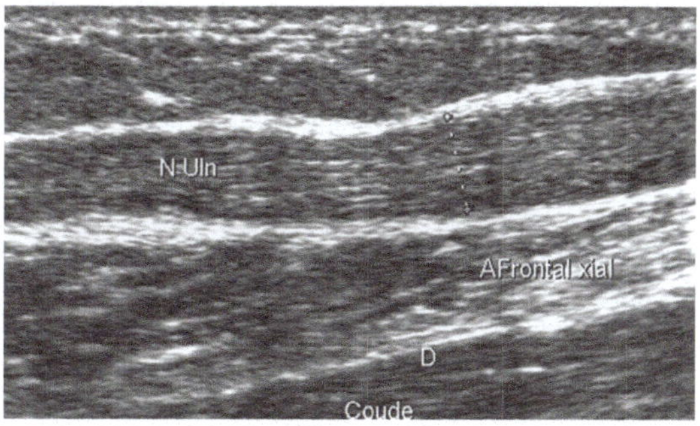

Fig. 8.24 Major and diffuse thickening of the ulnar nerve as part of leprosy

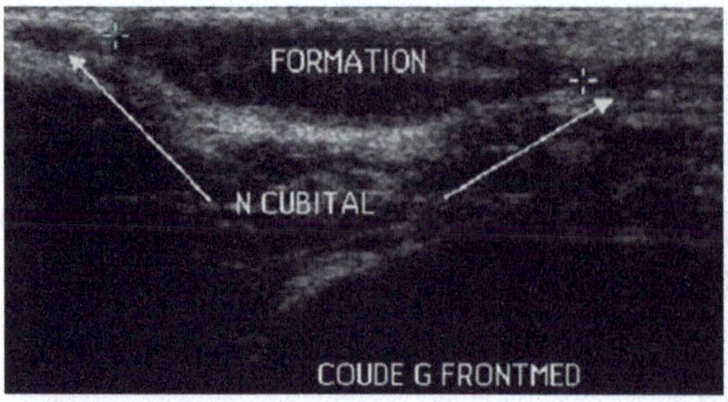

Fig. 8.23 Fusiform swelling of the ulnar nerve corresponding to a neuroma

8.4 Conclusion

Ultrasound of the ulnar nerve at the elbow is the essential asset of the clinician as it can guide a therapeutic procedure but first specify exactly the origin of the patient's symptomatology. In addition, the appearance of the nerve can also be monitored to assess the return to normal after treatment and in particular surgical release [40, 41].

References

1. Jacobson JA, Fessell DP, Lobo Lda G, Yang LJ. Entrapment neuropathies I: upper limb (carpal tunnel excluded). Semin Musculoskelet Radiol. 2010;14(5):473–86. https://doi.org/10.1055/s--0030-1268068. Epub 2010 Nov 11.
2. Bianchi S, Martinoli C. Elbow. In: Ultrasound of the musculoskeletal system. Springer; 2007. p. 349–407.
3. Jacob D, Lambert A. Ultrasound of the posterior side of the elbow. In: Brewer JL, Fustier A, Mercy G, Monzani Q, Lucidarme O, editors. News in ultrasound of the locomotor appareil, vol. 14. Montpellier: Medical Sauramps; 2017. p. 281–98.
4. Coraci D, Giovannini S, Loreti C, Di Sante L, Santilli V, Padua L. Ultrasonographic appearance of ulnar nerve at different points of elbow. Eur J Radiol. 2018;102:228–30. https://doi.org/10.1016/j.ejrad.2017.12.023. Epub 2017 Dec 28.
5. Okamoto M, Abe M, Shirai H, Ueda N. Diagnosis ultrasonography of the ulnar nerve in cubital tunnel syndrome. J Hand Surg Br. 2000;25(5):499–502.
6. Beekman R, Visser LH, Verhagen WI. Ultrasonography in ulnar neuropathy at the elbow: a critical review. Nerve Muscle. 2011;43(5):627–35. https://doi.org/10.1002/mus.22019.
7. Schertz M, Mutschler C, Masmejean E, Silvera J. High-resolution ultrasound in etiological evaluation of ulnar neuropathy at the elbow. Eur J Radiol. 2017;95:111–7. https://doi.org/10.1016/j.ejrad.2017.08.003. Epub 2017 Aug 7.
8. Shen PC, Chern TC, Wu KC, Tai TW, Jou IM. The assessment of the ulnar nerve at the elbow by ultrasonography in children. J Bone Joint Surg Br. 2008;90(5):657–61. https://doi.org/10.1302/0301-620X.90B5.19820.
9. Yoon JS, Hong SJ, Kim BJ, Kim SJ, Kim JM, Walker FO, Cartwright MS. Ulnar nerve and cubital tunnel ultrasound in ulnar neuropathy at the elbow. Arch Phys Med Rehabil. 2008;89(5):887–9. https://doi.org/10.1016/d.apmr.2007.10.024.
10. Volpe A, Rossato G, Bottanelli M, Marchetta A, Caramaschi P, Bambara LM, et al. Ultrasound evaluation of ulnar neuropathy at the elbow: correlation with electrophysiological studies. Rheumatology (Oxford). 2009;48(9):1098–101. https://doi.org/10.1093/rheumatology/kep167. Epub 2009 Jun 30.
11. Jacob D, Lambert A, Cohen M. The ulnar nerve at the elbow and elsewhere. In: The peripheral nerve. Montpellier: Sauramps; 2015. p. 237–55.
12. Jacob D, Lambert A, Cohen M. Ultrasound of struthers arcade. In: Brasseur JL, Mercy G, Monzani Q, Benayan E, Grenier P, editors. News in ultrasound of the musculoskeletal system, vol. 12. Montpellier: Medical Sauramps; 2015. p. 103–12.
13. Tubbs RS, Deep A, Shoja MM, Mortazavi MM, Loukas M, Cohen-Gadol AA. The arcade of Struthers: an anatomical study with potential neurosurgical significance. Surg Neurol Int. 2011;2:184.
14. Camerlinck M, Vanhoenacker FM, Kiekens G. Ultrasound demonstration of Struthers' ligament. J Wink Ultrasound. 2010;38(9):499–502.
15. Gelberman HR, Yamaguchi K, Hollstien SB, Winn SS, Heidenreich FP Jr, Bindra RR, et al. Changes in interstitial pressure and cross-sectional area of the cubital tunnel and of the ulnar nerve with flexion of the elbow. An experimental study in human cadavera. J Bone Joint Surg Am. 1998;80(4):492–501.
16. Michelin P, Leleup G, Duparc F. Ligamentous biomechanics of the cubital tunnel. In: Brewer JL, Fustier A, Mercy G, Monzani Q, Lucidarme O, editors. News in ultrasound of the musculoskeletal system, vol. 14. Montpellier: Medical Sauramps; 2017. p. 339–52.
17. Michelin P, Leleup G, Ould-Slimane M, Merlet MC, Dubourg P, Duparc F. Ultrasound biomechanical anatomy of the soft structures in relation to the ulnar nerve in the cubital tunnel of the elbow. Surg Radiol Anat. 2017;39(11):1215–21.
18. James J, Sutton LG, Werner FW, Basu N, Allison MA, Palmer AK. Morphology of the cubital tunnel: an anatomical and biomechanical study with implications for treatment of ulnar nerve compression. J Hand Surg Am. 2011;36(12):1988–95. https://doi.org/10.1016/jhsa.2011.09.014. Epub 2011 Nov 3.
19. Yang SN, Yoon JS, Kim SJ, Kang HJ, Kim SH. Movement of the ulnar nerve at the elbow: a sonographic study. J Ultrasound Med. 2013;32(10):1747–52. https://doi.org/10.7863/ultra.32.10.1747.

20. Okamoto M, Abe M, Shirai H, Ueda N. Morphology and dynamics of the ulnar nerve in the cubital tunnel. Observation by ultrasonography. J Hand Surg Br. 2000;25(1):85–9.
21. Jacob D, Creteur V, Courthaliac C, Bargoin R, Sassus B, Bacq C, Rozies JL, Casket JP, Brewer JL. Sonoanatomy of the ulnar nerve in the cubital tunnel: a multicentre study by the GEL. Eur Radiol. 2004;14(10):1770–3. Epub 2004 Jul 17.
22. Yoon JS, Walker FO, Cartwright MS. Ultrasonographic swelling ratio in the diagnosis of ulnar neuropathy at the elbow. Nerve Muscle. 2008;38(4):1231–5. https://doi.org/10.1002/mus.21094.
23. Pompe SM, Beekman R. Which ultrasonographic measure has the upper hand in ulnar neuropathy at the elbow? Clin Neurophysiol. 2013;124(1):190–6. https://doi.org/10.1016/j.clinph.2012.05.030. Epub 2012 Oct 1.
24. Chang KV, Wu WT, Han DS, Ozçakar L. Ulnar nerve cross-sectional area for the diagnosis of cubital tunnel syndrome: a meta-analysis of ultrasonographic measurements. Arch Phys Med Rehabil. 2018;99(4):743757. https://doi.org/10.1016/j.apmr.2017.08.467. Epub 2017 Sep 6.
25. Assmus H, Antoniadis G, Bischoff C, Hoffmann R, Martini AK, Preissler P, Scheglmann K, Schwerdtfeger K, Wessels KD, Wüstner-Hofmann M. Cubital tunnel syndrome a review and management guidelines. Cent Eur Neurosurg. 2011;72(2):90–8. https://doi.org/10.1055/s-0031-1271800. Epub 2011 May 4.
26. Bayrak AO, Bayrak IK, Turker H, Elmali M, Nural MS. Ultrasonography in patients with ulnar neuropathy at the elbow: comparison of cross-sectional area and swelling ratio with electrophysiological severity. Nerve Muscle. 2010;41(5):661–6. https://doi.org/10.1002/mus.21563.
27. Terayama Y, Uchiyama S, Ueda K, Iwakura N, Ikegami S, Kato Y, Kato H. Optimal measurement level and ulnar nerve cross-sectional area cutoff threshold for identifying ulnar neuropathy at the elbow by MRI and ultrasonography. J Hand Surg Am. 2018;43(6):529–36. https://doi.org/10.1016/j.jhsa.2018.02.022. Epub 2018 Apr 3.
28. Paluch Ł, Noszczyk B, Nitek Z, Walecki J, Osiak K, Pietruski P. Shear-wave elastography: a new potential method to diagnose ulnar neuropathy at the elbow. Eur Radiol. 2018;28(12):4932–9. https://doi.org/10.1007/s00330-018-5517-9. Epub 2018 Jun 1.
29. Paluch Ł, Noszczyk BH, Walecki J, Osiak K, Kiciński M, Pietruski P. Shear-wave elastography in the diagnosis of ulnar tunnel syndrome. J Plast Reconstr Aesthet Surg. 2018;71(11):1593–9. https://doi.org/10.1016/d.bjps.2018.08.018. Epub 2018 Sep 4.
30. Bjerre JJ, Johannsen FE, Rathcke M, Krogsgaard MR. Snapping elbow-a guide to diagnosis and treatment. World J Orthop. 2018;9(4):65–71. https://doi.org/10.5312/wjo.v9.i4.65. eCollection 2018 Apr 18.
31. Steinert AF, Goebel S, Rucker A, Barthel T. Snapping elbow caused by hypertrophic synovial plica in the radiohumeral joint: a report of three cases and review of literature. Arch Orthop Trauma Surg. 2010;130(3):347–51. https://doi.org/10.1007/s00402-008-0798-0. Epub 2008 Dec 17.
32. Spinner RJ, Goldner RD. Snapping of the medial head of the triceps and recurrent dislocation of the ulnar nerve. Anatomical and dynamic factors. J Bone Joint Surg Am. 1998;80(2):239–47.
33. Bozkurt MC, Tağil SM, Ozçakar L, Ersoy M, Tekdemir I. Anatomical variations as potential risk factors for ulnar tunnel syndrome: a cadaveric study. Clin Anat. 2005;18(4):274–80.
34. Uscetin I, Bingol D, Ozkaya O, Orman C, Akan M. Ulnar nerve compression at the elbow caused by the epitrochleoanconeus muscle: a case report and surgical approach. Turk Neurosurg. 2014;24(2):266–71. https://doi.org/10.5137/1019-5149.JTN.6913-12.0.
35. Erdem Bagatur A, Yalcin MB, Ozer EU. Anconeus epitrochlearis muscle causing ulnar neuropathy at the elbow: clinical and neurophysiological differential diagnosis. Orthopedics. 2016;39(1):988–91.
36. Li P, Lou D, Lu H. The cubital tunnel syndrome caused by intraneural ganglion cyst of the ulnar nerve at the elbow: a case report. BMC Neurol. 2018;18(1):217. https://doi.org/10.1186/s12883-018-1229-7.
37. Chang WK, Li YP, Zhang DF, Liang BS. The cubital tunnel syndrome caused by the intraneural or extraneural ganglion cysts: case report and review of the literature. J Plast Reconstr Aesthet Surg. 2017;70(10):14041408. https://doi.org/10.1016/j.bjps.2017.05.006. Epub 2017 Jul 6.
38. Bathala L, Krishnam VN, Kumar HK, Neladimmanahally V, Nagaraju U, Kumar HM, Telleman JA, Visser LH. Extensive sonographic ulnar nerve enlargement above the medial epicondyle is a characteristic sign in Hansen's neuropathy. PLoS Negl Trop Dis. 2017;11(7):e0005766. https://doi.org/10.1371/journal.pntd.0005766. eCollection 2017 Jul.
39. Gallon A, Pérignon R, Lhoste-Trouilloud A. Imaging the nerve damage of leprosy. In: Brasseur JL, Mercy G, Monzani Q, Benayan E, Grenier P, editors. News in ultrasound of the musculoskeletal system, vol. 12. Montpellier: Medical Sauramps; 2015. p. 143–58.
40. Lucchina S, Fusetti C, Guidi M. Sonographic follow-up of patients with cubital tunnel syndrome undergoing in situ open neurolysis or endoscopic release: the SPECTRE study. Hand (N Y). 2021;16(3):385–90. https://doi.org/10.1177/1558944719857816. [Epub ahead of print].
41. Simon NG, Ralph JW, Poncelet AN, Engstrom JW, Chin C, Kliot M. A comparison of ultrasonographic and electrophysiologic 'inching' in ulnar neuropathy at the elbow. Clin Neurophysiol. 2015;126(2):391–8. https://doi.org/10.1016/j.clinph.2014.05.023. Epub 2014 Jun 4.

9 Ultrasound Radial Nerve of the Elbow

G. Morvan and V. Vuillemin

The radial nerve (NR), the large nerve of the posterior surface of the upper limb (MS), the face of the extension, manages the extension and supination. It is mainly a motor nerve that controls the extensor muscles of the elbow (the powerful triceps and the small anconeus), the supinators (supinator and brachioradialis), the extensors of the wrist (short and long radial carpal extensors, extensor carpi ulnaris), and the fingers (short and long extensor of the thumb, common extensor of the fingers, proper extensors of 2 and 5) and even the long abductor of the thumb.

It is also the sensory nerve of the posterior faces of the arm and posterolateral of the elbow, the median region of the posterior surface of the forearm, and the dorsal part of the radial edge of the hand (Fig. 9.1).

Clinical signs of an RN lesion depend on the level of the lesion. Above all, it is a deficit of extension: drooping hand and lack of extension of the first phalanges of the four long fingers that remain flexed due to the uncompensated action of the interosseous muscles. The thumb, extended by the adductor alone, remains stuck to the index finger, and the first commissure no longer opens. The extension of the elbow is usually preserved due to the high origin of the nerves of the triceps.

G. Morvan (✉) · V. Vuillemin
Centre d'imagerie de l'appareil moteur Léonard de Vinci, Paris, France

9.1 Radial Nerve Above the Elbow

The origin of the RN is very logical, fully in line with its function: intended for the posterior side of the MS, it originates from the posterior half of the brachial plexus [1] (Fig. 9.2) and contains fibers from all the roots that make up the latter. It is the only big nerve coming from the posterior plexus. It vertically crosses the axillary hollow and joins the posterior compartment of the arm through the humero-tricipital slit, passing under the tendons of the teres major and the latissimus dorsi, accompanied by the deep brachial artery (Fig. 9.3).

As soon as it enters the posterior compartment, it provides motor branches to the three heads of the triceps (the high origin of these branches explains that they are usually preserved during fractures of the humeral diaphysis, more distally).

A little further, the RN rejoins the humerus. Covered by the lateral head of the triceps, it intersects the posterior side of the diaphysis from top to bottom and from inside to outside in an elongated X, directly in contact with the bone, within a shallow groove, the spiral groove. From medial as it was, it gradually becomes lateral (Fig. 9.4).

Approximately 15 cm above the lateral epicondyle, the RN reaches the lateral intermuscular

T. Apard, J. L. Brasseur (eds.), *Ultrasonography for the Upper Limb Surgeon*,
https://doi.org/10.1007/978-3-030-84234-5_9

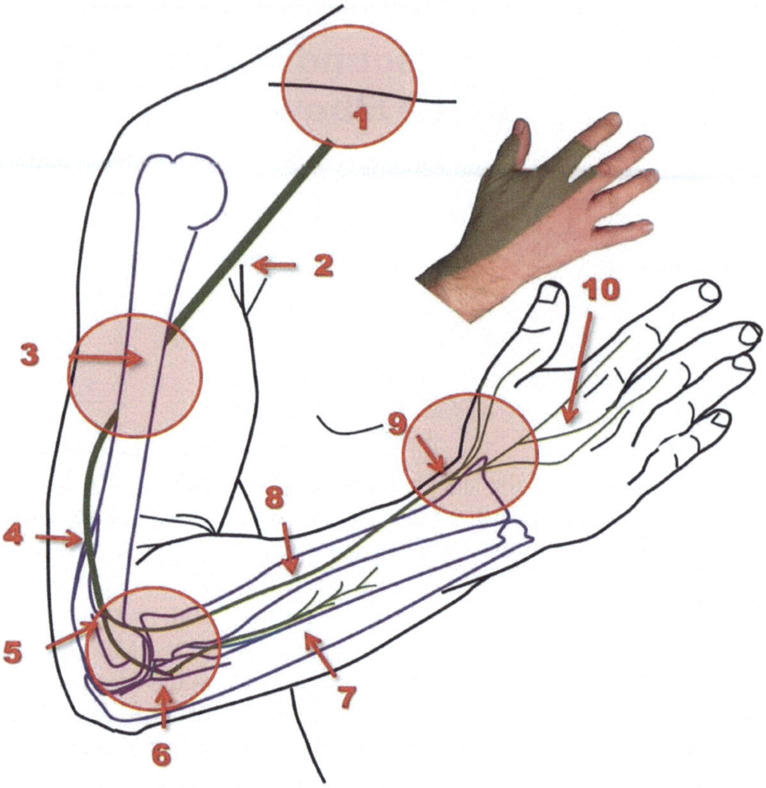

Fig. 9.1 The sites crossed by the RN and its sensory territory on the back of the hand. (1) brachial plexus; (2) axillary hollow; (3) posterior surface of arm; (4) crossing of the lateral intermuscular septum; (5) division into two anterior sensory and posterior motor branches at the anterior aspect of the elbow; (6) radial tunnel; (7) posterior motor branches in posterior compartment of forearm; (8) anterior sensory branch in anterior compartment of forearm; (9) crossing; (10) back of the hand

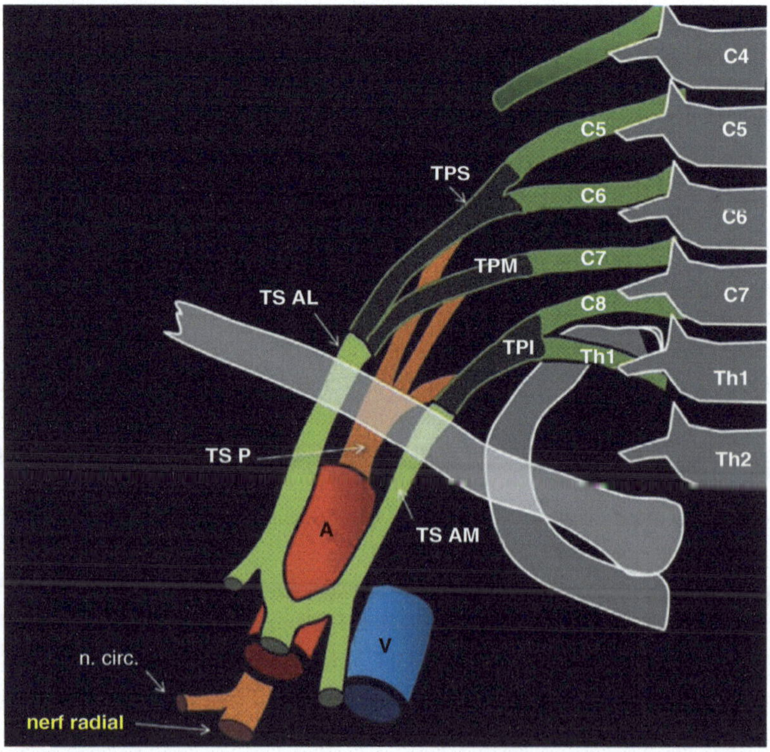

Fig. 9.2 Brachial plexus. RN is the only large nerve to be born in the posterior brachial hemiplexus (orange). TPS, TPM, TPI: upper, middle, and lower primary trunks. TSAL, TSAM, TSP: anterolateral, anteromedial, and posterior secondary trunks

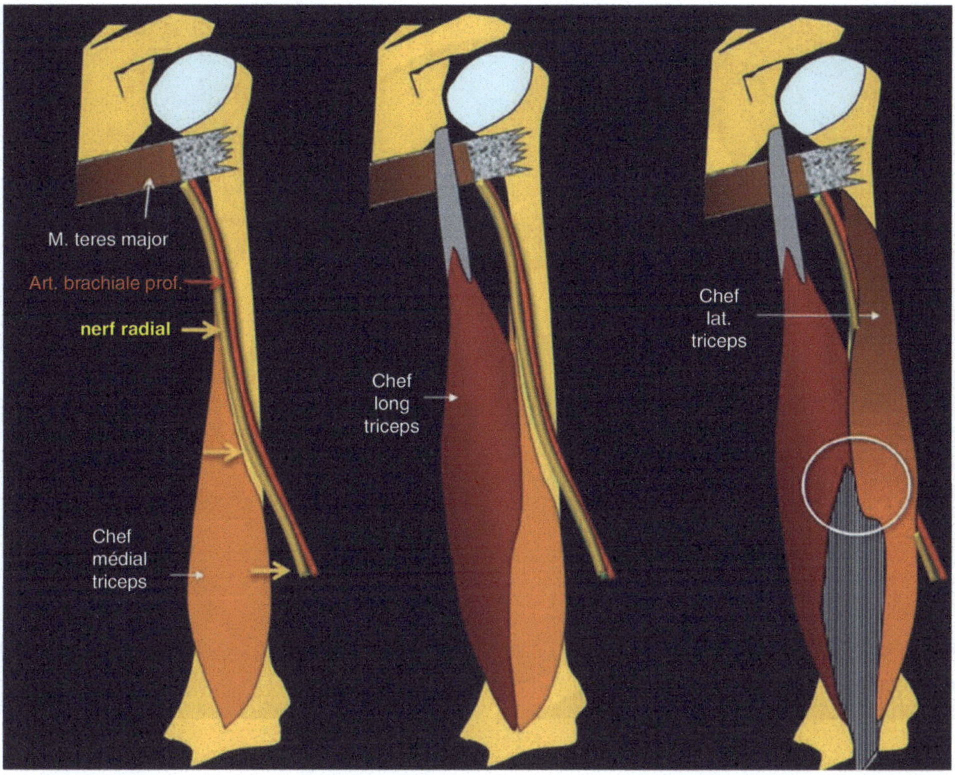

Fig. 9.3 The RN at the posterior surface of the arm, in the spiral groove at immediate contact with the humeral diaphysis, covered by the triceps heads

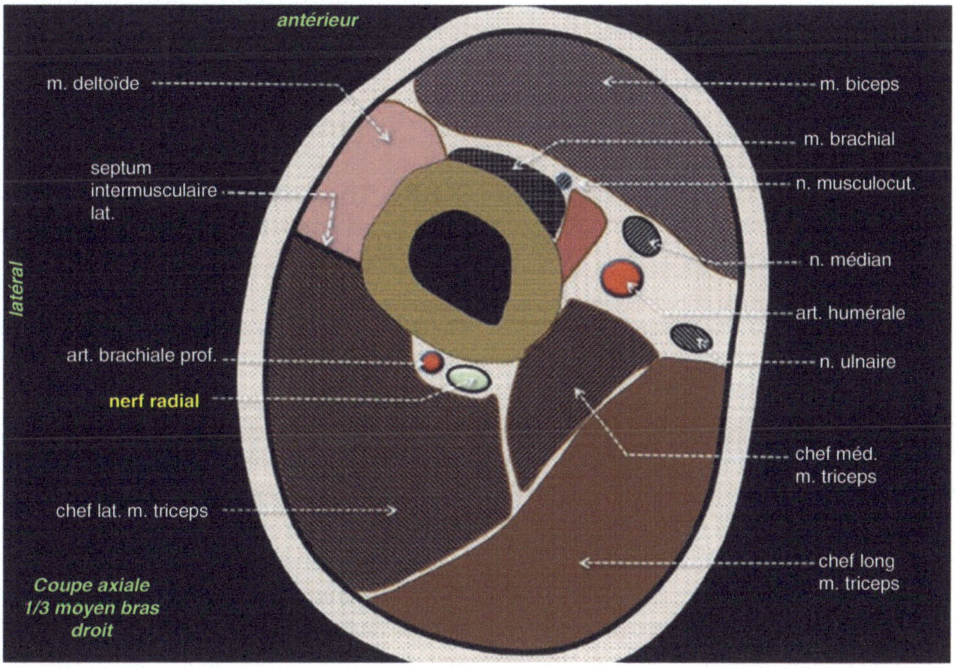

Fig. 9.4 Axial cut at the median third of the right arm (upper segment of the cut). The RN is in contact with the posterior surface of the humerus, under the triceps, accompanied by the deep brachial artery

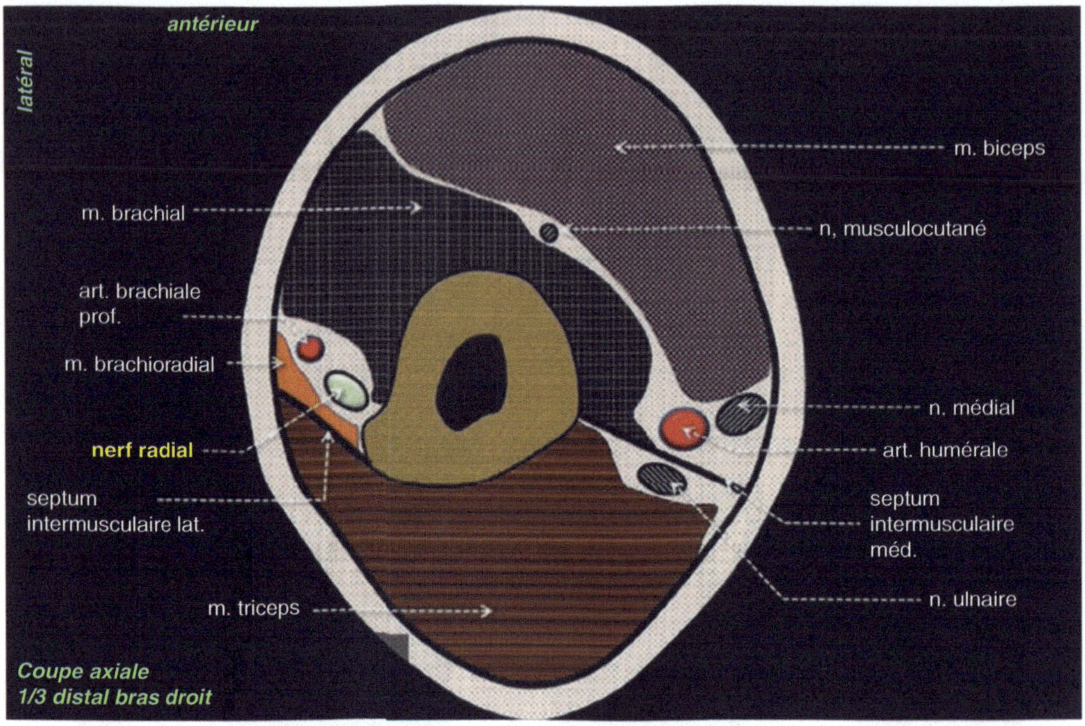

Fig. 9.5 The same axial cut at the distal third of the arm. The RN has just passed through the lateral intermuscular septum and is found in the anterior compartment, under the brachialis muscle, accompanied by the deep brachial artery

Table 9.1 Etiology of RN neuropathies on the posterior side of the arm

• Fractures of the humeral diaphysis, especially spiroid and displaced
• Impingement between RN and osteosynthesis material [2]
• Humeral lengthening osteotomies [3]
• Prolonged compression of the RN between the humerus and the head of a partner resting on the arm of the other ("honeymoon" syndrome)
• Prolonged compression of the RN between the humerus and a hard plane (chair backrest, bath edge) or by swinging arm out of bed, favored by the abuse of alcohol, sleeping pills, or narcotics ("Saturday evening" syndrome)
• Compression of the RN between the humerus and the anterior surface of the contralateral knee (milititary shooters in the knee-to-ground position) [4]
• RN compression by muscle hypertrophy in bodybuilders [5]
• Intraoperative compression of the RN (thorax surgery) [6]

septum, crosses it (Fig. 9.5), and thus passes from the posterior compartment of the arm to the anterolateral surface of the elbow.

This posterior region of the arm is rich in potential pathologies, the main ones of which are listed in Table 9.1.

9.2 Radial Nerve at the Elbow

9.2.1 The Radial Nerve in Front of the Humeral Pallet and Its Division

Once the septum is crossed, the RN descends to the anterior surface of the distal humerus, then from the capitellum through the lateral bicipital groove, between the biceps tendon and the brachialis muscle medially and behind, and the brachioradialis and extensor carpi radialis longus laterally and in front (Fig. 9.6).

At varying height, it divides in this zone into its two terminal branches: the anterior sensory branch and the posterior motor branch. The RN and its splitting branches are easily visible at this level in E° and in MRI (Fig. 9.7).

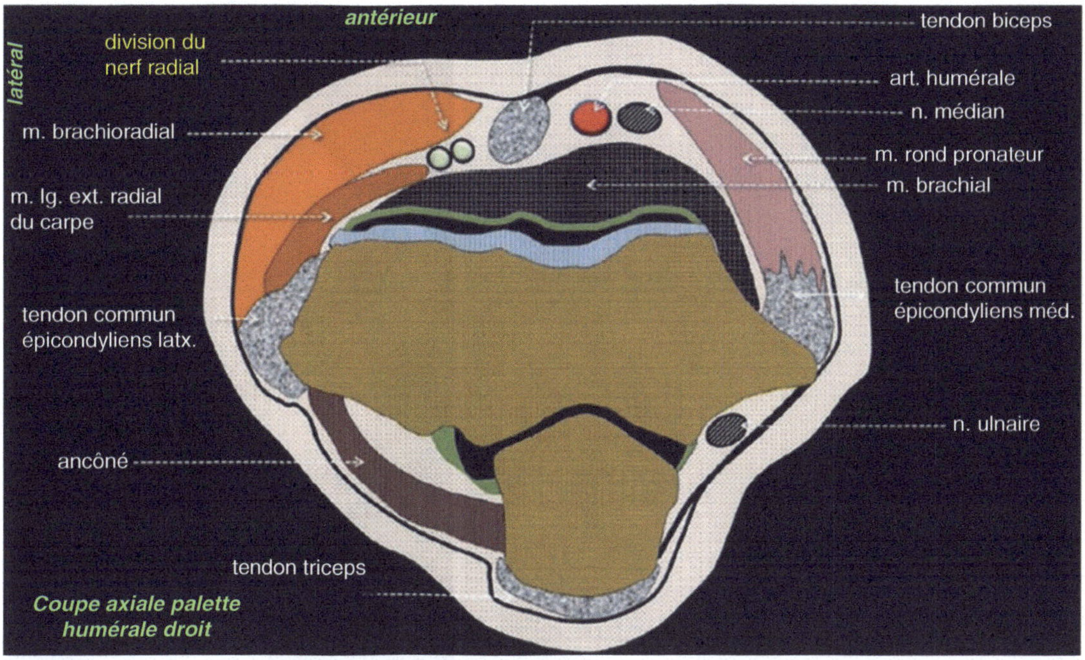

Fig. 9.6 The same axial cut passing through the distal humerus. The RN is dividing

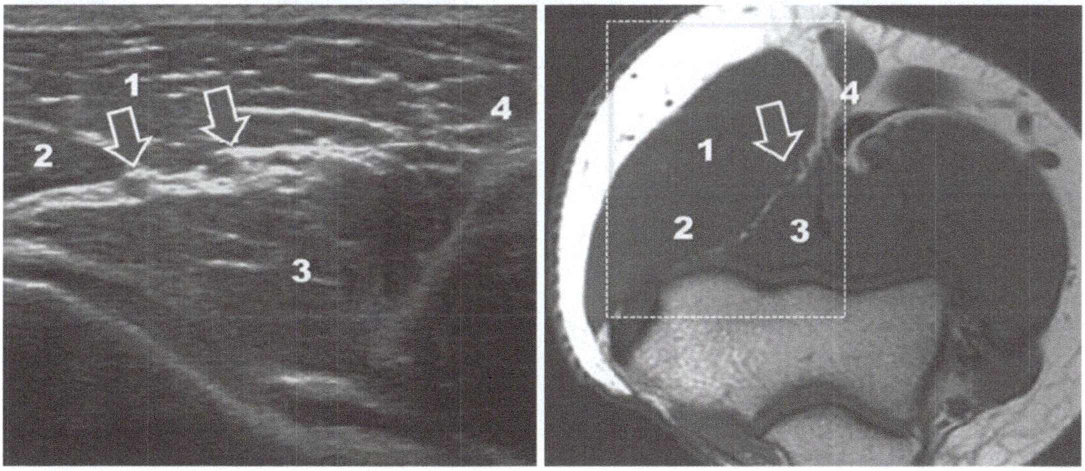

Fig. 9.7 Axial E° and MRI T1 passing through the RN bifurcation. (1) brachioradialis m.; (2) extensor carpi radialis longus ECRL m.; (3) brachialis m.; (4) biceps tendon; (5) RN bifurcation

In this site, the RN can be lesioned during displaced fractures of the pallet (Fig. 9.8), by orthopedic equipment necessary for their treatment and due to joint pathologies of the elbow. Table 9.2 lists the main etiologies of lesions. The neurological deficit then concerns the extensors of the wrist and fingers and the brachioradialis, with the triceps remaining normal.

9.2.2 The Two Branches of the Radial Nerve

The superficial branch, essentially sensory, continues the course of the nerve and runs under the brachioradialis muscle along the lateral part of the anterior surface of the forearm (Figs. 9.9 and 9.10).

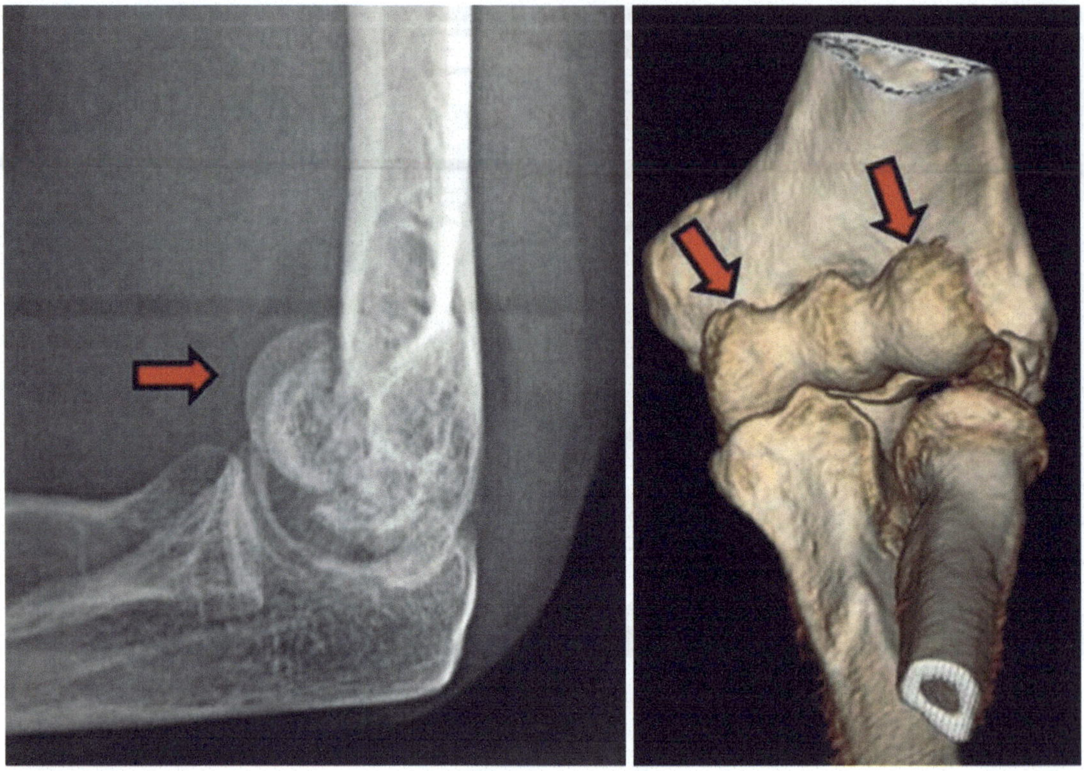

Fig. 9.8 Displaced supracondylar fracture (arrows) with radial deficit

Table 9.2 Etiology of RN neuropathies just above the elbow

• Supracondylar fractures, mostly displaced (Fig. 9.8)
• Fasciculated osteosynthesis or by broach for diaphyseal or supracondylar fracture of the humerus
• Repetitive flexion-extension movements (pushups, mountain biking)
• Humero-radial joint lesions (synovial cysts, synovial tumors, rheumatoid nodule)
Local masses
Recurrent vessels in front of lateral epicondylar mass

The deep branch, mostly motor, but not exclusively, penetrates between the two heads of the supinator muscle wrapped around the neck of the radius (Figs. 9.9, 9.10, and 9.11). It takes the name of the posterior interosseous nerve (PIN) upon leaving this muscle and then goes lower to the posterior surface of the forearm along the posterior surface of the interosseous membrane. This deep branch, wrongly called motor, is actually a mixed nerve that contains some sensory fibers [7], which explains the possibility of confusion between neurogenic pain and lateral epicondylar enthesopathy (both of which can be combined).

In addition to the muscles of the six dorsal compartments of the wrist, the deep branch of the RN innervates the anconeus, the supinator, and the brachioradialis. The motor branch of the extensor carpi radialis brevis, contrary to the classical notion, can come from the trunk of the nerve before its bifurcation (20% of cases), from its deep motor branch before crossing the supinator (32%), but also from its superficial branch in its first centimeters (48% of cases) [8].

The immediate subcutaneous and protruding character of the elbow makes this joint particularly susceptible to trauma. The same applies to the vasculo-nervous elements that pass through it.

The majority of nerve lesions at the elbow are neuropraxias or axonotmesis (lesion of axons without complete nerve section) linked to stretching or transient compressions [9].

Displaced supracondylar humerus fractures account for almost one-third of the limb fractures in young children [10]. Their usual treatment consists of reduction followed by broaching. In Babal's meta-analysis [10], which studied 5194 fractures,

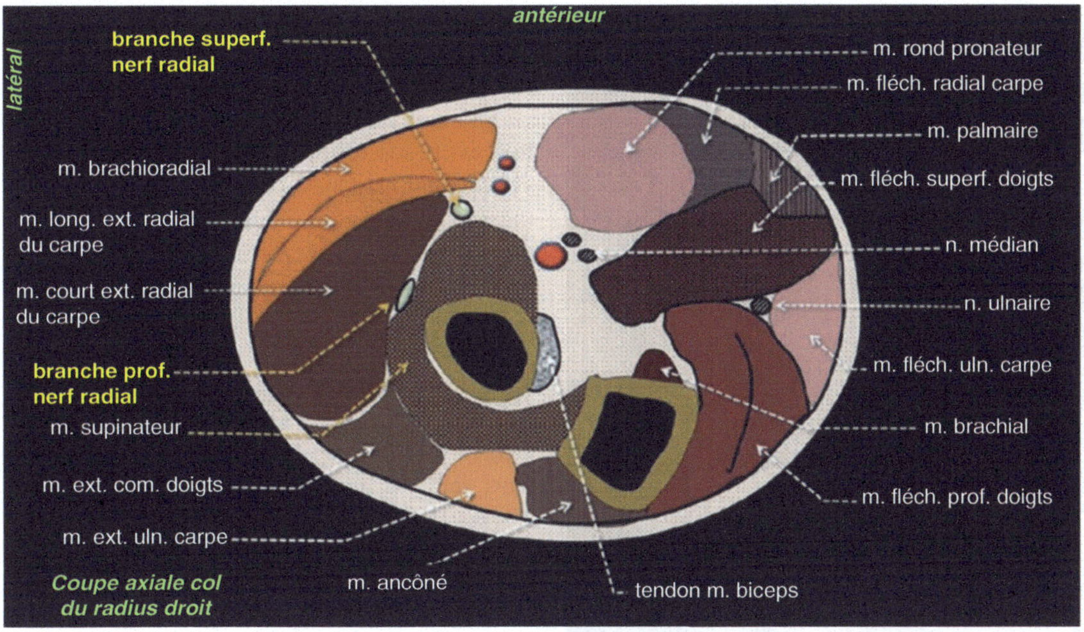

Fig. 9.9 The same axial section as Figs. 9.4, 9.5, and 9.6, passing through the neck of the radius and through the supinator muscle between the two heads of which we see the deep branch of the RN

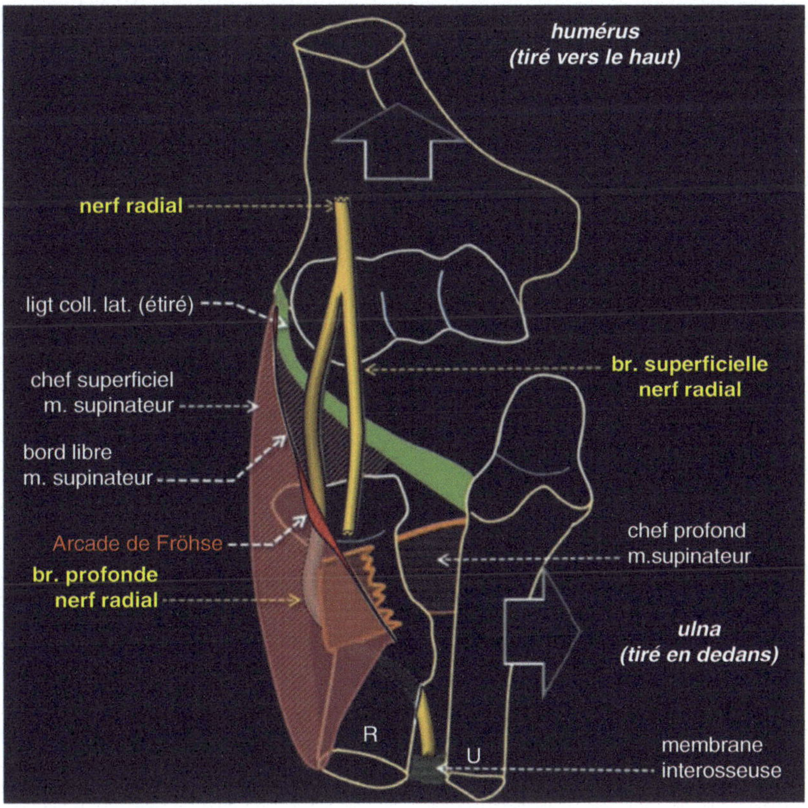

Fig. 9.10 Radial tunnel and its nerve content. Exposure of the contents necessitated artificially pulling the elbow bones away from each other, as if the ligaments joining them were elastic

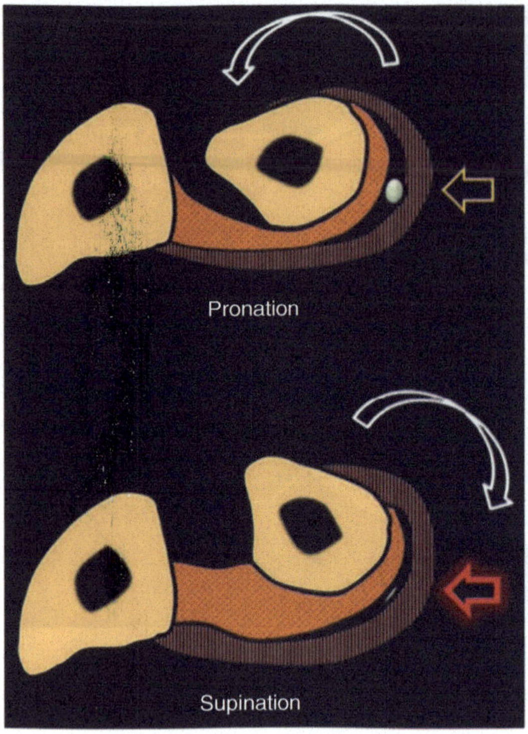

Fig. 9.11 In pronation, the posterior branch of the RN is free between the two heads of the supinator (yellow arrow). In supination, contraction thickens the muscle and compresses the nerve (red arrow)

traumatic neuropraxia was present in 13% of extended fractures (by far the most frequent) and 17% of flexion fractures, of which 5% were RN or PIN lesions. Other studies place RN at the forefront of lesioned nerves [11, 12]. Broaching itself would cause 4% of iatrogenic neuropraxias [10] most often reaching the median or ulnar nerves.

9.2.3 Radial Tunnel

The radial tunnel lies between the lateral epicondyle of the humerus and the distal part of the supinator muscle [13], about 5 cm [14] (Figs. 9.9 and 9.10).

Its lateral face consists of the brachioradialis muscle and the short and long carpi radialis muscles and its medial face by the brachialis muscle and the tendon of the biceps. Its floor is formed by the capsule of the radiohumeral joint and the deep head of the supinator muscle [15] and its ceiling by the superficial head of the supinator and by the tense aponeurotic expansions from the lateral epicondyle, the insertion of the short radial extensor carpi radialis brevis muscle, and the superficial head of the supinator [13].

The motor branch of the RN creeps between the two heads of the supinator to which it provides motor branches. In this gap, it goes around the neck of the radius to find itself in the posterior compartment of the forearm, just behind the interosseous membrane.

Two out of three times [16], the proximal edge of the superficial head of the supinator muscle appears as a fibrous band. This resistant fibrous edge forms the arch of Fröhse, the main traumatic element of the deep branch of the RN upon its entry into the supinator muscle (Fig. 9.10) [14]. The distal edge of the supinator can also be fibrous.

In pronation, the nerve flows comfortably between the two heads of the supinator, relaxed. In contrast, during supination, which strains the muscle and swells it, it is cramped, especially in case of muscle hypertrophy (Fig. 9.11).

The incessant alternations of pronation and supination implied by certain activities (conductor, musician) can generate repeated microtraumas of the nerve stuck between two inextensible structures: most often the arcade of Fröhse and the radius.It is not just this arcade that can compress the nerve in the radial tunnel. Table 9.3 lists the other potentially aggressive structures that sit there [13].

Table 9.3 Etiology of RN neuropathies in the radial tunnel

• Proximal fibrous border of supinator muscle (Fröhse arch)
• Hypertrophy of the supinator muscle by overuse (athletes, violinists, drummers)
• Thickened cranial border of the ECRB extensor carpi radialis brevis, especially in case of enthesopathy of the common tendon of the lateral epicondylar muscles [14]
• Adhesions or flanges of the anterior capsule of the radiohumeral joint
• Abnormal recurrent vessels tying the posterior interosseous nerve (Henry's bridle)
• Intermuscular septum between ulnar extensor carpi ulnaris and proper extensor of the fifth finger
• Distal border of the supinator muscle [17]
• Extrinsic compression by a rod, fracture of the head of the radius, tumor or pseudotumor of soft parts (cysts (Fig. 9.12), lipoma (Fig. 9.13)), and synovitis (septic arthritis, synovial chondromatosis, rheumatoid arthritis) [17]

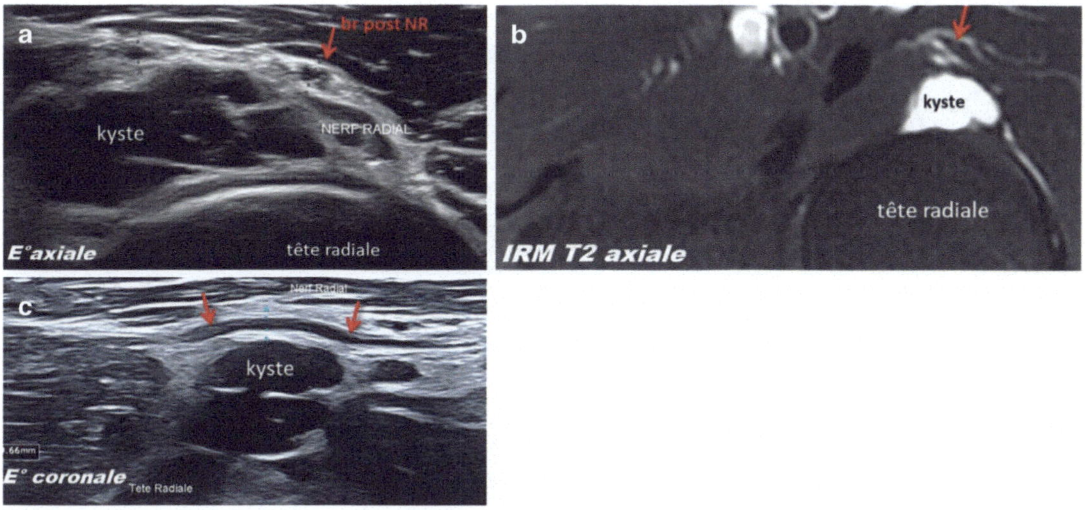

Fig. 9.12 Compression of the motor branch of the RN by an arthrosynovial cyst from the humero-radial joint. Axial E° and T2 MRI. E coronal. We perfectly see the RN (red arrow), pushed back and flattened by the cyst

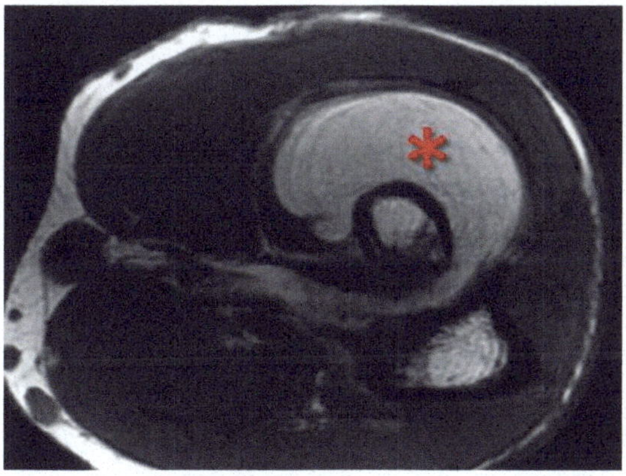

Fig. 9.13 Compression of the motor branch of the RN by a lipoma surrounding the neck of the radius (red asterisk). Axial MRI T1

This syndrome of the deep branch of the NR, also called the syndrome of the PIN, the supinator, and the radial tunnel, results in muscle pain and/or weakness. It is usually pain in the lateral edge of the forearm that can radiate to the first interdigital commissure. Unspecific, sometimes reproduced by the aggravated supination or the aggravated extension of the third finger, they are similar to those of lateral epicondylalgia, with which they can be confused.

The fairly frequent coexistence of these two lesions (enthesopathy and neuropathy) may lead to misdiagnosis (5% of recurrent epicondylalgia are actually PIN syndromes) [18]. There is no sign of Tinel. The EMG may be equivocal or normal due to the lack of well-established criteria. The E° usually resolves the problem provided that the nerve damage is sought even in the case of enthesopathy (Fig. 9.14).

The deep branch of the RN can be followed in static and dynamic extension (during winding movements of pronosupination) and in MRI in its path within the supinator. Sometimes the arcade of Fröhse can be seen in MRI as a hypointense band at the proximal edge of the supinator muscle.

An increase in the caliber of the nerve at its entry into the muscle is sought in extension (Figs. 9.15 and 9.16) and, on T2 MRI, a muscle hypersignal, an indirect but early sign of muscle denervation, downstream of the compression level [19] (Fig. 9.17).

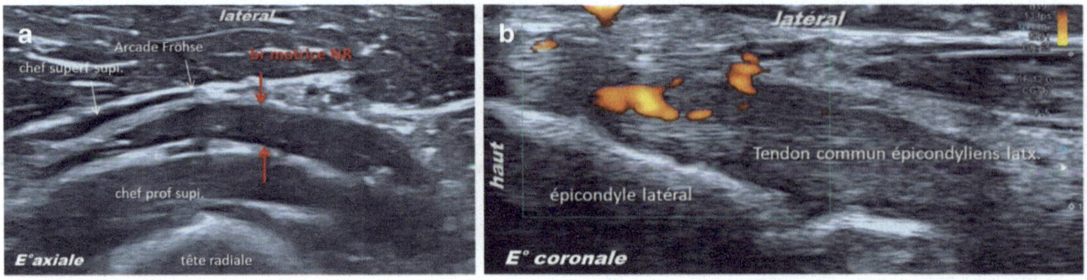

Fig. 9.14 Coexistence of compression of the motor branch of the RN under the arcade of Fröhse (red arrows) and enthesopathy of the common tendon of the lateral epicondyle, in which power Doppler mode hyperemia is noted

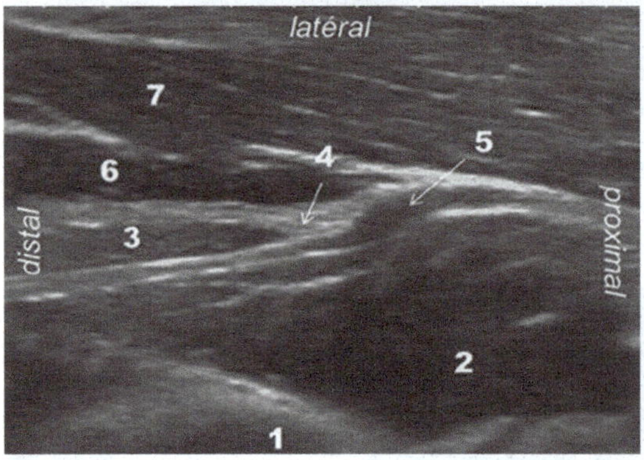

Fig. 9.15 Compression of the deep branch of the RN by a hypertrophied supinator muscle (professional percussionist). Coronal ultrasound. (1) radius; (2) deep head of the supinator M., very thickened; (3) superficial head; (4) arcade of Fröhse; (5) deep branch of the RN with an increased focal caliber; (6) m. extensor carpi radialis brevis; (7) long extensor and brachioradialis

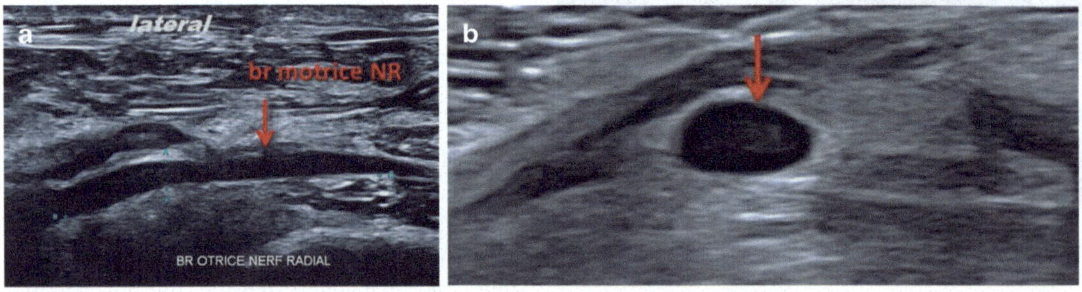

Fig. 9.16 Compression of the posterior branch of the RN at the level of the supinator. Coronal and axial E°. The nerve is increased in volume on 18 mm and hypoE°. The traumatic element is the arcade of Fröhse

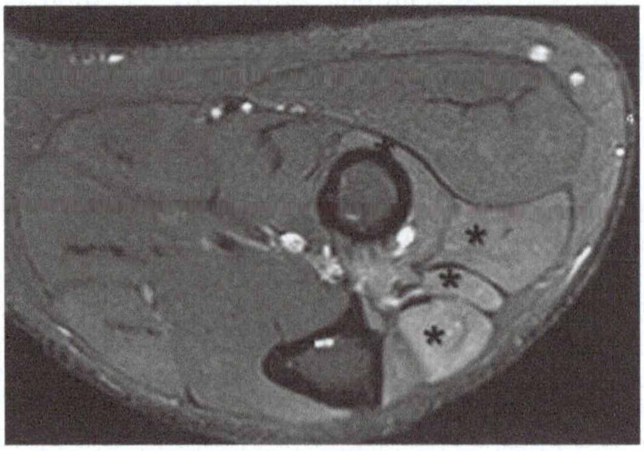

Fig. 9.17 Compression of the posterior branch of the RN at the level of the supinator. Axial MRI T2 FS. No direct sign of compression, but presence of an indirect sign: hypersignal of supinator muscle and extensors (black asterisks)

9.3 The Radial Nerve Beyond the Elbow

9.3.1 Distribution of Motor Branches in the Posterior Compartment of the Forearm

At the posterior compartment of the arm, as soon as the supinator exits, the posterior branch of the RN leaves a bunch of branches for the extensor muscles of the fingers and wrist, the extensor carpi radialis brevis muscle sometimes receiving its innervation directly from the trunk of the RN or even its anterior branch. After giving off these branches, the nerve, reduced to a thread, descends behind the interosseous membrane until branching on the dorsal surface of the wrist.

At this level, its pathology boils down to a few rare extrinsic compressions.

9.3.2 The Path of the Sensory Branch in the Anterior Compartment of the Forearm

The superficial sensory branch of the radial nerve descends vertically along the lateral region of the anterior surface of the forearm, within the sheath of the brachioradialis muscle that covers it (Figs. 9.18 and 9.19). It is flanked medially by the radial artery, good ultrasound reference (Fig. 9.19), and crosses the pronator teres muscles and superficial flexor of the fingers.

At the distal third of the forearm, it passes under the tendon of the brachioradialis and then pierces the superficial fascia, a little behind this tendon to continue its path into the subcutaneous fat of the posterolateral region of the forearm. At this time, it approaches a new critical area: the crossing region, which is outside the scope of our subject.

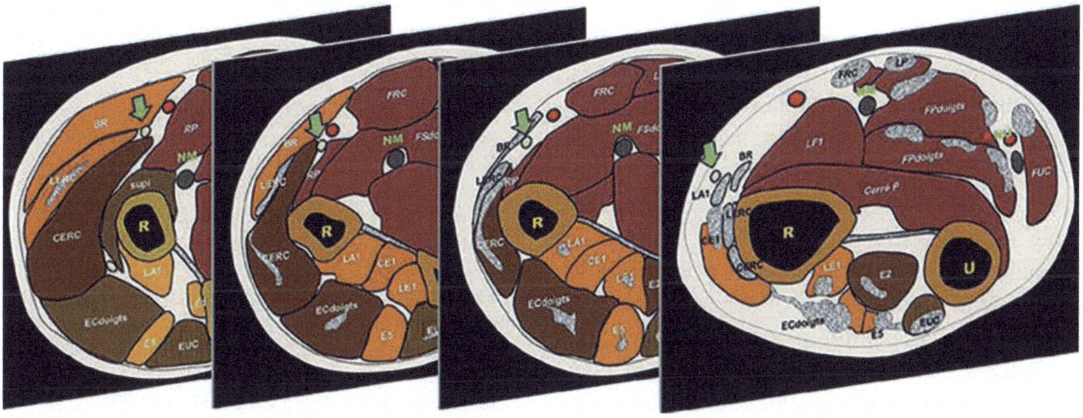

Fig. 9.18 Path of the superficial branch of the RN (green arrow) to the anterior surface of the forearm accompanied inside the radial artery (red arrow). Axial cuts from top to bottom (upper segment) passing through the upper 1/3, the middle part, the lower 1/3, and the lower quarter of the forearm. *BR* brachioradial m., *square P* pronator quadratus m., *CERC* extensor carpi radialis brevis m., *EC1* extensor digitorum brevis m., *EC fingers* common extensor of fingers m., *E2* proper extensor of index finger m., *E5* extensor of fifth finger m., *EUC* extensor carpi ulnaris m., *FP fingers* flexor digitorum profundus m., *FRC* flexor carpi radialis muscle, *FS fingers* superficial flexor of fingers m., *FUC* flexor carpi ulnaris m., *LA1* m. long abductor of thumb m., *LE1* long extensor of thumb m., *ECRL* extensor carpi radialis longus m., *LP* long palmar m., *NM* median nerve, *NU* ulnar nerve, *R* radius, *RP* pronator teres m., *supi* supinator m., *U* ulna

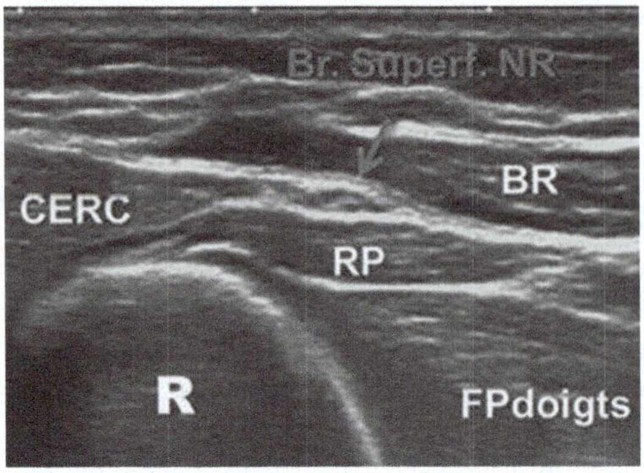

Fig. 9.19 Sensory branch of the RN to the forearm and its relations with the muscles and radial artery (for legends *see* Fig. 9.18)

In its path to the forearm, mechanical damage to the anterior branch of the RN is infrequent, apart from a few displaced fractures or penetrating wounds.

9.4 Conclusion

RN, the nerve of extension and supination, arises from the posterior part of the brachial plexus. This nerve or its two branches of division pass through three dangerous zones: the posterior side of the arm, the radial tunnel, and the radial edge of the wrist. The E° allows you to track the RN along its entire route and to highlight intrinsic anomalies or compressive factors. MRI may also show an early indirect sign of denervation: muscle edema. The painful manifestations of this nerve have the distinction of being often confused with two tendinopathies, lateral epicondylalgia and de Quervain's tenosynovitis, with which they can also be associated.

References

1. Morvan G, Vuillemin V, Guerini H, et al. The radial nerve. In: Lhoste-Trouilloud A, et al. editors. Le nerf périphérique. Montpellier: Sauramps médical; 2015.
2. Lefèvre CH, Gérard R, Le Cour Grandmaison F, Jacq JJ, Le Nem D. Anatomical risks of osteosyndiaphyseal theses of the humerus. Maîtrise orthopédique. 2007;164.
3. Rozbruch SR, Fryman C, Bigman D, Adler R. Use of ultrasound in detection and treatment of nerve compromise in a case of humeral lengthening. HSSJ. 2011;7:80–4. https://doi.org/10.1007/s11420-010-9182-z.
4. Shyu WC, Linn JC, Chang MK, Tsao WL. Compressive radial nerve palsy induced by military shooting training: clinical and electrophysiological study. J Neurol Neurosurg Psychiatry. 1993;56:890–3.
5. Ng AB, Borhan J, Ashton HR, Misra AN, Redfern DRM. Radial nerve palsy in an elite bodybuilder. Br J Sports Med. 2003;37:185–6.
6. Papadopoulou M, Spengos K, Papapostolou A, Tsivgoulis G, Karandreas N. Intraoperative radial nerve injury during coronary artery surgery. Report of two cases. J Brach Plexus Periph Nerve Injury. 2006;1:7. https://doi.org/10.1186/17497221-1-7.
7. Masmejean E, Bauer B, Alnot JY. Injury of radial nerve trunk at arm. In: Alnot JY, Chammas M, editors. Injuries of peripheral nerves: from direct nerve repair to palliative interventions. Paris: Elsevier Masson; 2007.
8. Messrs A-Q. The nerve supply to extensor carpi radialis brevis. J Anat. 1996;188:249–50.
9. Adams EA, Steinmann SP. Nerve injury about the elbow. Curr Opin Orthop. 2006;17:348–54.
10. Babal JC, Mehlman CT, Klein GB. Nerve injuries associated with pediatric supracondylar humeral fracture: a meta-analysis. J Pediatr Orthop. 2010;30:253–63.
11. Iobst CA, Spurdle C, King WF, et al. Percutaneous pinning of pediatric supracondylar humerus fractures with the semisterile technique: the Miami experience. J Pediatr Orthop. 2007;27:17–22.
12. Lipscomb PR. Vascular and neural complications in supracondylar fractures of the humerus in children. J Bone Joint Surg Am. 1955;37A:487–92.
13. Clavert P, Lutz JC, Adam P, Wolfram-Gabel R, Liverneaux P, Kahn JL. Frohse's arch is not the only seat of compression of the radial nerve in its tunnel. RCO. 2009;95:2131–6.
14. Ferdinand BD, Sadka Rosenberg Z, Schweitzer ME, et al. MR imaging features of radial tunnel syndrome: initial experience. Radiology. 2006;240:161–8.
15. Barnum M, Mastey RD, Weiss AC, Akelman E. Radial tunnel syndrome. Hand Clin. 1996;12:679–89.
16. Koudougou C. Fröhse's arcade. Memory for the certificate of anatomy, imaging and morphogenesis. Nantes. 2006.
17. Andreisek G, Crook DW, Burg D, Marincek B, Weishaupt D. Peripheral neuropathies of the median, radial, and ulnar nerves: MR imaging features. Radiographics. 2006;26:1267–87.
18. Werner CO. Lateral elbow pain and posterior interosseous nerve entrapment. Acta Orthop Scand Suppl. 1979;174:1–62.
19. Dog AJ, Jamadar DA, Jacobson JA, Hayes CW, Louis DS. Sonography and MR imaging of posterior interosseous nerve syndrome with surgical correlation. AJR. 2003;181:219–21.

Part III

Forearm

Ultrasound of the Interosseous Membrane of the Forearm

10

Marc Soubeyrand

10.1 Introduction

The interosseous membrane (IOM) is stretched between the two bones of the forearm. It participates in the dynamic stabilization of the antebrachial frame, in the transverse but also longitudinal plane. It can be torn by a longitudinal shear mechanism and, in this case, combined with a fracture-impaction of the radial head and a tear of the triangular fibrocartilaginous complex (TFCC) of the wrist resulting in Essex-Lopresti syndrome (Fig. 10.1) [1]. Incomplete tears can also occur in distal radioulnar dislocation (isolated or associated with fracture of the radius: Galeazzi-type lesion) or proximal radioulnar dislocation (in Monteggia-type lesion) (Fig. 10.2).

In the acute phase of trauma to the forearm, the diagnosis of rupture of the IOM is sometimes evident before the displacement of the radius from the ulna, but often the diagnosis is missed at the initial stage. IOM rupture induces major destabilization of the antebrachial framework, and this diagnosis will affect surgical management: contraindication to isolated resection of the radial head, stabilization of the radial ulnar joint, and ligamentoplasty of the forearm [2].

M. Soubeyrand (✉)
Conservative and Traumatological Surgeon Service, Bicêtre Hospital, Le Kremlin-Bicêtre, France

Two imaging tests are proposed to explore IOM: ultrasound [3–5] and magnetic resonance (MRI) imaging [6, 7]. The purpose of this chapter is to describe the use of ultrasound as a means of exploring the IOM.

10.2 Anatomo-pathological Reminders

Anatomy and Biomechanics: The IOM consists of two layers of fibers, the most important of which are oriented up and out (radial) (Fig. 10.3). Some of these fibers are rather strained in supination and others in pronation. This positional fiber recruitment allows continuous operation of the IOM regardless of the rotation of the forearm without impeding the rotation of the radius around the ulna. The orientation of the fibers explains the double stability of the IOM: transverse (prevents the two bones from moving away) and longitudinal/vertical (prevents the relative ascent of the radius relative to the ulna). In addition to the IOM, longitudinal stability of the forearm is ensured by the TFCC (which also participates in transverse stability) and by the radial head (which prevents the rise of the radius by buttressing against the humeral capitellum) [8].

Anatomical studies distinguish three different parts of the IOM: proximal, medial, and distal. The middle portion is the strongest and most

T. Apard, J. L. Brasseur (eds.), *Ultrasonography for the Upper Limb Surgeon*,
https://doi.org/10.1007/978-3-030-84234-5_10

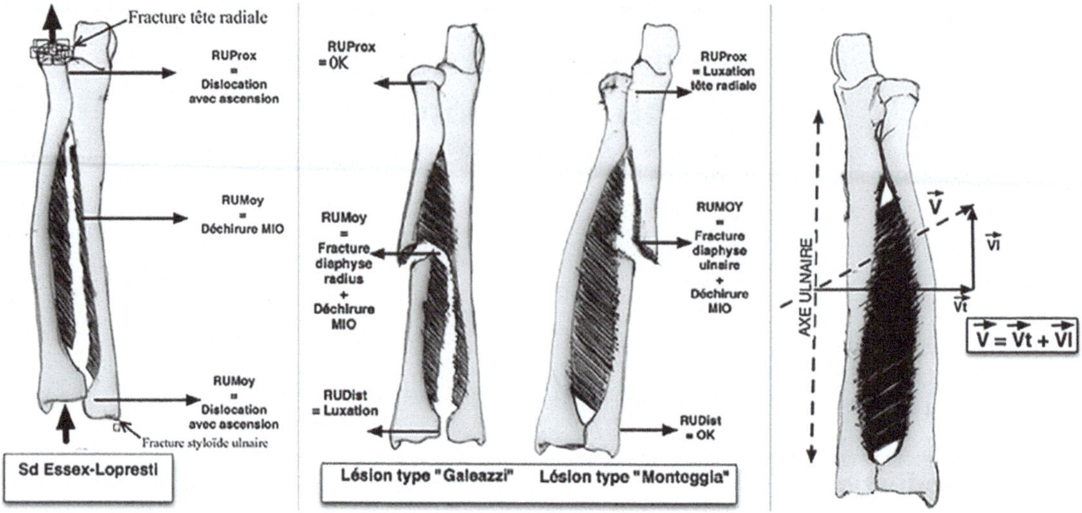

Fig. 10.1 Essex-Lopresti syndrome in its complete form: IOM tear, radial head fracture, ascension of the radius with inversion of the radioulnar index

functionally important. It occupies the widest portion of the interosseous space and stretches rather in neutral rotation. In pronation it is relaxed because the two bones are crossed, and the interosseous space is reduced.

10.3 Traumatic Lesions of the IOM

IOM tears can be partial or complete (full height) and are the result of indirect mechanisms of longitudinal translation/separation of both forearm bones. It appears that the rupture occurs preferentially in the middle of the interosseous space, where the IOM is finer. Three names are to be remembered to describe the traumatic lesions of the IOM: Essex-Lopresti, Monteggia, and Galeazzi.

Essex-Lopresti Syndrome is the complete form with longitudinal and transverse destabilization. Standard radiographs always have the same lesion association: fracture of the radial head usually comminuted and inversion of the distal radioulnar index, which in summary corresponds to a proximal migration of the radius relative to the ulna. This ascent is due to the transmission of stresses from the carpus to the radius at the time of a fall on the palm. Because the IOM is completely ruptured, it no longer holds the proximal migration of the radius. Subsequently, this ascent is maintained by the action of muscles and especially the biceps brachii. Naturally the radius does not "go down," and the evolution is toward a limitation of pronosupination (proximal radioulnar injury as a result of fracture of the radial head +/distal radioulnar dislocation), wrist pain (distal radioulnar damage and ulnocarpal impingement: long pseudo-ulna), and elbow (proximal radioulnar injury).

Lesions of the "Monteggia" type conventionally associate a fracture of the ulna with a complete dislocation of the proximal radioulnar joint. In the manner of Maisonneuve fractures of the leg, the lesion necessarily implies a partial tearing of the proximal part of the IOM: in fact it is impossible to completely dislocate the proximal radioulnar without damage to the IOM.

Galeazzi-type lesions associate a fracture of the radius with a distal radioulnar dislocation. Again, distal radioulnar dislocation is not possible without tearing of TFCC and IOM.

It is accepted that the IOM cannot heal spontaneously for two mechanical reasons. First, the IOM is composed of elastin fibers, and once severed, there is an immediate retraction to its radial and ulnar bone inserts that prevents spontaneous

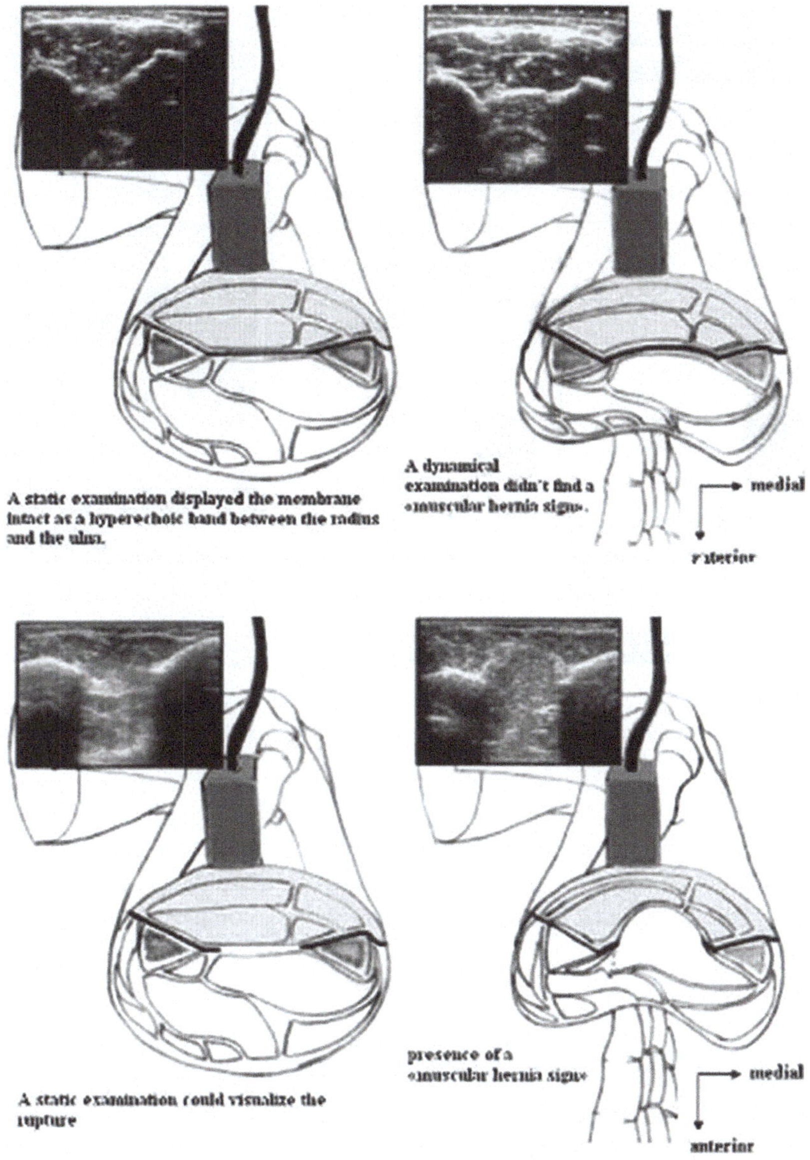

Fig. 10.2 The two classical lesion syndromes depending on whether the IOM tear is associated with an injury of the proximal (Monteggia) or distal (Galeazzi) radial ulnar

re-confrontation of the ruptured banks. Secondly, the surrounding muscles (deep flexors) naturally tend to enter the IOM gap and thus a mechanical obstacle to the confrontation of the banks. The natural evolution is therefore toward a lack of IOM healing while the interosseous space is filled with cicatricial fibrosis that no longer has the mechanical properties of the native IOM ("ligament elongation callus"). In addition, scar processes lead to a gradual fixation of the radius in the upper position relative to the ulna.

Diagnostic means of IOM rupture: X-ray examinations, computed tomography (CT), and standard radiographs don't allow you to see the satellite lesions of IOM rupture: fracture of the radial head, ascent of the radius, and fracture of the ulnar styloid. In some cases, these signs are not visible at the outset, which may lead to the omission of the diagnosis. Direct observation of IOM is possible only with MRI and ultrasound. MRI has the advantage of providing functional information (tissue edema) and not being a

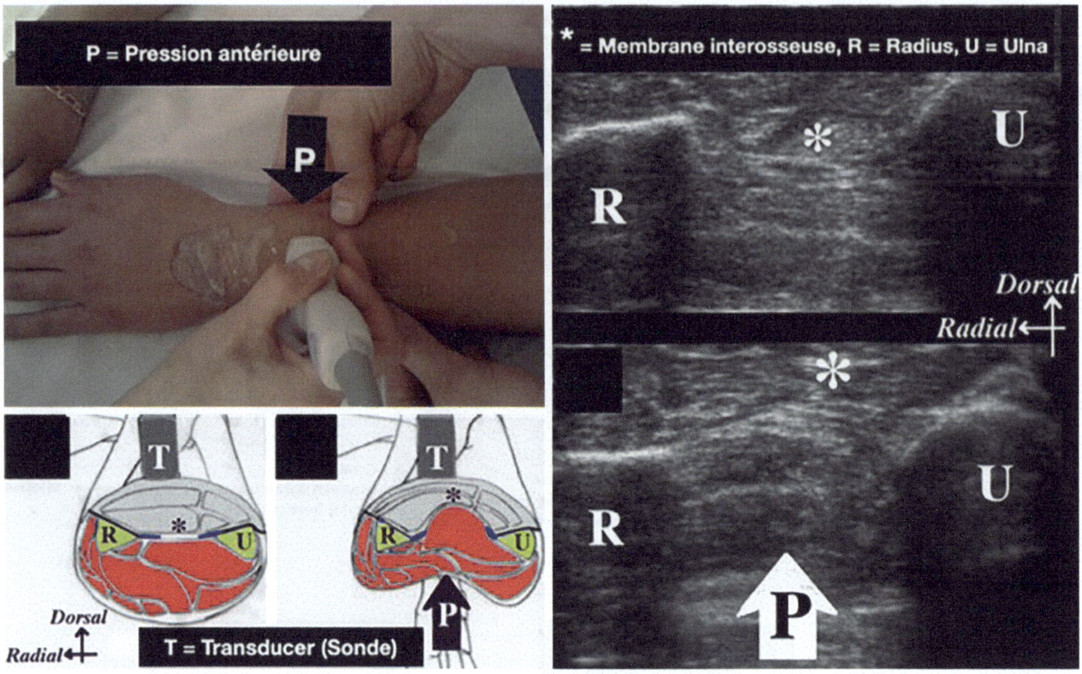

Fig. 10.3 The most important fibers in the IOM are oriented from the ulna to the radius and from the bottom to the top. Thus the force vector corresponding to them can be broken down into a horizontal vector (transverse stability: prevents the separation of the two bones) and vertical vector (longitudinal stability: prevents the rise of the radius)

dependent operator. However, it also has several limitations in this context: difficult to access in emergency, degraded images from the moment the metal material (osteosynthesis plates, screws, radial head prosthesis) was implanted, no dynamic examination possible, and high cost. In the acute phase, MRI can show the interruption of the membrane in T1 and T2 sequences as well as edema in the soft parts surrounding the IOM, signaling the reality of an acute traumatic process [7]. In the chronic phase, its interpretation is more complex because the inflammatory process has disappeared, and if there is no fiber healing with effective length, scar tissue can fill the rupture bank without ensuring the normal function of the IOM ("ligament elongation callus").

Treatments and issues of diagnosis of IOM rupture: All authors conform to the fact that chronic phase treatment has poor functional outcomes [9]. One of the reasons is that once the rise of the radius is "frozen" at the chronic phase, it is technically almost impossible to descend the radius. The ulna should usually be shortened by osteotomy to correct the distal radioulnar index. Confirmation of a complete IOM rupture indicates that the radial head has become the site of significant longitudinal stresses, which can be considered a risk factor for failure of head osteosynthesis. Carrying out arthroplasty will then be preferable. For the same reasons, isolated resection of the radial head would be contraindicated. Finally, the diagnosis of complete rupture could be an argument for the complementary execution of an IOM ligamentoplasty to stabilize the forearm.

10.4 Ultrasound of the Interosseous Membrane

10.4.1 When to Perform an Ultrasound of the IOM?

After trauma to the forearm, in the acute or chronic phase, and in the presence of the satellite lesions described above (fracture of the radial head, inversion of the distal radioulnar index, ulnar styloid tearing), a lesion of the IOM should be evoked and ultrasound performed. Ultrasound can also be performed after surgery even if metal equipment has been implanted.

10.4.2 What Is the Normal Ultrasound Appearance of the IOM?

When the IOM is intact, it is very easy to visualize in ultrasound: it appears as a hyperechogenic structure stretched between the interosseous edges of the two bones. When the forearm rotates, the interosseous space opens and closes, the IOM stretching and relaxing accordingly. The upper part of the IOM is narrower and deeper and therefore harder to observe, but its functional importance is less. The medial part is the most important and is ideally observed in neutral rotation where it is stretched. The distal portion is rather tense in supination. The ideal is to position yourself in front of the patient who is sitting with both elbows on the examination table, in neutral rotation of the forearms. This allows easy access to both forearms.

10.4.3 What Is the Ultrasound Appearance of the Disrupted IOM?

The review must be bilateral and comparative. It is necessary to begin with a morphological examination and then to conduct a dynamic evaluation. In the acute phase, asymmetry can be seen, a continuity solution signaling the tear or the presence of a hematoma in the interosseous space. In the chronic phase, it is much more difficult to diagnose the rupture on the morphological examination alone because scar (nonfunctional) fibrous tissue usually takes place in the interosseous space and gives an appearance of continuity of the fibers between the two bones. This scar is usually a little thicker and may even mistakenly suggest that the IOM is more resistant on the lesioned side.

We recommend performing dynamic IOM testing using the dynamic "muscle hernia sign." We initially described this test on the basis of anatomical work, and it was originally intended for acute ruptures. However, in the chronic phase there is an asymmetry between the two sides. The principle is very simple and is based on the fact that when there is a rupture, one can pass part of the deep flexor muscles through the rupture, toward the posterior compartment of the forearm. The operator places the probe on the back side of the forearm and presses the anterior side at the same time. If the IOM is intact, then the flexor muscles cannot pass through the interosseous space. If the IOM is broken, one manages to generate a real muscle hernia through the interosseous space (test for provoked muscle hernia [3]).

10.5 Conclusion

There is an important stake in making a diagnosis of IOM rupture. Ultrasound is a valuable tool, especially since the lesion will be recent. The surgeon will be able to visualize the rupture, especially by testing for the provoked muscle hernia.

References

1. Essex-Lopresti P. Fractures of the radial head with distal radio-ulnar dislocation; report of two cases. J Bone Gasket Surg Br. 1951;33B:244–7.
2. Soubeyrand M, Lafont C, De Georges R, Dumontier C. [Traumatic pathology of antibrachial interosseous membrane of forearm]. Chir Hand. 2007;26:255–277. S1297-3203 (07) 00122-9 [pii] https://doi.org/10.1016/d.hand.2007.09.004.
3. Soubeyrand M, Lafont C, Oberlin C, France W, Maulat I, Degeorges R. The "muscular hernia sign": an original ultrasonographic sign to detect lesions of the forearm's interosseous membrane. Surg Radiol Anat. 2006;28:372–8. https://doi.org/10.1007/s00276-006-0100-5.
4. Jaakkola JI, Riggans DH, Lourie GM, Lang CJ, Elhassan BT, Rosenthal SJ. Ultrasonography for the evaluation of forearm interosseous membrane disruption in a cadaver model. J Hand Surg Am. 2001;26:1053–7. S0363502301160144 [pii].
5. Failla JM, Jacobson J, van Holsbeeck M. Ultrasound diagnosis and surgical pathology of the torn interosseous membrane in forearm fractures/dislocations. J Hand

Surg Am. 1999;24:257–66. S03635023(99)82539-8 [pii]. https://doi.org/10.1053/ddhsu.1999.0257.
6. Fester EW, Murray PM, Sanders TG, Inmari JV, Leyendecker J, Leis HL. The efficacy of magnetic resonance imaging and ultrasound in detecting disruptions of the forearm interosseous membrane: a cadaver study. J Hand Surg Am. 2002;27:418–24. S0363502302759637 [pii].
7. Wallace AL. Magnetic resonance imaging or ultrasound in assessment of the interosseous membrane of the forearm. J Bone Joint Surg Am. 2002;84-A:496–7.
8. Moritomo H. The distal interosseous membrane: current concepts in wrist anatomy and biomechanics. J Hand Surg Am. 2012;37:1501–7. S0363-5023(12)00593-X [pii]. https://doi.org/10.1016/j.ddhsa.2012.04.037.
9. Wegmann K, Dargel J, Burkhart KJ, Bruggemann GP, Muller LP. The Essex-Lopresti lesion. Strategies Trauma Limb Reconstr. 2012;7:131–9. https://doi.org/10.1007/s11751-012-0149-0.

Ultrasound of the Pronator Quadratus PQ

11

Jean Louis Brasseur

11.1 Introduction

The pronator quadratus PQ muscle was a muscle often overlooked by imaging, and only the fat border bordering its palmar face received attention in standard radiology as it could be an indirect sign of damage to the distal end of the radius [1]. Thanks to cross section imaging and especially the development of ultrasound, other indications appeared. Let's see in this chapter the main ones among them.

11.2 Anatomy and Sonoanatomy

The pronator quadratus PQ muscle is a flat muscle, located transversely to the deep palmar face of the distal end of the forearm, in contact with the interosseous membrane and deep into the flexor muscles. It is located in a specific compartment identified by a fascia, bordered superficially by a greasy border [2–4].

It is innervated by the anterior interosseous nerve (AION) and is about 6 cm long and slightly more than 3 cm high and consists of two bundles: one superficial and one deep. These bundles contribute to the gripping force: their direction is different as well as some of their functions [5]:

- The superficial bundle acts on the pronosupination of the distal radioulnar.
- The deep beam is a stabilizer of this joint with the triangular complex and the interosseous membrane.

On average, the thickness of these muscles is slightly larger in men than in women [6] but is also (as well as force) more important on the dominant side [7], which is important to take into account in the search for atrophy.

In ultrasound, the two bundles are well identified in both planes of space deep to the flexor muscles and in the area of the interosseous membrane (Fig. 11.1).

The appearance of the cut differs between pronation and supination. In particular, the contour of the ulnar cortex is more flattened in pronation (Fig. 11.2), and the radioulnar distance decreases (Fig. 11.3).

The superficial fascia of the pronator quadratus PQ muscle merges with the fatty space that shapes the muscle in other imaging techniques (Fig. 11.4).

J. L. Brasseur (✉)
G.H. Pitié-Salpêtrière, Service de Radiologie, Paris, France
e-mail: jlbrasseur@impf.fr

T. Apard, J. L. Brasseur (eds.), *Ultrasonography for the Upper Limb Surgeon*,
https://doi.org/10.1007/978-3-030-84234-5_11

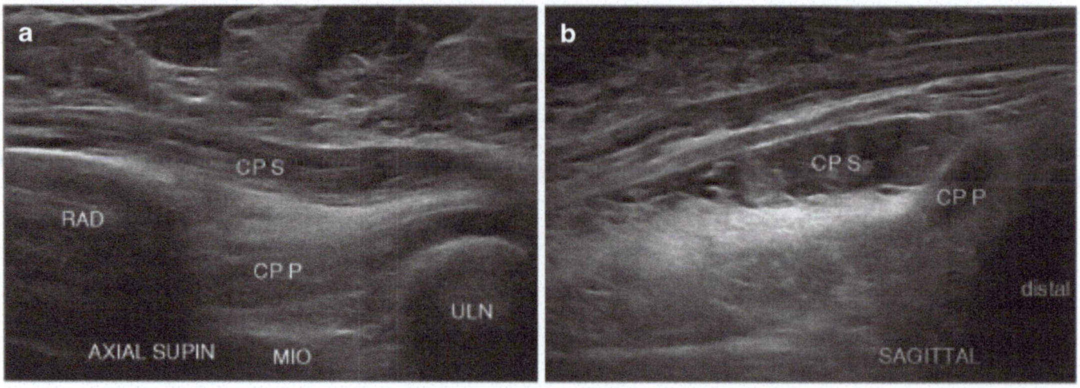

Fig. 11.1 Axial (**a**) and sagittal (**b**) ultrasound section of the pronator quadratus PQ whose surface bundle (CP S) and deep bundle (CP P) are clearly visible on the palmar face of the interosseous membrane (IOM)

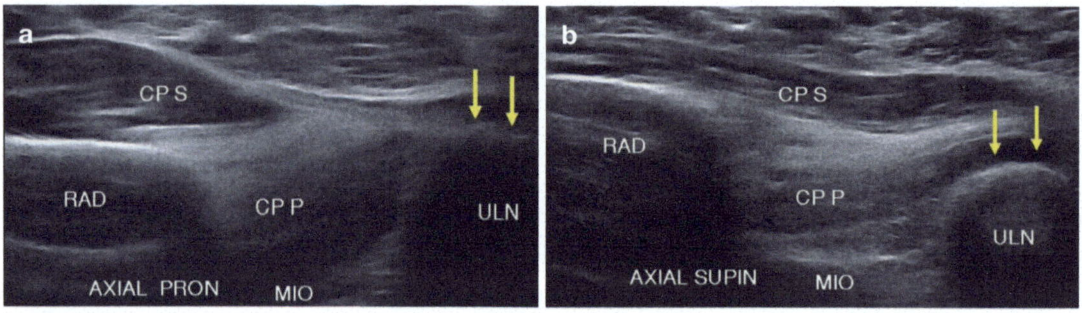

Fig. 11.2 Axial section of the pronator quadratus showing a more flattened ulnar cortex (arrows) in pronation (**a**) than in supination (**b**)

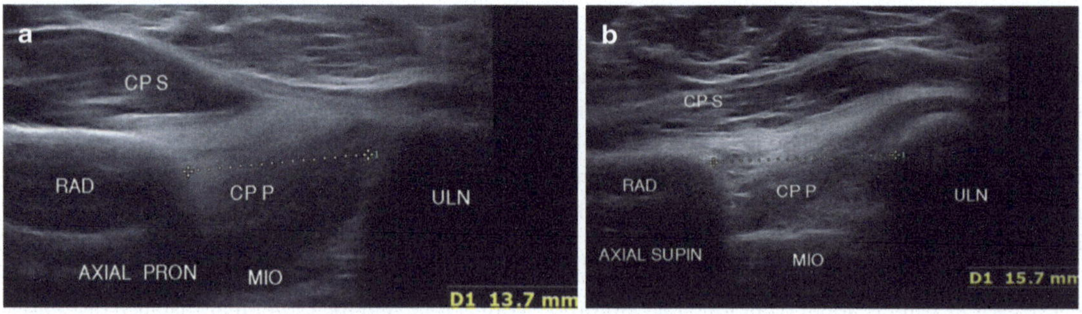

Fig. 11.3 Axial ultrasound section showing a decrease in the radioulnar space in pronation (**a**) compared to the measure in supination (**b**)

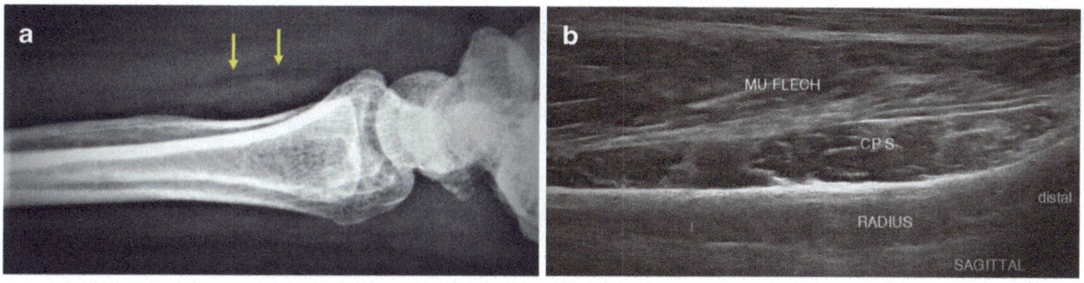

Fig. 11.4 Radiographic sagittal view of the wrist (**a**) showing the fatty border (arrow) on the palmar face of the pronator quadratus muscle; ultrasound sagittal view at radius (**b**) in which the border merges with the muscle fascia

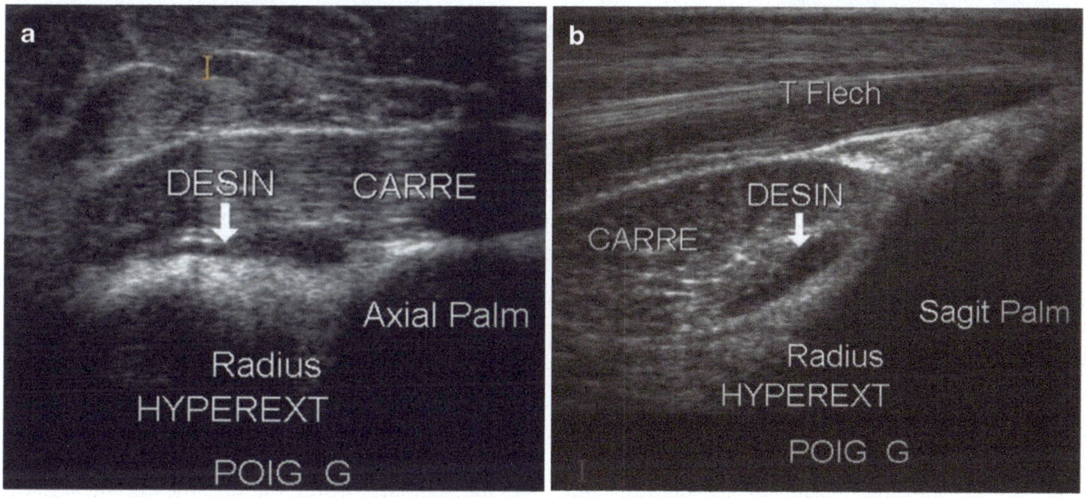

Fig. 11.5 Peripheral disinsertion of the pronator quadratus muscle well seen in hyperextension of the wrist in the axial (**a**) and sagittal (**b**) plane

11.3 The Pronator Quadratus in Pathology

Lesions of the pronator quadratus PQ are rare, but its analysis is important because some pathologies may cause a change in its appearance and may be detected by its analysis. In addition, it is at the height of this pronator quadratus PQ that it is interesting to spot the median nerve.

11.3.1 Lesions of the Pronator Quadratus PQ

Intrinsic lesions of the pronator quadratus PQ may occur in case of brutal hyperextension of the wrist resulting in peripheral disinsertion, limited in our experience; lesions are best seen in hyperextension [3] (Fig. 11.5).

Due to the deep topography of the muscle, direct contusions are rare, but the deep surface of

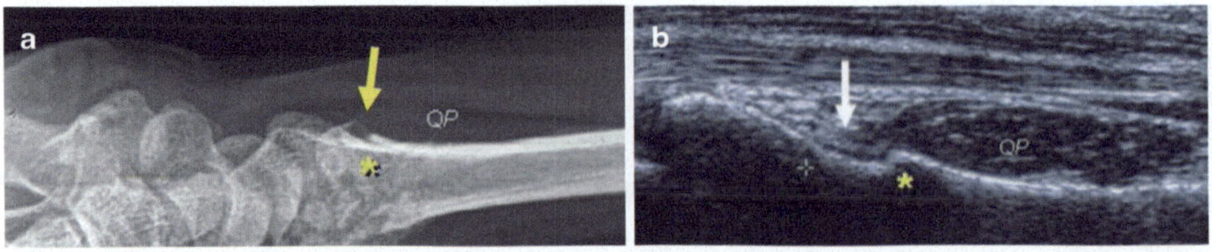

Fig. 11.6 Partial incarceration of the pronator quadratus PQ muscle in the callus of a fracture of the palmar surface of the radius on the X-ray profile (**a**) and in ultrasound (**b**) (from 3 with permission)

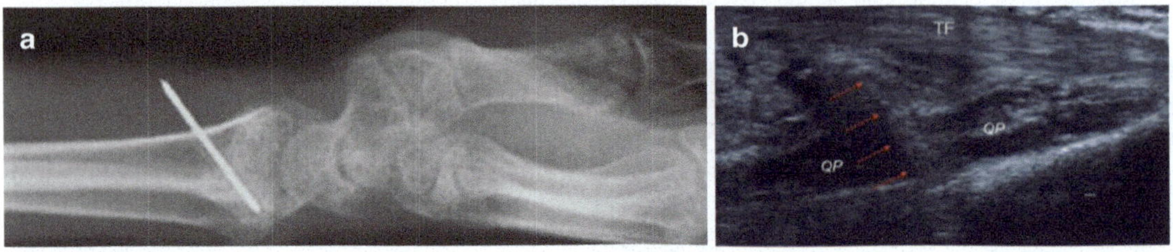

Fig. 11.7 Reshaping of the pronator quadratus PQ muscle after placing a pin on the wrist image profile (**a**) and in ultrasound (**b**) (from 3 with permission)

the muscle can be incarcerated in the event of a fracture of an adjacent cortex (most often the radius) or partially incarcerated in the callus of a complex fracture (Fig. 11.6) [3].

Postsurgical changes can be detected (Fig. 11.7), and the value of evaluating and repairing the pronator quadratus PQ after placing a palmar synthesis plate has been the source of several publications [8–12].

Ultrasound may also facilitate the placement of a palmar plaque [13].

Given the small expansion of the anatomical compartment in which the pronator quadratus PQ is located, these traumas and postsurgical remodeling, especially in the case of protruding material, are likely to cause a compartment syndrome [2]. Elastography could play a role in detecting these syndromes [14].

Also noteworthy is the use as a flap of this pronator quadratus PQ in some cases of pseudarthrosis or neuroma (aspirin flap) [15–17].

11.3.2 The Pronator Quadratus PQ: Indirect Sign of Lesion

11.3.2.1 Thickening of the Pronator Quadratus PQ

On the standard profile picture, the classic sign of compression of the fat border in the event of an occult fracture of the adjacent radius [1] is known; this sign has been questioned [18].

The hypertrophy of the pronator quadratus PQ on a comparative axial section is another factor in detecting these occult fractures [19, 20] taking into account the variations in thickness previously described [6, 7].

11.3.2.2 Hyperechogenic Changes of the Pronator Quadratus PQ

The pronator quadratus PQ is innervated by the anterior interosseous nerve, and in case of damage to this nerve (Kiloh and Nevin syndrome) neurogenic edema (hyperechogenic hypertro-

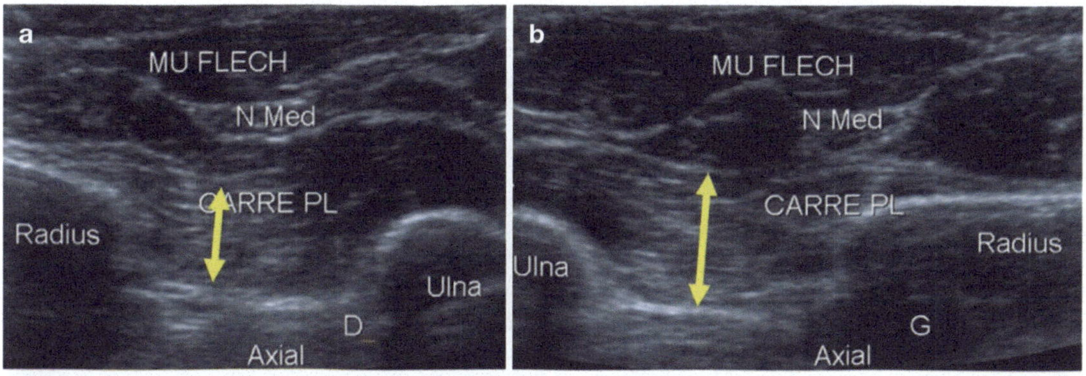

Fig. 11.8 AION pain resulting in hyperechogenic hypotrophy of the pronator quadratus PQ (**a**) clearly visible compared to the opposite side (**b**)

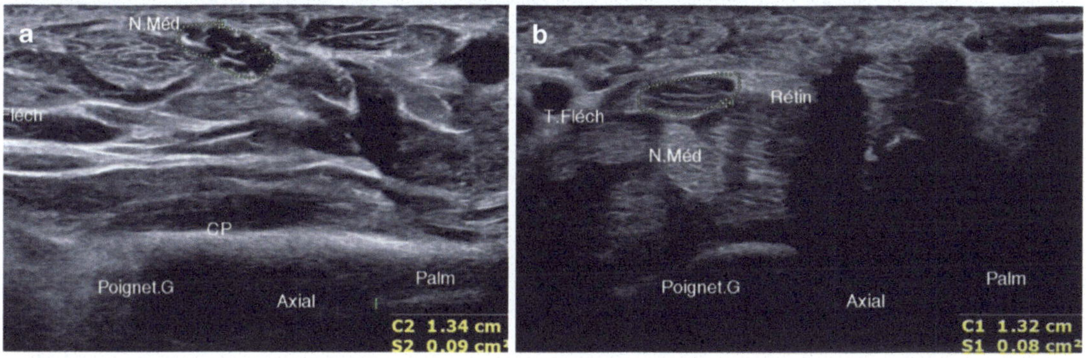

Fig. 11.9 Measurement of the median nerve at the height of the pronator quadratus PQ muscle (**a**) and within the carpal tunnel (**b**). No significant differences were observed in this patient

phy) followed by fibro-fatty degeneration (hyperechogenic hypotrophy) is an often valuable indirect sign (Fig. 11.8) [21, 22]. It is earlier and easier to detect in MRI, but regardless of the technique used, one should be wary of hyperechogenicity (or hypersignal) sometimes found in asymptomatic patients [2, 3, 23, 24]; moreover, due to the orientation of its fibers, the pronator quadratus PQ is often more in hypersignal than neighboring muscles [2]. Comparing the opposite side is, of course, the solution to this difficulty.

11.3.3 The Pronator Quadratus PQ Used as a Marker

The interest of measuring the surface of the median nerve at the height of the pronator quadratus PQ has caused this muscle to be covered by many imagers (Fig. 11.9). This measurement should be compared with that carried out in the carpal tunnel. Klauser [25, 26] showed that a difference of more than 2 mm^2 between the surface of the nerve in relation to the pronator quadratus PQ and that of the swelling in the canal is the

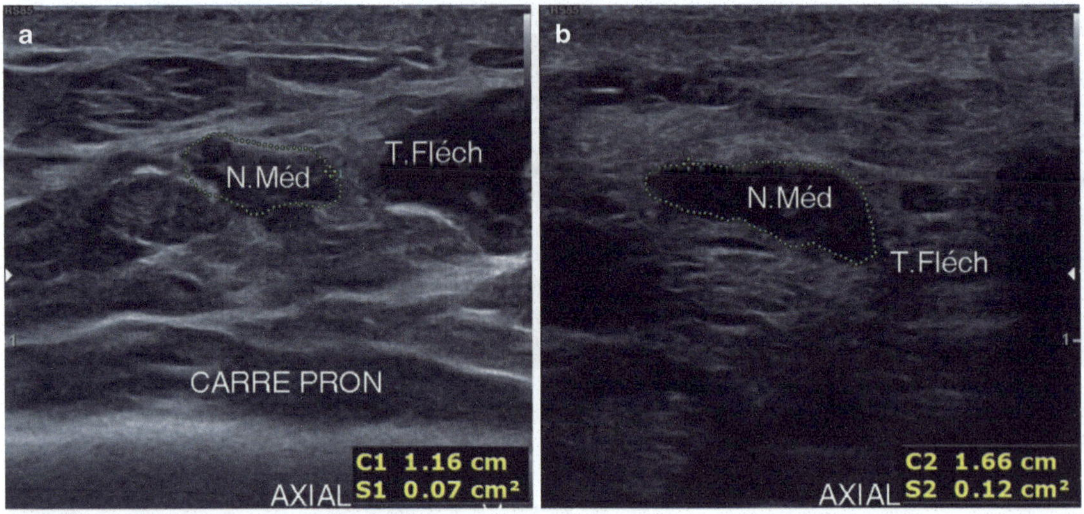

Fig. 11.10 Measurement of the median nerve at the height of the pronator quadratus PQ muscle (image on the left (**a**)) and within the carpal tunnel (image on the right (**b**)) showing a surface difference greater than 2 mm^2 which is a sensitive and specific element in favor of carpal tunnel syndrome

most sensitive and specific imaging sign of detection of compression of the median nerve (Fig. 11.10). This sign is also valid in case of bifid nerve [27].

11.4 Conclusion

In addition to the problems that this muscle may pose in the event of wrist surgery, the pronator quadratus is important to study in ultrasound mainly because it may be an indirect sign of a lesion (distal fracture of the radius or damage to the AION) but also because it is the main measuring point in case of suspicion of compression of the median nerve.

References

1. Moosikasuwan JB. The pronator quadratus sign. Radiology. 2007;244:927–8.
2. Morvan G, Vuillemin V, Guerini H. Square muscle pronator in ultrasound of wrist and hand. Montpellier: Sauramps Medical; 2017. p. 69–73.
3. Créteur V, Madani A, Brasseur JL. Pronator quadratus imaging. Diagn Interv Imaging. 2012;93:22–9.
4. Sotereanos DG, McCarthy DM, Towers JD, Britton CA, Herndon JH. The pronator quadratus: has separate forearm space? J Hand Surg. 1995;20A:496–9.
5. Shin WJ, Kim JP, Kim JS, Park HJ. Sonographic quantification of pronator quadratus activity during gripping effort. J Ultrasound Med. 2015;34(12):2269–78. https://doi.org/10.7863/ultra.15.02038. Epub 2015 Nov 16.
6. Sato J, Ishii Y, Noguchi H, Takeda M, Toyabe S. Sonographic appearance of the pronator quadratus muscle in healthy volunteers. J Ultrasound Med. 2014;33(1):111–7.
7. Ok N, Agladioglu K, Gungor HR, Kitis A, Akkaya S, Akkoyunlu NS, Demirkan F. Relationship of side dominance and ultrasonographic measurements of pronator quadratus muscle along with handgrip and pinch strength. Med Ultrasound. 2016;18(2):170–6.
8. Sonntag J, Hern J, Woythal L, Branner U, Lange BS. The pronator quadratus muscle after volar plating: ultrasound evaluation of anatomical changes correlated to patient-reported clinical outcome. Hand (N Y). 2019:1558944719840737. https://doi.org/10.1177/1558944719840737. [Epub ahead of print].
9. Nho JH, Gong HS, Song CH, Wi SM, Lee YH, Baek GH. Examination of the pronator quadratus muscle during hardware removal procedures after volar plating for distal radius fractures. Wink Orthop Surg. 2014;6(3):267–72.
10. Huang HK, Wang JP, Chang MC. Repair of pronator quadratus with partial muscle split and distal transfer for volar plating of distal radius fractures. J Hand Surg Am. 2017;42(11):935.e1–5.
11. Goorens CK, Van Royen K, Grijseels S, Provyn S, De Mey J, Scheerlinck T, Goubau JF. Ultrasonographic evaluation of the distance between the flexor pollicis longus tendon and volar prominence of the plate as a function of volar plate positioning and pronator

quadratus repair a cadaver study. Hand Surg Rehabil. 2018;37(3):171–4.
12. Walch A, Erhard L, Vogels J, Pozzetto M, Gibert N, Locquet V. Ultrasound evaluation of the protector role of the pronator quadratus suture in volar plating. J Ultrasound Med. 2019;38(10):2785–91. https://doi.org/10.1002/jum.14968. [Epub ahead of print].
13. Kinoshita M, Naito K, Goto K, Sugiyama Y, Nagura N, Obata H, Iwase Y, Kaneko K. Anatomical-positional relationship between the bone structure of the distal radius and flexor pollicis longus tendon using ultrasonography. Surg Radiol Anat. 2019;41(7):785–9. https://doi.org/10.1007/s00276-019-02216-9. [Epub ahead of print].
14. Burke CJ, Babb JS, Adler RS. Shear wave elastography in the pronator quadratus muscle following distal radial fracture fixation: a feasibility study comparing the operated versus nonoperated sides. Ultrasound. 2017;25(4):222–8.
15. Belmahi A, Amrani A, Gharib N, Abbassi A. The pronator quadratus PQ: a flap "aspirin" in analgesic surgery of painful neuromas on the wrist. Chir Main. 2002;21(3):188–93.
16. Papp C, Moor H, Ausserlechner WD. Reconstruction of pseudarthritis of the scaphoid bone utilizing an osteomuscular pronator quadratus transposition flap. Anatomical and clinical considerations. Eur J Plast Surg. 1993;16:257–62.
17. Fontaine C, Millot F, Blancke D, Mestdagh H. Anatomic basis of pronator quadratus flap. Surg Radiol Anat. 1992;14:295–9.
18. Fallahi F, Jafari H, Jefferson G, Jennings P, Read R. Explorative study of the sensitivity and specificity of the pronator quadratus fat pad sign as a predictor of subtle wrist fractures. Skeletal Radiol. 2013;42(2):249–53.
19. Sato J, Ishii Y, Noguchi H, Toyabe S. Sonographic swelling of pronator quadratus muscle in patients with occult bone injury. BMC Med Imaging. 2015;15:9.
20. Sun B, Zhang D, Gong W, Huang S, Luan Q, Yang J, Wang D, Tian J. Diagnostic value of the radiographic muscle-to-bone thickness ratio between the pronatorquadratus and the distal radius at the same level in undisplaced distal forearm fracture. Eur J Radiol. 2016;85(2):452–8.
21. Andreisek G, Crook DW, Burg D, Marincek B, Weishaupt D. Peripheral neuropathies of the median, radial, and ulnar nerves: MR imaging features. Radiographics. 2006;26:1267–87.
22. Sibileau E, Vuillemin V. In: Brasseur JL, Mercy G, Fustier A, Lucidarme O, editors. Ultrasound news of the musculoskeletal system, vol. 14. Montpellier: Sauramps Médical; 2017.
23. Tagliafico A, Perez MM, Padua L, Klauser A, Zicca A, Martinoli C. Increased reflectivity and loss in bulk of the pronator quadratus muscle does not always indicate anterior interosseous neuropathy on ultrasound. Eur J Radiol. 2013;82(3):526–9.
24. Gyftopoulos S, Rosenberg ZS, Petchprapa C. Increased MR signal intensity in the pronator quadratus muscle: does it always indicate anterior interosseous neuropathy? AJR Am J Roentgenol. 2010;194(2):490–3.
25. Klauser AS, Halpern EJ, DeZordo T, et al. Carpal tunnel syndrome assessment with US: value of additional cross-sectional area measurements of the median nerve in patients versus healthy volunteers. Radiology. 2009;250:171–7.
26. Klauser AS, Faschingbauer R, Bauer T, Wick TM, Gable M, et al. Entrapment neuropathies II: carpal tunnel syndrom. Semin Musculoskelet Radiol. 2010;14:487–500.
27. Klauser AS, Halpern EJ, Faschingbauer R, Guerra F, Martinoli C, Gabl MF, Arora R, Bauer T, Sojer M, Löscher WN, Jaschke WR. Bifid median nerve in carpal tunnel syndrome: assessment with US cross-sectional area measurement. Radiology. 2011;259(3):808–15.

Part IV

Wrist/Hand

Ultrasound of the Extensor Carpi Ulnaris

12

Jean Louis Brasseur

12.1 Introduction

Multiple pathologies can cause pain in the ulnar side of the carpus, and their clinical differentiation is often difficult mainly because of the close relationship of anatomical elements present at this level [1–5]. Pathologies can be tendon (extensor carpi ulnaris tendon (ECU) and extensor of V) but also ligamentous (ulnocarpal, radioulnar, ulnotriquetral), articular (lower radioulnar), from the fibrocartilaginous complex (TFCC), or even from underlying bone damage. These lesions can also coexist, which further complicates the diagnostic problem.

The role of imaging is therefore to define, as a first step, the pathological structure(s), knowing that there are asymptomatic variants and changes. Each of these elements, and in particular the ECU, may have different lesions; imaging must recognize them, define their severity, and specify whether the lesion is evolutionary or sequellary [1–6].

Since only ECU lesions are discussed in this chapter, it should be borne in mind that they often fit into a broader framework and that other structures also need to be evaluated to determine the exact causes of pain on surface of the carpi ulnaris.

J. L. Brasseur (✉)
G.H. Pitié-Salpêtrière, Service de Radiologie, Paris, France
e-mail: jlbrasseur@impf.fr

12.2 Anatomical Presentation [7–9]

The ECU has a dual origin: the posterior part of the common tendon of the lateral epicondyle on the one hand and the dorsal side of the ulnar diaphysis on the other. Its muscle sits on the ulnar surface of the posterior compartment of the forearm and is innervated by the posterior interosseous nerve. Its myotendinous junction is located at the distal third of the forearm forming a tendon forming the sixth dorsal column of the wrist. It passes through an osteofibrous tunnel 15–20 mm long, whose floor consists of a groove of variable depth located on the dorsal side of the ulnar epiphysis (between the head and the styloid), and it is inserted distal to the dorsal side of the base of the fifth metacarpal.

A clean synovial sheath surrounds the tendon until it is inserted to facilitate sliding under the retinaculum.

The mobility of the lower radioulnar joint in pronosupination is responsible for that of the ECU. The elements that stabilize it and hold it in place against the ulna are

- The proper retinaculum of the ECU formed by an aponeurotic splitting which is inserted on the walls of the groove; physiological variations may be present in part at the level of its lateral insertion; it is sometimes loose or even absent at the origin of subluxation or

T. Apard, J. L. Brasseur (eds.), *Ultrasonography for the Upper Limb Surgeon*,
https://doi.org/10.1007/978-3-030-84234-5_12

asymptomatic tendon dislocation [10–13]; the tendon comes in this case to "climb" the ulnar styloid in supination to find itself on its palmar side. Longitudinal fibrous elements (linea jugata) reinforce the insertion of this retinaculum, some of which join the epimysium of the tendon itself, which is another additional factor of stability [7].

- The dorsal retinaculum is the thickening of the fascia that lines the surface side of the preceding one; it is inserted on the radius and then bypasses the head of the ulna, without inserting on it (to allow pronosupination), to attach palmar to the pisiform and triquetrum (Fig. 12.1).

The depth of the groove is an element in the stability of the ECU; the groove may not be present or may be slightly dug, facilitating abnormal mobility (Fig. 12.2).

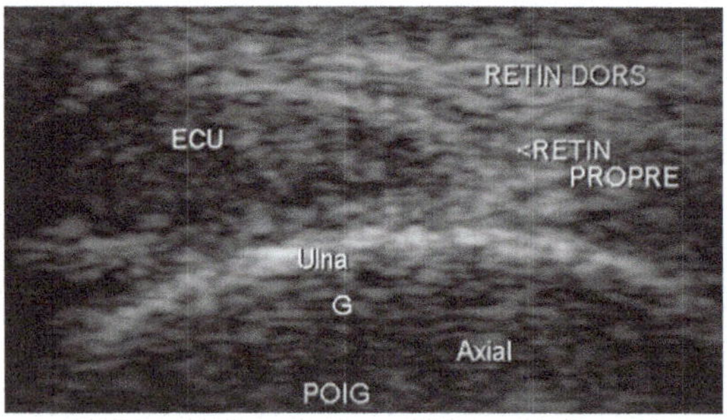

Fig. 12.1 Ultrasonographic axial section at the height of the furrow showing the two superimposed retinacula; the superficial strip corresponds to the common retinaculum of the extensor tendons and the deep strip to the proper retinaculum of the ECU

Ulna length and styloid morphology are other variables that can also affect tendon stability [14].

Morphological variants are described, complicating the study and detection of pathological elements of the ECU:

- Tendon duplication is not uncommon especially at the distal insertion level; one of these replicas described by Barfred [15] unites the end of the ECU with that of the extensor of the 5 and is considered pathogenic, causing more frequent lesions of the ECU.
- Tendon cracking (dividing the tendon into two equal parts) are often found in the absence of symptomatology especially in athletes (morphological variants or asymptomatic acquired cracking?) [1, 11, 12] (Fig. 12.3).
- The nonunion of the ulnar styloid (congenital or sequellary of trauma), which favors the appearance of tendinopathies and partial ruptures [16].

12.3 Imaging Techniques and Normal Appearance

The two imaging techniques suitable for tendon study are ultrasound [17–21] and MRI [21–25] because they both have a density resolution

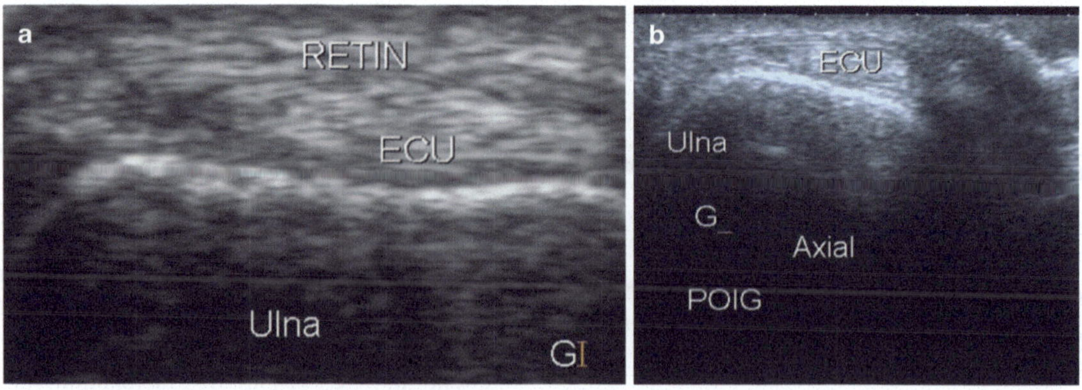

Fig. 12.2 Morphological variant with the presence of a shallow groove consisting of a factor favoring tendon dislocation (**a**); absence of groove in another patient (**b**)

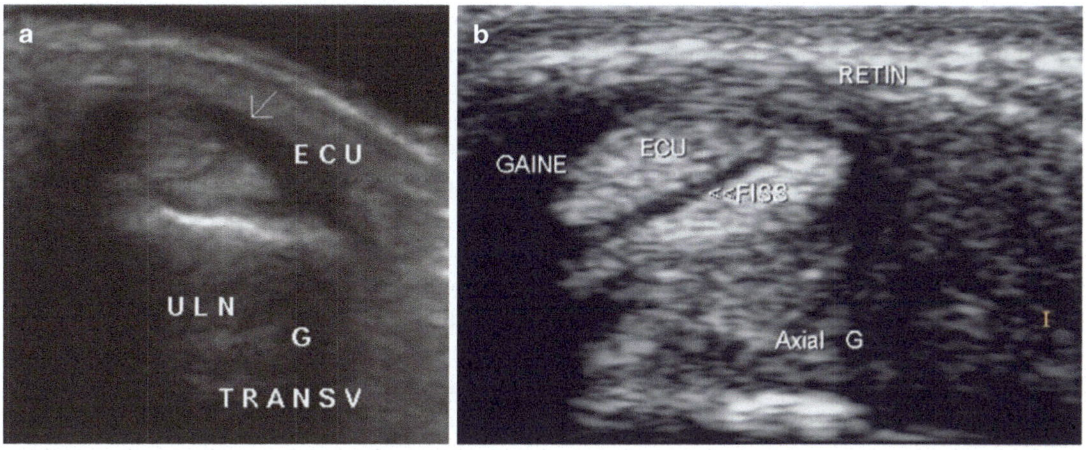

Fig. 12.3 Non-symptomatic cracking of the tendon in the axial plane; frequent variant in the athlete (**a**); the appearance is similar to that of a crack occurring in a painful context (**b**)

allowing the tendon and its environment to be identified in the normal state but especially in pathology (which cannot be scanned).Ultrasound has great advantages:

- Systematic bilateral study
- Dynamic specificity
- Spatial resolution allowing analysis of the fibrillar structure of the tendon
- Possibility of bilateral (comparative) vascular analysis without injecting contrast medium
- Availability
- Price (10–15 times cheaper than an MRI)

The big black spot of ultrasound is its difficulty (and the need to have a high-end device) due to its operator-dependent character.

The MRI also has great advantages:

- Better contrast resolution through the use of various sequences
- Analysis of bone structures adjacent to the tendon
- An appreciable "cartographic" appearance preoperatively
- Excellent vascular sensitivity after injection of gadolinium
- On the other hand, the examination has a less precise spatial resolution, is one-sided, more expensive, and static, and requires a puncture for vascular study.

12.4 Ultrasound Technique and Normal Appearance

Ultrasound study is systematically comparative and dynamic. It is carried out with high-end equipment given the delicacy of the lesions to explore. A bag of water or other interposition material (condom filled with ultrasound gel) is useful for axial cuts and in particular for the dynamic study carried out in this plane. The operator is seated in front of the patient; the examination begins with the elbows in extension for the pronation study and then the flexed elbows resting on thighs or on a table in front of the patient for pronosupination maneuvers [17–19].

Comparative frontal sections are performed as well as axial sections in pronation and supination.

In the frontal plane we find the usual hyperechogenic fibrillar structure of the tendon, which is clearly visible in ultrasound in the normal state from its myotendinous junction to its insertion on the base of M5. On the surface of the tendon is the tendon sheath covered by the thickened fascia of the extensor retinaculum (Fig. 12.4); the retinaculum of the ECU is visible in the normal state, especially in case of effusion (this increases the contrast between the structures). At the deep side of the tendon, the hyperechoic line of the capsular plane is observed, reinforced by the ulnar collateral ligament and deeper to the TFCC and ulnar recess of the radio-carpal joint.

Axial cuts are performed in pronation, first at the height of the groove, then facing the styloid, and then at the ulnar side of the carpus. The tendon has a spotty appearance; it is hyperechogenic but subject to anisotropic artefact [17]. Its sectional surface is most often oval facing of the groove to round off more distally. Recall the frequent asymptomatic cracking of this tendon in two parts, visible in ultrasound in the form of a thin hypoechogenic line passing through the tendon thickness.

This tendon is surrounded by a synovial sheath whose thickness is appreciated by comparison with the opposite side, and the elements described above are found on its deep slope; the lift technique allows it to be well followed until its distal insertion. The supination maneuver shows in the normal state the tendon that deforms "in comma" but does not extend beyond the edge of the styloid from which it remains separated by a small hypoechogenic border; the clean retinaculum is raised during this maneuver, and its insertion is often well visualized suppression of **233;e**. In addition, some cracks are best detected in supination (Fig. 12.5). Important variants can be viewed. They are often bilateral at the origin of subluxation (especially on the tip of the styloid) (Fig. 12.6) or palmar dislocation in supination (Fig. 12.7). During this maneuver, the appearance of the proper retinaculum on the lateral surface of the groove is studied, since it is then perfectly visualized (Fig. 12.8).

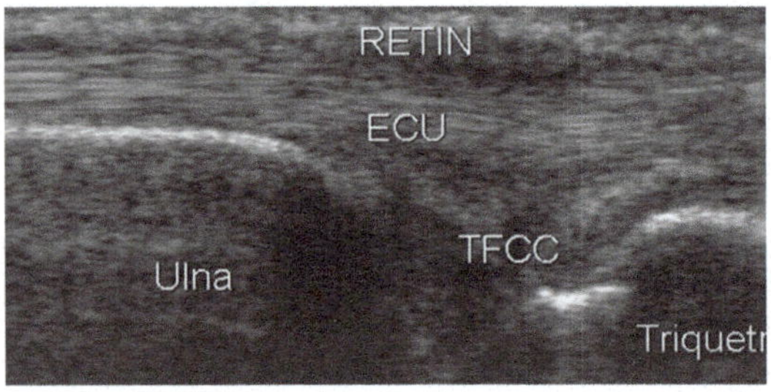

Fig. 12.4 Normal frontal section showing the normal picture of the thickening of the two retinacula in the area of tendon fibers; the use of anisotropic artefact made these retinacula hypoechogenic for tendon differentiation

The search for a dislocation or subluxation also involves other maneuvers: aggravated pronation, supination accompanied by possibly antagonized extension, but the most effective maneuver in our experience is to ask the patient to reproduce the painful movement (sports gesture by example) with the probe placed against the groove in search of abnormal mobilization.

The anisotropic artifact, a generator of hypoechogenic false images, is the enemy of tendon ultrasound, but it can be useful for detecting tendon contours in hyperechogenic enlargement. Therefore, small angulation movements of the

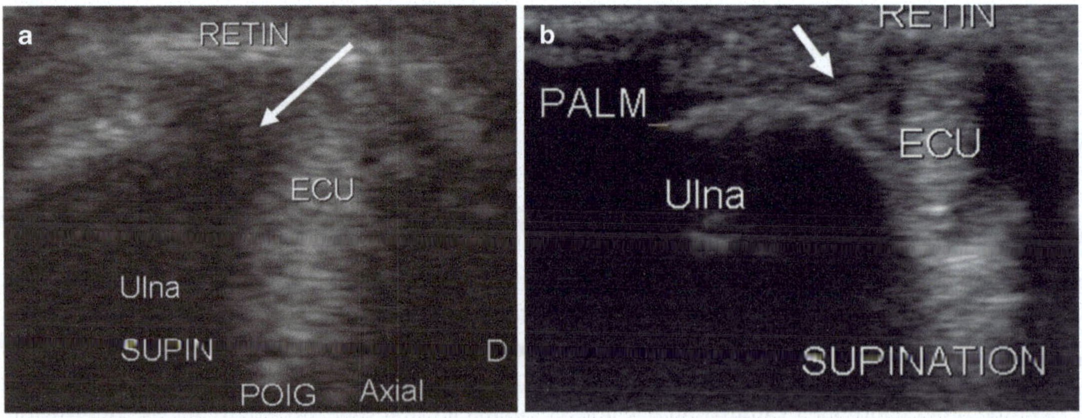

Fig. 12.5 In supination, the normal tendon remains separated from the cortex by a hypoechogenic triangle (arrow) (**a**); the tendon lifts the retinaculum and clearly shows its insertion on the lateral edge of the groove (arrow) (**b**)

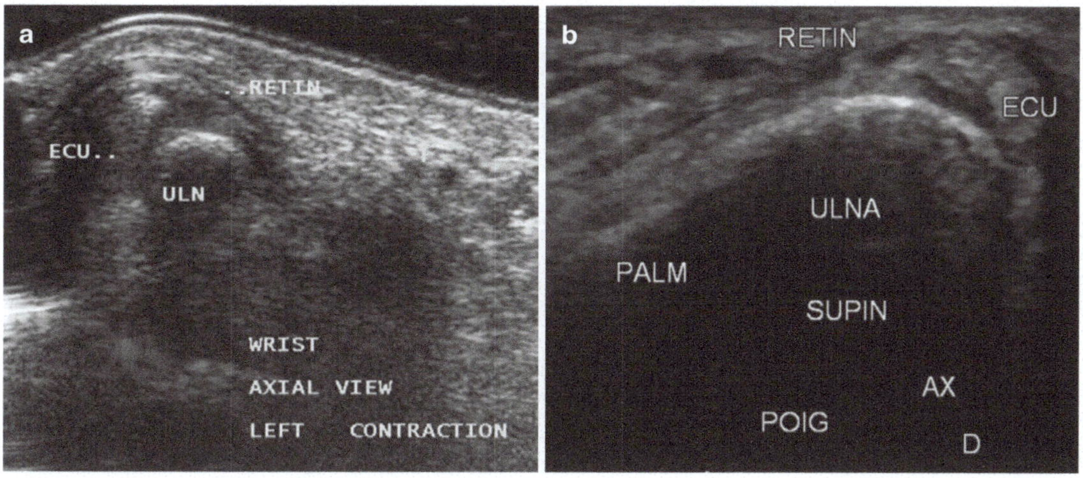

Fig. 12.6 Minimal asymptomatic subluxation of the tendon in relation to the tip of the styloid with partial detachment of the proper retinaculum (**a**); greater subluxation in another patient (**b**)

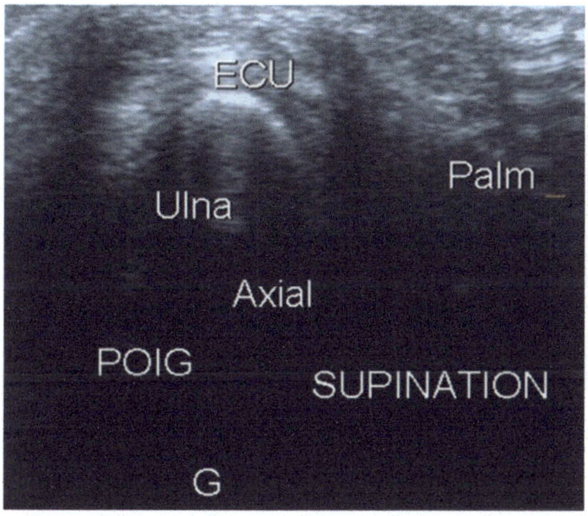

Fig. 12.7 Complete dislocation of the ECU in an asymptomatic patient

probe should be carried out at all times when these axial sections are carried out.

12.5 Pathological Appearances

The ECU shows several pathological changes especially in athletes (especially instability problems) [1–4, 6, 21] but also in patients with rheumatoid arthritis (RA) who will mainly develop tenosynovitis and ruptures [26].

12.5.1 Instabilities, Subluxation, and Dislocation

Pronosupination movements cause mobility of the ECU tendon whose supporting structures are subjected to tension forces sometimes leading to reactional thickening of the retinaculum. In addition, the friction forces generated by the tendon climbing on the styloid give rise to tenosynovitis (see below). However, some people present with completely asymptomatic subluxations or dislocations [10, 11, 17]; therefore, one should always compare the appearance on both sides and compare imaging with clinical symptomatology.

These pathologies should also be separated according to their occurrence: acute injury and chronic lesion. Racket sports, especially tennis, are often at the root of this pathology because they lead to sudden movements of radial inclination and aggravated pronation. These constraints are accentuated by the practice of the forehand lift and the backhand with two hands. The kinetics of the gestures of tennis ensure that the hand farthest from the sieve is subjected to stress and during the reverse, the hand that is closest to the sieve. A right-handed player will therefore have pain in the right wrist during forehands and in the left hand on backhands (the opposite is for the left-handed player) [1, 6, 17].

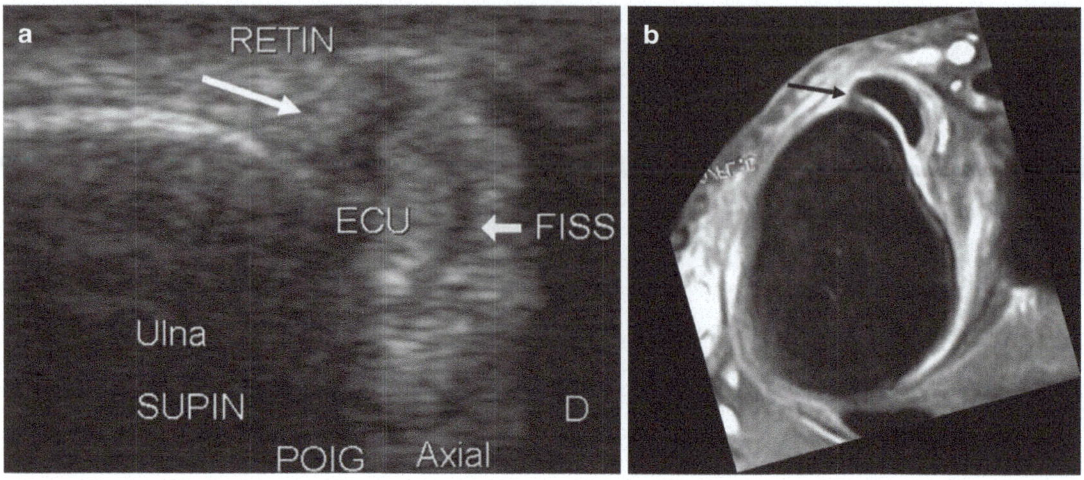

Fig. 12.8 In supination, the tendon deforms, a crack may "open," but the proper retinaculum remains well inserted and takes on a "comma" appearance well seen in ultrasound (**a**) as in dynamic MRI (**b**) (Pr Drapé shot)

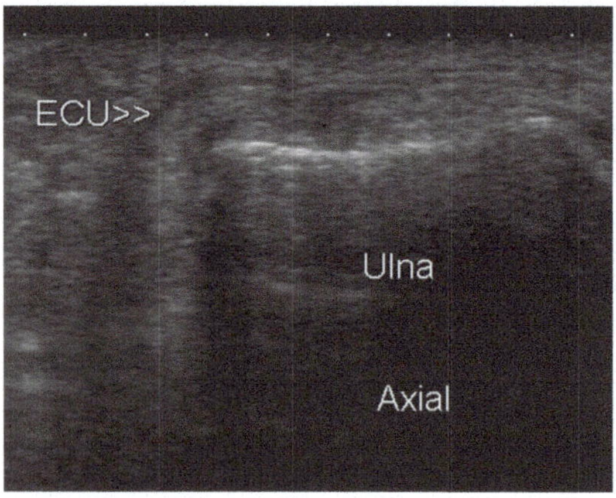

Fig. 12.9 Permanent dislocation of the tendon after an acute accident

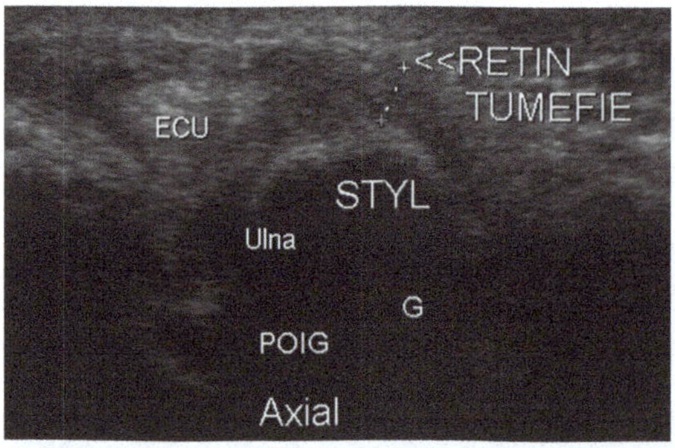

Fig. 12.10 Tendon returned to normal position in pronation; only hypoechogenic thickening of the retinaculum should attract attention

12.5.1.1 Acute Dislocation of ECU

It occurs mainly in sports pathology, but palmar dislocations have also been described in RA in patients with rupture of the extensor tendon of the fingers [26]. Acute dislocation of the ECU leads to sudden pain and functional impairment leading to immediate cessation of activities. This may be a rupture of the proper retinaculum of the ECU, a disinsertion of its radial attachment (the retinaculum may then be subverted under the tendon), but most often of its ulnar insertion with palmar dislocation of the ECU tendon below the dorsal carpal retinaculum [1, 17, 21] (Fig. 12.9).

One should never lose sight of the fact that the tendon often returns to place after the acute episode requiring the realization of dynamic maneuvers to highlight this dislocation knowing that they are mild and that the athlete often hesitates to perform these movements, making it more difficult to diagnose (Fig. 12.10) [17].

The rupture or disinsertion of the retinaculum is detected in ultrasound, but it is the abnormal mobility of the tendon that confirms the diagnosis during supination. Partial ruptures of the retinaculum are most common with the preservation of tendon stability or simple subluxation. Only complete ruptures lead to frank palmar dislocation of the ECU.

Associated lesions of the tendon, mainly tenosynovitis, occur almost systematically in the acute phase. A hypoechogenic range is also sought at the periphery of the head of the ulna, below the reflection zone of the dorsal retinaculum; this image corresponds to the detachment pocket formed by the tendon when it dislocates (Fig. 12.11); it sometimes extends to the palmar reaching the pronator quadratus.

This area exhibits reactive vascularization during the healing phase to be studied with power Doppler mode (Fig. 12.12); in the healing phase it transforms into a hyperechogenic cicatricial thickening. The disappearance of reactive vascularization is therefore important to identify in order to assess the stage of healing (Fig. 12.13).

12.5.1.2 Subluxation and Chronic Lesions

It is also in athletes especially in racket sport that these injuries occur most frequently. Chronic tensile forces on retinaculum insertion following repeated movements possibly associated with increased tendon mobilization may cause chronic tendinopathies (see below) but also chronic retinacular lesions associated with a gradually formed detachment pocket.

The changes to be sought in imaging (pocket, abnormal mobilization, and tense lesions) are therefore identical to this phase except for the retinaculum, which exhibits thickening without rupture or disinsertion (Fig. 12.14).

To assess the effectiveness of treatment, the following are analyzed:

- The modification of this pocket and its vascularization
- The disappearance of the abnormal hypoechogenicity of the retinaculum
- The abnormal mobility of the tendon in dynamics before allowing the athlete to replay

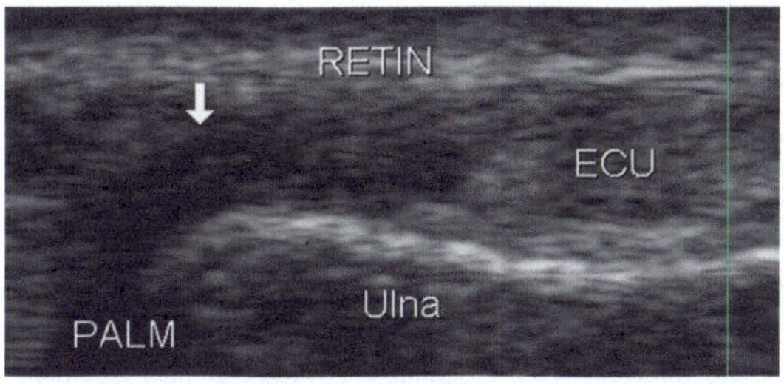

Fig. 12.11 Presence of a detachment pocket resulting from a history of dislocation

12.5.2 Tendon Ruptures

Total rupture of the ECU is a symptom known for its frequency in patients with RA causing sudden pain and functional impairment; it is the interruption of tendon fibers that provides ultrasound diagnosis; the extent of the retraction and the appearance of a more or less regular appearance of the edges of the rupture are also determined (Fig. 12.15). An effusion in the tendon sheath is systematically present, sometimes associated with synovitis. The synovial pannus, rubbing

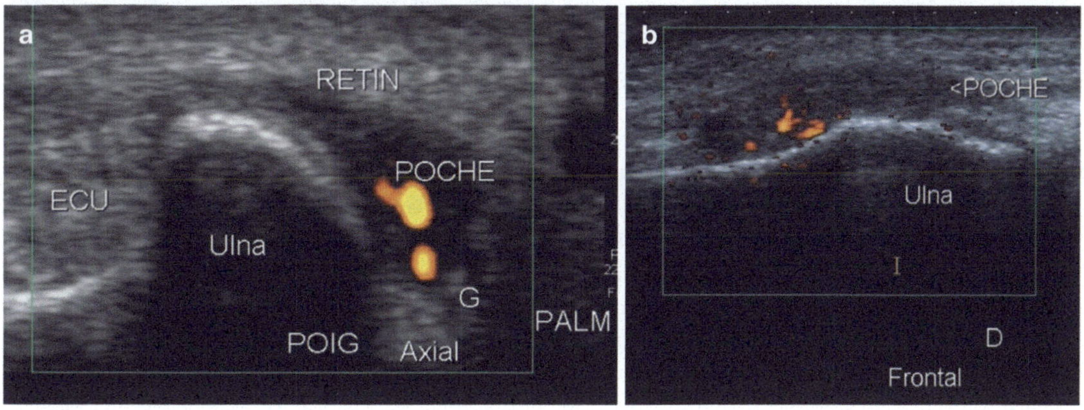

Fig. 12.12 Vascularization of the Doppler detachment pocket in the axial (**a**) and sagittal (**b**) plane

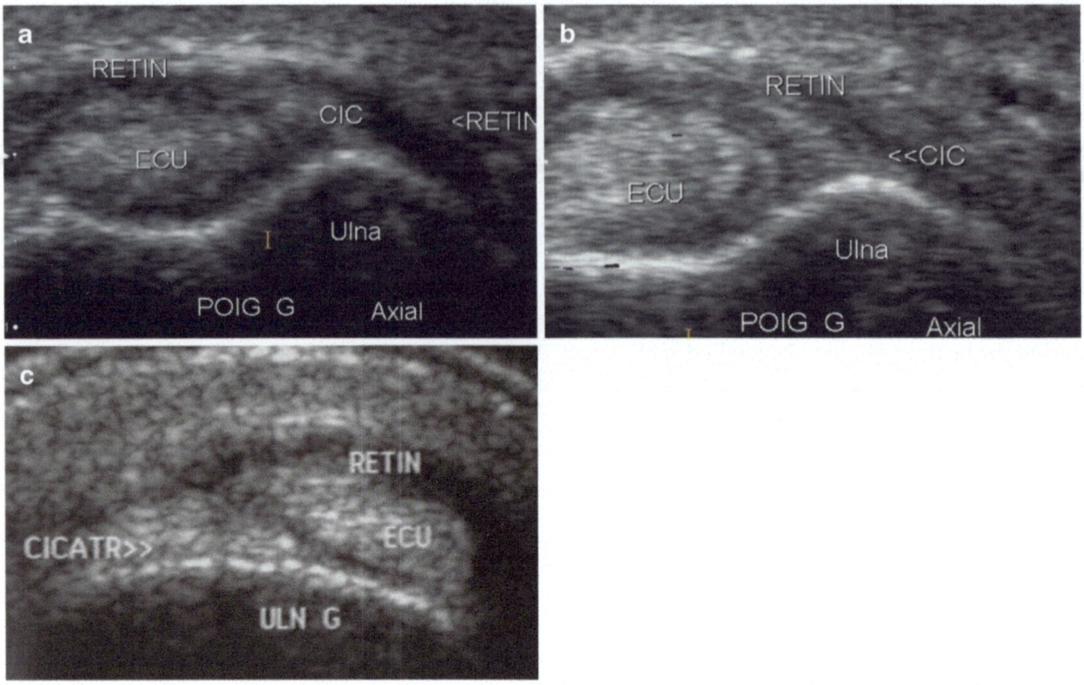

Fig. 12.13 Scar remodeling in place of the detachment zone (**a**) with progressive disappearance of the hypoechogenic zones (**b**) and (**c**)

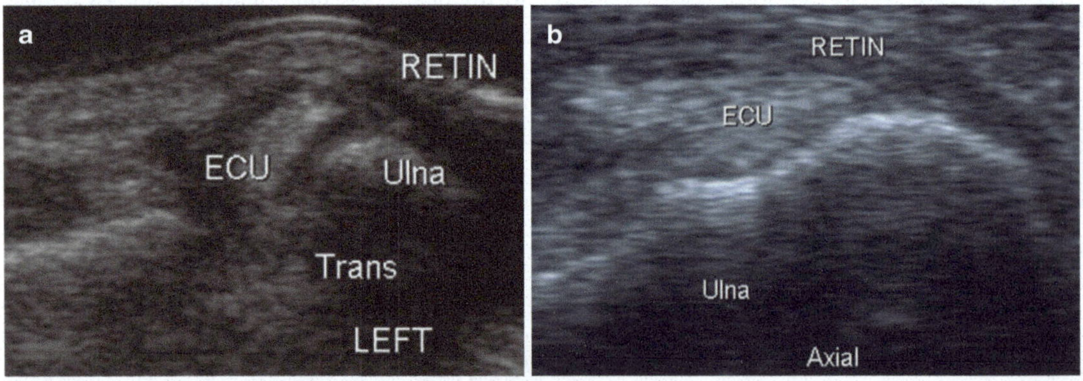

Fig. 12.14 Thickening of retinaculum and rough outline of detachment in chronic pain (**a**); simple thickening in another patient (**b**)

against an ulnar styloid made irregular by erosions, and instability of the lower radioulnar are the factors contributing to these ruptures [26, 27].

The implications of corticosteroid injections are also known, especially when they are not carried out strictly in the peritendineum.

Partial rupture is rarer and is mainly found in patients with identification of the ulnar styloid [16, 17].

12.5.3 Tenosynovitis and Tendinopathy

A synovial sheath surrounds the tendon and promotes its sliding under the retinaculum.

Reactive synovitis may occur as part of an inflammatory disease (it is present in 30% of patients with RA) but also as a result of mechanical irritation causing peritendinous effusion or

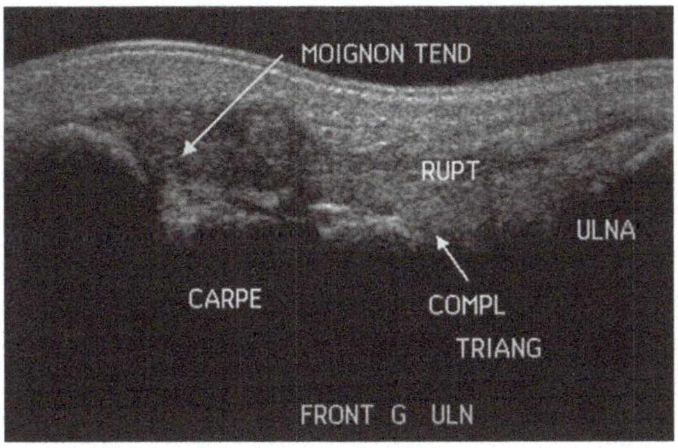

Fig. 12.15 ECU rupture with retraction of thickened proximal stump

synovitis whose inflammatory character is assessed in Doppler [18] (Fig. 12.16).These disorders may benefit from an ultrasound-guided infiltration (Fig. 12.17).

A scar thickening of the sheath may also be observed as a result of stenosing damage, which is similar to that of de Quervain's tenosynovitis.

The tendon itself can be the site of an added tendinopathy, possibly fissure, keeping in mind the number of asymptomatic cracks (Fig. 12.18). The comparison between the two sides is therefore very important in determining the importance of a change in size or structure.

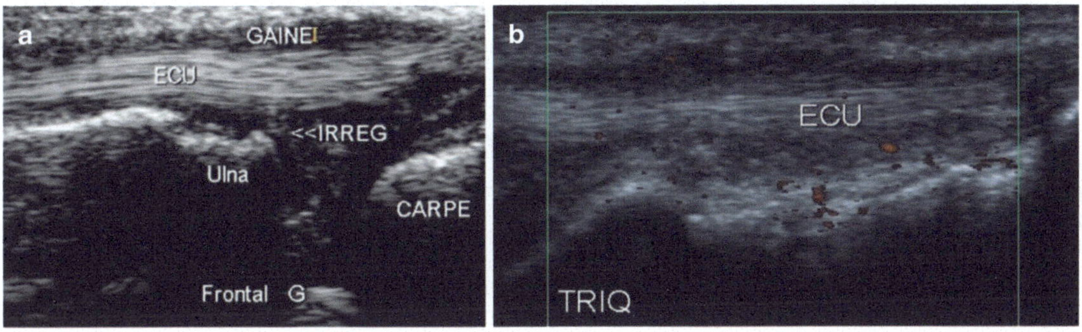

Fig. 12.16 Tenosynovitis resulting from ulnar cortical irregularity (**a**); vascularized peritendinous synovitis with Doppler in a patient with RA (**b**)

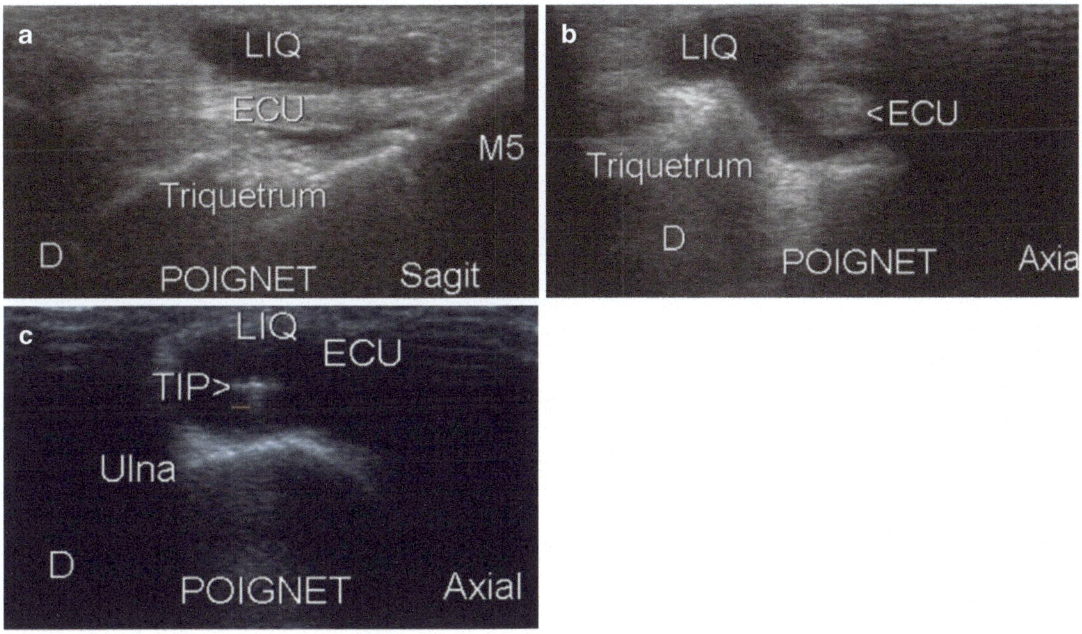

Fig. 12.17 Tenosynovitis with peritendinous effusion well visualized in the sagittal (**a**) and axial plane (**b**); this patient benefited from an ultrasound-guided infiltration (tip) respecting tendon fibers (**c**)

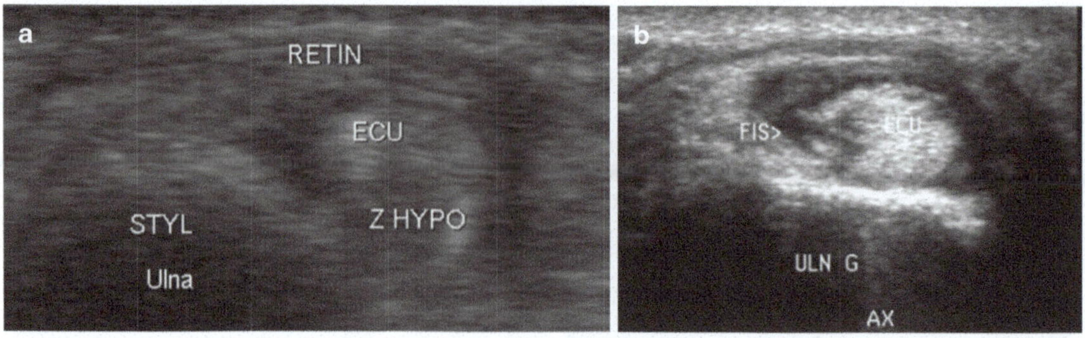

Fig. 12.18 Hypoechogenic nodular area of a painful tendon in a tennis player (**a**): tendon thickened and cracked in another player (**b**)

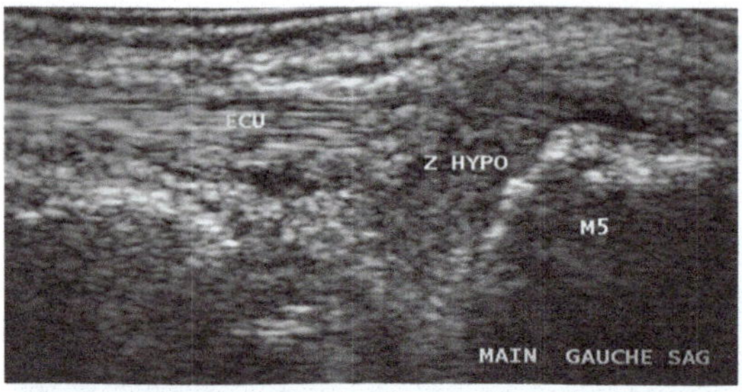

Fig. 12.19 Diffuse hypoechogenic swelling of distal enthesopathy of the ECU at its attachment on the base of the fifth metatarsal

12.5.4 Enthesopathy

The insertion of the ECU tendon on the base of the fifth metacarpal may be the site of an overuse causing hypoechogenic swelling of the distal tendon attachment. These enthesopathies are essentially of mechanical origin in our experience. They can cause fine calcifications to occur in the center of the insertion zone in the chronic stage [17] (Fig. 12.19).

12.6 Conclusion

Imaging plays an important role in detecting, analyzing, and determining the severity of ECU lesions. Ultrasound and MRI have specific advantages that make the two techniques complement each other and are systematically combined in difficult cases. The dynamic nature of the ultrasound study is crucial in the analysis of instabilities, but MRI is irreplaceable for showing frequently associated lesions and particularly spongy disease.

References

1. Montalvan B, Bet J, Brewer JL, Le Viet D, Drape JL. Extensor carpi ulnaris injuries in tennis players: a study of 28 cases. Br J Sports Med. 2006;40(5):424–9; discussion 429.
2. Pang EQ, Yao J. Ulnar-sided wrist pain in the athlete (TFCC/DRUJ/ECU). Curr Rev Musculoskelet Med. 2017;10(1):53–61.
3. Graham TJ. Pathologies of the extensor carpi ulnaris (ECU) tendon and its investments in the athlete. Hand Clin. 2012;28(3):345–56, ix.
4. Campbell D, Campbell R, O'Connor P, Hawkes R. Sports-related extensor carpi ulnaris pathology: a review of functional anatomy, sports injury and management. Br J Sports Med. 2013;47(17):1105–11.
5. Coggins CA. Imaging of ulnar-sided wrist bread. Clin Sports Med. 2006;25:505–26.
6. Guerini H, Drapé JL, Leviet D, Thevenin F, Roulot E, Pessis E, et al. Imaging the athlete's wrist. J Radiol. 2007;88:11–28.
7. Iwamoto A, Morris RP, Andersen C, Patterson RM, Viegas SF. An anatomic and biomechanic study of the wrist extensor retinaculum septa and tendon compartements. J Hand Surg Am. 2006;31:896–903.
8. Taleisnik J, Gelberman HR, Miller BW, Szabo RM. The extensor retinaculum of the wrist. J Hand Surg Am. 1984;9:495–501.
9. Palmer AK, Skahen JR, Werner FW, Glisson RR. The extensor retinaculum of the wrist: an anatomical and biomechanical study. J Hand Surg Br. 1985;10:11–6.
10. Petchprapa CN, Meraj S, Jain N. ECU tendon "dislocation" in asymptomatic volunteers. Skeletal Radiol. 2016;45(6):805–12.
11. Sole JS, Wisniewski SJ, Newcomer KL, Maida E, Smith J. Sonographic evaluation of the extensor

carpi ulnaris in asymptomatic tennis players. PM R. 2015;7(3):255–63.
12. Erickson J, Kwart A, Steven YS. Extensor carpi ulnaris tendon anatomy may mimic tears. J Hand Surg Asian Pac. 2019;24(2):175–9.
13. Pratt RK, Hoy GA, Bass FC. Extensor carpi ulnaris subluxation or dislocation? Ultrasound measurement of tendon excursion and normal values. Hand Surg. 2004;9:137–43.
14. Allende C, Le Viet D. Extensor carpi ulnaris problems at the wrist-classification, surgical treatment and results. J Hand Surg Br. 2005;30:265–72.
15. Barfred T, Adamsen S. Duplication of the extensor carpi ulnaris tendon. J Hand Surg Am. 1986;11:423–5.
16. Kiyono Y, Nakatsuchi Y, Saitoh S. Ulnar-styloid nonunion and partial rupture of extensor carpi ulnaris tendon: two case reports and review of the literature. J Orthop Trauma. 2002;16:674–7.
17. Brewer JL, Zeitoun-Eiss D, Bach G, Renoux J, Montalvan B, Drape JL. Ulnar carp extender. In: Drapé JL, Blum A, Cyteval C, Pham T, Dautel G, Boutry N, Godefroy D, editors. Wrist and hand. Montpellier: Sauramps Médical; 2009. p. 69–80.
18. Spicer PJ, Romesberg A, Kamineni S, Beaman FD. Ultrasound of extensor carpi ulnaris tendon subluxation in a tennis player. Ultrasound Q. 2016;32(2):191–3.
19. Bianchi S, Martinoli C. Wrist. In: Bianchi S, Martinoli C, editors. Ultrasound of the musculoskeletal system. Berlin: Springer; 2007. p. 425–94.
20. Robertson BL, Jamadar DA, Jacobson JA, Kalume-Brigido M, Caoili EM, Margaliot Z, et al. Extensor retinaculum of the wrist: sonographic characterization and pseudosynovitis appearance. AJR Am J Roentgenol. 2007;188:198–202.
21. Guerini H, Drape JL, Brasseur JL, Montalvan B, Le Viet D, Chevrot A. Recurrent dislocation of the ulnar extensor tendon of the carp in tennis player: ultrasound and MRI evaluation. In: Brasseur JL, Zeitoun-Eiss D, Dion E, editors. News in ultrasound of the musculoskeletal system. Montpellier: Sauramps Médical; 2004. p. 135–42.
22. Zanetti M, Saupe N, Nagy L. Role of MR imaging in chronic wrist pain. Eur Radiol. 2007;17:927–3.
23. Santo S, Omokawa S, Iida A, Shimizu T, Hasegawa H, Tanaka Y. Magnetic resonance imaging analysis of the extensor carpi ulnaris tendon and distal radioulnar joint in triangular fibrocartilage complex tears. J Orthop Sci. 2018;23(6):953–8.
24. Kaiser P, Kellermann F, Arora R, Henninger B, Rudisch A. Diagnosing extensor carpi ulnaris tendon dislocation with dynamic rotation MRI of the wrist. Clin Imaging. 2018;51:323–6.
25. Egi T, Inui K, Goto H, Takaoka K, Kasuki K. Volar dislocation of the extensor carpi ulnaris tendon on magnetic resonance imaging is associated with extensor digitorum communis tendon rupture in rheumatoids wrists. J Hand Surg Am. 2006;31:1454–60.
26. Valeri G, Ferrara C, Ercolani P, De Nigris E, Giovagnoni A. Tendon involvement in rheumatoid arthritis of the wrist: MRI findings. Skeletal Radiol. 2001;30:138–43.
27. Garcia-Elias M. Tendinopathies of the extensor carpi ulnaris. Handchir Mikrochir Plast Chir. 2015;47(5):281–9.

Ultrasound of the Scapholunate Ligament

13

Thomas Apard

Rupture of the scapholunate ligament is a frequent but often neglected lesion in common traumatology. Left to hazardous symptomatic treatment, it leads to a complete and inevitable progressive destabilization of the entire carpus, causing intracarpal arthritis [1, 2]. Its diagnosis is difficult, and a thorough and targeted exploration is needed. Conventionally, the clinical examination looks for a forced scaphoid projection and pain on palpation of the scapholunate interval [3]. Radiological examinations then look for signs of static instability (scapholunate diastasis, scaphoid horizontalization, and ring sign). But these examinations reveal very little or very poorly the predynamic or dynamic instabilities [4]. Some authors even recommend the use of arthrography and arthroscopy to ensure diagnosis [5].

Ultrasound is a simple, noninvasive, comparative, and dynamic tool. With the development of high-frequency linear probes, ultrasound allows a fine study of surface structures. Some authors already use it in combination with clinical examination of the wrist [6–8].

We describe a specific dynamic ultrasound sign of the scapholunate ligament rupture in the same way as stress tests for other ligaments (e.g., varus for the lateral collateral ligament of the ankle or for an anterior drawer for the anterolateral cruciate ligament of the knee).

T. Apard (✉)
Hand Sonosurgery Center, Versailles, France

13.1 How to Carry Out Ultrasound Examination?

The clinical examination in consultation is the “pivot shift test” of the scaphoid known as Watson’s test: search for the protrusion felt by the examiner or the patient.

Ultrasound examination of the dorsal portion of the scapholunate ligament is performed in consultation in a comparative way. The patient’s wrist is closed in pronation, and the elbow is placed on the table, in a slight palmar flexion thanks to a gel vial placed below (Fig. 13.1). The high-frequency probe (between 12 and 18 MHz) is arranged on the wrist for a cross section on Lister’s tubercle. The hockey-stick probe is not wide enough to allow dynamic examination.

The probe then shifts slightly distally to show the scapholunate ligament that is measured (Fig. 13.2): it must be hyper- or isoechogenic and measured between 2 and 4 mm. A “V”-shaped anechogenic space is suspected of rupture.

There should be no hypoechogenic border on the bone because the scaphoidian and lunarian view cannot see cartilage physiologically. If a border is visualized, then one must think about an image of the head of the capitate revealed by the semilunar palmar tilt *(dorsal intercalated segmental instability)*.

The examiner then exerts pressure on the head of the third metacarpal without moving the probe. In case of scapholunar lesion, the capitate

T. Apard, J. L. Brasseur (eds.), *Ultrasonography for the Upper Limb Surgeon*,
https://doi.org/10.1007/978-3-030-84234-5_13

"herniates" between the two bones on the screen of the ultrasound graph (Fig. 13.3) because it interposes between the two bones. Figure 13.4 **illustrates** the desired behavior of carpal bones.

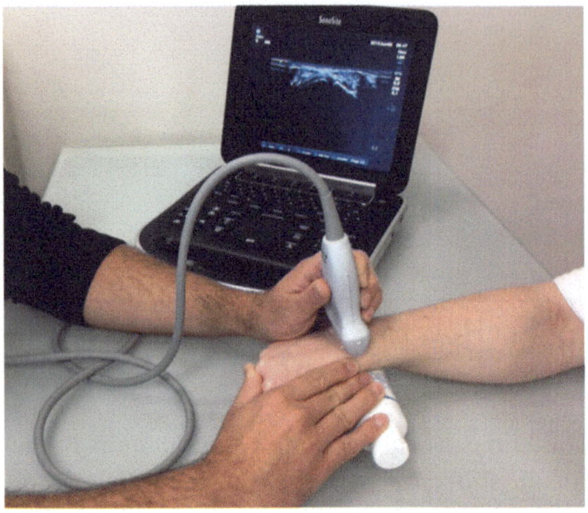

Fig. 13.1 Installation of the examiner and patient

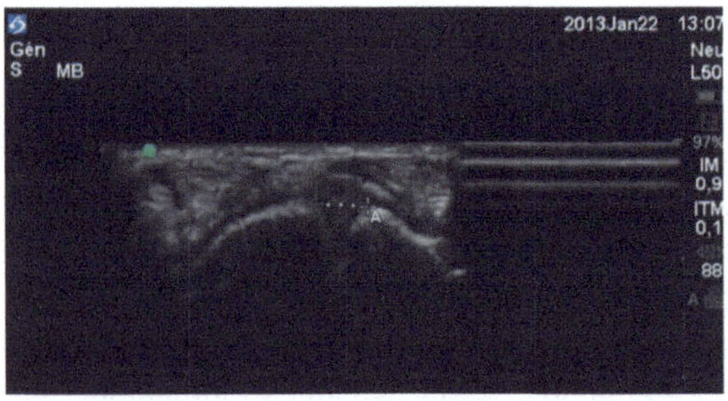

Fig. 13.2 Ultrasound cross section of the scapholunate ligament (Edge, Sonosite 6–15 MHz)

The following radiological assessment is systematically carried out in the radiology department: frontal and strict profile radiography, ulnar inclination radiography [9], and radiography of the closed fist face of both wrists [10].

The normal length of the dorsal part of the scapholunate ligament is 1.7 mm (±0.4) according to Boutryl et al. [7]. This measure is useful for static stages but does not have a range in dynamic stages. A ligament stress test is therefore useful for the scapholunate ligament as is available for lateral ankle sprain (forced varus) or for the anterolateral cruciate ligament of the knee (Lachman test).

In the test described, the slight bending of the wrist allows the clearing of the dorsal part of the scapholunate, which is the thickest and strongest part; it is stretched in extension making it more

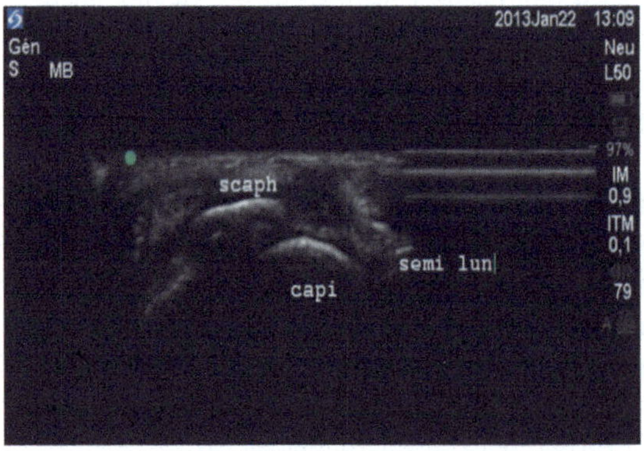

Fig. 13.3 The same cut with axial compression on the third metacarpal

Fig. 13.4 Diagram of the behavior of carpal bones before and with compression

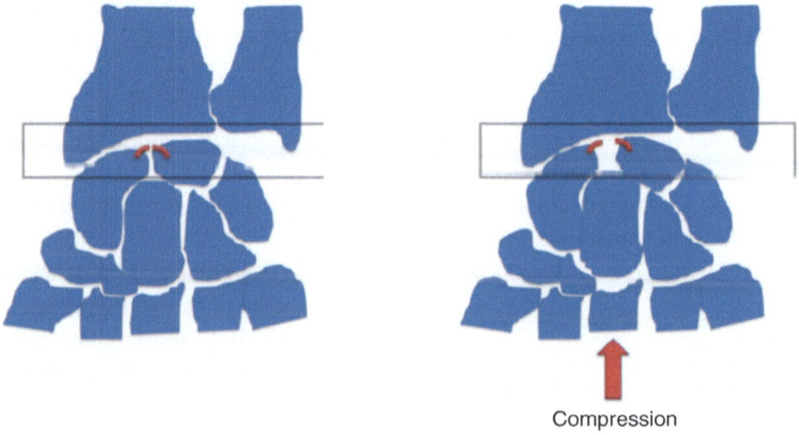

exposed during trauma [2] and is fully visualized in 97% of cases [7].

Jacobson et al. [11] analyzed in a cadaveric study that the scapholunate ligament was not visualized in the event of rupture and the interosseous space became hypoechogenic; ultrasound scanners cannot quantitatively measure echogenicity, making this test unreproducible.

The test described is dynamic and allows to explore all stages of scapholunar rupture especially the sprain stage which is the most difficult to diagnose. It can be used in consultation with ease as the ultrasound is easily accessible and feasible by the clinician.

The test is painless, and the patient also looks at the screen: one easily understands the difference in the behavior of the carpal bones by comparing the dynamic images of the two wrists.

This test is also applicable to the operating room under general or local-regional anesthesia since the compression is carried out passively by the examiner. Thus, it can be used notably after repair of a joint fracture of the distal radius or after repair of the scapholunate ligament.

Acknowledgements No conflicts of interest for authors.

References

1. Definition of carpal unstable. The anatomy and biomechanics Committee of the International Federation of Societies for Surgery of the Hand. J Hand Surg. 1999; 24A:866–867.
2. Laulan J. Rotatory subluxation of the scaphoid: pathology and surgical management. Chir Hand. 2009;28(4):192–206. https://doi.org/10.1016/j.main.2009.04.005. Epub 2009 May 13. English.
3. Watson HK, Ashmead D 4th, Makhlouf MV. Examination of the scaphoid. J Hand Surg Am. 1988;13(5):657–60.
4. Berdia S, Wolfe S. Anatomy, biomechanics, and natural history of scapholunate interosseous ligament injuries. Atl Hand Clin. 2003;8:191–9.
5. Kitay A, Wolfe SW. Scapholunate instability: current concepts in diagnosis and management. J Hand Surg Am. 2012;37(10):2175–96. https://doi.org/10.1016/jhsa.2012.07.035.
6. Taljanovic MS, Sheppard JE, Jones MD, Switlick DN, Hunter TB, Rogers LF. Sonography and sonoarthrography of the scapholunate and lunotriquetral ligaments and triangular fibrocartilage disk: initial experience and correlation with arthrography and magnetic resonance arthrography. J Ultrasound Med. 2008;27(2):179–91.
7. Boutry N, Lapegue F, Masi L, Claret A, Demondion X, Cotten A. Ultrasonographic evaluation of normal extrinsic and intrinsic carpal ligaments: preliminary experience. Skeletal Radiol. 2005;34(9):513–21. Epub 2005 Jul 12.
8. Dao KD, Solomon DJ, Shin AY, Puckett ML. The efficacy of ultrasound in the evaluation of dynamic scapholunate ligamentous instability. J Bone Joint Surg Am. 2004;86-A(7):1473–8.
9. Kuo CE, Wolfe SW. Scapholunate instability: current concepts in diagnosis and management. J Hand Surg. 2008;33A:998–1013.
10. Lawand A, Foulkes GD. The "clenched pencil" view: a modified clenched fist scapholunate stress view. J Hand Surg Am. 2003;28(3):414–8; discussion 419–20.
11. Jacobson JA, Oh E, Propeck T, Jebson PJL, Jamadar DA, Hayes CW. Sonography of the scapholunate ligament in four cadaveric wrists: correlation with MR arthrography and anatomy. RDA Am J Roentgenol. 2002;179:523–7.

14 Ultrasound of the Carpal Tunnel

Thomas Apard

14.1 Introduction

Carpal tunnel ultrasound is not a very popular examination by orthopedists with regard to the number of patients affected: approximately 600,000 patients are affected by carpal tunnel syndrome each year, and 130,000 are operated on.

However, ultrasound analysis of the carpal tunnel is very useful for exploring the median nerve (carpal tunnel syndrome), flexor tendons (tenosynovitis or rupture), the anterior surface of the carpus (synovitis), and the retinaculum of the flexors (especially if it has been opened surgically); it is also useful to explain to the patient the anatomy of the carpal tunnel before operating. Anatomical variations of carpal tunnel are very frequent and then, must be analyzed before treating it [1].

14.2 Anatomy of the Median Nerve

The median nerve is located on the wrist between the long palmar tendon and flexor carpi radialis. It has an ovoid and flattened appearance under the carpi volare. Its entry into the carpal tunnel under the flexor retinaculum (RF) is made by diving at about 30° forward and down with the nine flexor tendons of the fingers. The examiner must therefore tilt the probe a lot to counter the anisotropic artefact. It is advisable to place a ball (or gel tube) under the wrist to obtain an extension of the wrist, stabilize the hand, and allow the movement of the probe.

In transverse view, the anisotropic artifact is an aid in distinguishing the median nerve from the tendons: the tendons (fibrillar structure) are very sensitive to this artefact and therefore disappear faster than the median nerve when the probe tilts slightly. Patients with carpal tunnel syndrome may experience paresthesia within a few seconds if the probe presses hard and the wrist is extended (anti-Phalen position). The elevator movement is important to perform in order to appreciate the median nerve in three dimensions and evaluate its minimum and maximum diameter (comparative studies of cuts to assess compression).

An artery is rarely present with the median nerve. It is easy to spot if the examiner does not crush it with his probe: the power Doppler mode confirms its presence (Fig. 14.1).

The median nerve can be divided into two more or less equal parts: this is called a "bifid nerve." This division on ultrasound can be observed only for a few centimeters or during the entire crossing of the wrist and hand.

The median nerve must be examined dynamically by moving the fingers, thus assessing its possible adhesion to the RF and the presence of prominent or supernumerary lumbrical or flexor muscles.

T. Apard (✉)
Hand sonosurgery Center, Versailles, France

T. Apard, J. L. Brasseur (eds.), *Ultrasonography for the Upper Limb Surgeon*,
https://doi.org/10.1007/978-3-030-84234-5_14

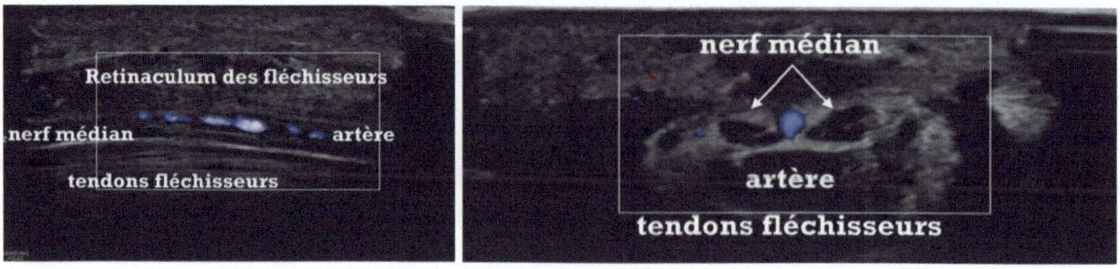

Fig. 14.1 Artery of the median nerve on bifid nerve in power Doppler mode. The top image is a transverse view, and the bottom image is a longitudinal view

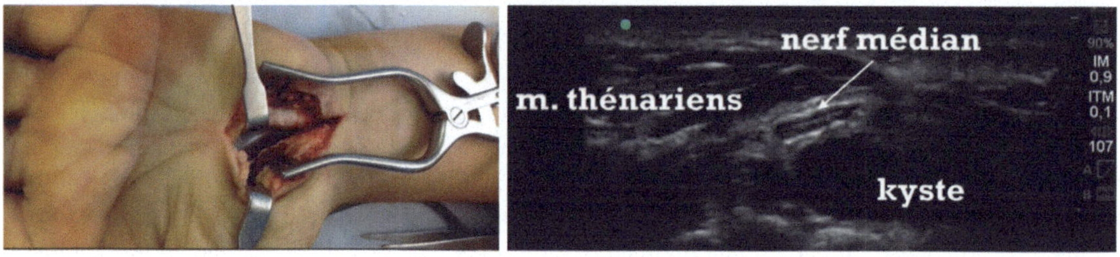

Fig. 14.2 Intracanal cyst. The upper image is a intraoperative image once the tendons and nerve have been pushed medially. The image below shows the cyst in the form of an anechoic mass pushing the median nerve forward and lateral

The thenar motor branch of the median nerve moves radially to innervate the opposing muscles of the thumb, the short abductor of the thumb, and part of the short flexor of the thumb: according to Henry et al., its position is most often extra-ligamentous (75.2%) and less rarely under the ligament (13.5%) or transligamentous (11.3%). Its ultrasound analysis requires a solid experience in ultrasound and appropriate equipment (18 MHz probe).

Regarding the diagnosis of carpal tunnel syndrome, ultrasound alone has not yet convinced the scientific community with a discordant literature on this subject [2]. Recent studies of elastographic ultrasound are trying to improve the performance of this examination to perhaps replace electromyographic analysis [3].

14.3 Anatomy of Tendon Flexors

Wrist flexor tenosynovitis is common in carpal tunnel syndrome but can also be isolated. It is presented as an anechoic halo on all or part of the nine flexor tendons. This halo should not be confused with a supernumerary muscle.

There are nine flexor tendons in the canal. The tendon of the long flexor of the thumb is the most radial. The median nerve is usually right next to it medially. The superficial and deep flexor tendons of long fingers are very difficult to isolate in static and even in dynamics.

The tendon rupture is seen in longitudinal view with a hyperechogenic tendon stump attached to the nearby hypoechogenic synovium. You have to mobilize your fingers passively in order to distinguish it. In these cases, it is necessary to continue the examination in more depth (adjustment of the focal length) and look for a radial or mediocarpal joint synovitis or even a carpal bone spur.

The presence of tenosynovitis should make you look for a hormonal disorder (diabetes, hypothyroidism, acromegaly) or rheumatic disorder (gout, chondrocalcinosis, polyarthritis).

Tendons are subject to anisotropic artifact. If, despite the inclinations of the probe, the tendons are still invisible, one should think about the exceptional presence of an intracanal cyst. It is presented as an anechoic mass that compresses all the contents of the carpal tunnel forward (Fig. 14.2).

14.4 Anatomy of the Anterior Surface of the Carpus

The dorsal part of the scapholunate ligament is the most mechanically competent. Ultrasound can explore the anterior scapholunate instability by dynamic maneuvers. The patient should be well placed in supination with a block under the wrist, and the examiner exhibits radioulnar tilt movements. In the acute phase, the joint synovitis is difficult to visualize. The anterior capsule is not visualized, and there will be no intra-articular effusion since the fluid will be transferred to the dorsal surface when the wrist is in extension (zone of low pressure). Ultrasound examination, like clinical examination, is always comparative.

In case of radial or mediocarpal osteoarthritis, chronic synovitis can be visualized in palmar without knowing its origin. Significant synovitis can be the site of joint pain but also neuropathic pain by compression of the median nerve: immobilization of the wrist will be effective in relieving nerve compression.

> Beware of the snap of the lunate that can hide the head of the capitate (in VISI) or on the contrary let it appear too much (in VISI). An X-ray of the wrist is essential to complete an ultrasound analysis of osteoarthritis.

14.5 Anatomy of the Retinaculum of Flexors

In cross section the tendon of the flexor carpi radialis is easily seen just above the tubercle of the scaphoid (before its diving with the trapezius). It indicates the radial edge of the RF, which is inserted below, excluding it from the canal. The Guyon tunnel is just in front of and medial of the carpal canal: the ulnar nerve is surrounded radially by the ulnar artery and medially by the pisiform.

RF is a slightly concave isoechogenic fibrous ligament behind. It is best visualized in case of tenosynovitis of the flexors.

In longitudinal section, RF corresponds to an isoechogenic mass pinning the median nerve and flexor tendons on the carpal floor. Distally, it ends a few millimeters before the superficial palmar arch (the power Doppler mode is recommended to visualize it).

14.5.1 Special Case of Carpal Tunnel Syndrome in Children

A nontraumatic carpal tunnel syndrome in children should be examined for a general pathology during a complete clinical examination: mucopolysaccharidosis and mucolipidosis, Déjerine-Sottas syndrome, Weill-Marchesani disease, Leri pleonostosis, melorheostosis, lipofibromatous hamartoma, and even hemophilia. An X-ray is systematic for bone dysplasia or intra-carpal synostosis.

The child's hand requires a narrower, higher-frequency probe (18 MHz hockey-stick probe). Growing carpus is visualizable by its anechogenic (physis) edges and not hyperechogenic as the adult bone cortex.

14.6 Carpal Tunnel Ultrasound Educational

In practice, patients who need carpal tunnel surgery often think that it is a "canal to unblock," and the surgeon tries to explain to them that "it's not about plumbing but about electricity!"

Ultrasound showing that it is really an osteofibrous canal allows the patient to understand their pathology and therefore the procedures and subsequent operative outcomes. The value of ultrasound is obvious for clearer preoperative information and therefore to reduce the medicolegal risk in this regard.

The possibility of capturing images/videos is also of scientific interest for the discussion of a clinical case between doctors.

14.7 Anatomy of the Operated Carpal Tunnel

The flexor RF appears hypoechogenic in its operated area. In the months following the procedure, in cross section, this area resembles a chimney going from the carpal canal to the dermis without Doppler effect. The patient reports pain under the probe. Over time the hypoechogenic surface decreases and becomes isoechogenic.

Ultrasound should analyze in longitudinal section the course of the median nerve in flexion/extension of the fingers [4]. Hunter's neurodesis is the adhesion of the nerve to the operated RF and may be the cause of recurrent carpal tunnel syndrome.

The examiner should consider analyzing the median nerve at the elbow for persistent postoperative pain after 6 months (see the chapter on ultrasound of the median nerve to the elbow) [5].

14.8 Conclusion

Ultrasound of the carpal tunnel allows us to analyze its anatomy entirely, in dynamics, in comparison. Its easy access and moderate cost make it a first-line examination before operating this anatomical area or to analyze postoperative anatomy.

References

1. Henry BM, Zwinczewska H, Roy J, et al. The prevalence of anatomical variations of the median nerve in the carpal tunnel: a systematic review and meta-analysis. PLoS One. 2015;10(8):e0136477.
2. Apard T. Ultrasonography for the orthopedic surgeon. Orthop Traumatol Surg Res. 2019;105(1S):S7–S14.
3. Lin CP, Chen IJ, Chang KV, Wu WT, Ozçakar L. Utility of ultrasound elastography in evaluation of carpal tunnel syndrome: a systematic review and meta-analysis. Ultrasound Med Biol. 2019;45(11):2855–65.
4. Apard T, Candelier G. Surgical ultrasound-guided carpal tunnel release. Hand Surg Rehabil. 2017;36(5):333–7.
5. Wang WL, Hanson T, Fowler JR. A comparison of 6 diagnostic tests for carpal tunnel syndrome using latent class analysis. Hand (N Y). 2020;15(6):776–9.

Ultrasound of the TFCC

15

Jean Louis Brasseur

The triangular complex (triangular fibrocartilage complex or TFCC) is one of the elements for which ultrasound study is insufficient [1–3]. The main reason for this limit is its horizontal arrangement forcing the ultrasound to approach it by its small side, which is an artifact generator. In addition, the superposition of the ulnar styloid and the curvature of the fibers inserted at this level further complicate its study (Fig. 15.1). Indications for the ultrasonic study of TFCC are traumatic injuries, but lesions are also detected in inflammatory pathology [4] and in chondrocalcinosis [5].

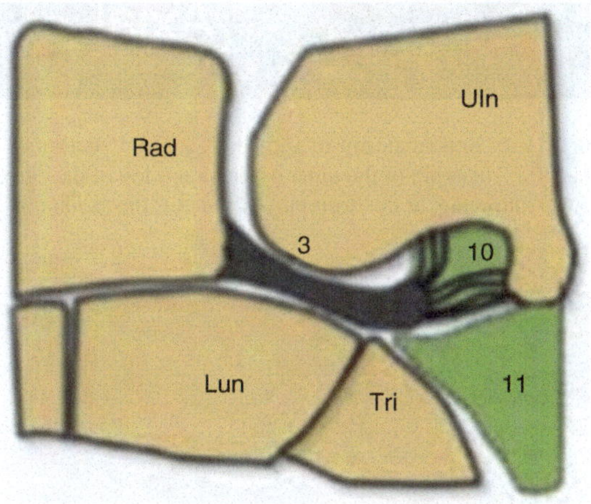

Fig. 15.1 Diagram showing the curvature of the styloid insertion (10) and the horizontal arrangement of the TFCC (3), distinct from the homologous meniscus (11) (according to Morvan [1] with permission)

15.1 Sonoanatomy

The most effective way to analyze TFCC is to perform an axial cut, with a relatively low frequency linear probe (as for a meniscus), by supination of the wrist and radial inclination to minimize the overlap of the styloid; a small inclination of the probe proximally is also necessary, and it is the visualization of the radial cortex in depth of the image which will be the criterion for success of the cut (Fig. 15.2).

One can then visualize a structure, more oval than triangular, limited in palmar, and dorsally by the radioulnar ligaments (Fig. 15.3). On the frontal section (Fig. 15.4) only a hypoechogenic rectangle with a small superficial axis "plunging" toward the radius is visualized; it can be differentiated from the homologous meniscus, which is much more echogenic, and the tendon of the extensor carpi ulnaris, but, except for the search for calcification, no anomaly can be clearly found in this incidence.

J. L. Brasseur (✉)
Department of Radiology, G.H. Pitié-Salpêtrière, Paris, France
e-mail: jlbrasseur@impf.fr

T. Apard, J. L. Brasseur (eds.), *Ultrasonography for the Upper Limb Surgeon*,
https://doi.org/10.1007/978-3-030-84234-5_15

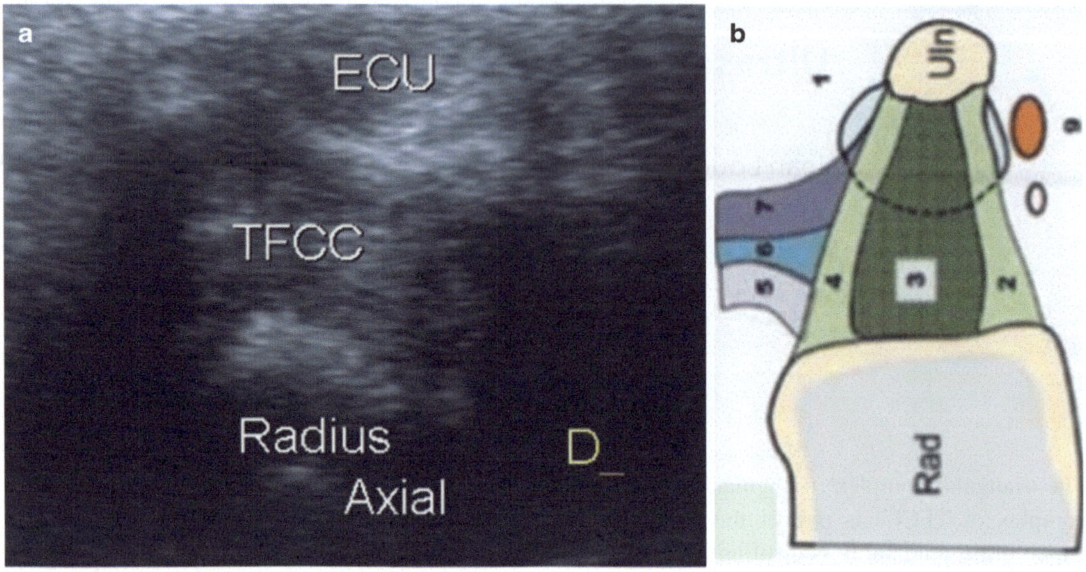

Fig. 15.2 Sonoanatomy of the TFCC. Axial section of the "disc" in depth of the ulnar extensor tendon of the carp (ECU) showing, at the deep part of the cut, the radial cortex (**a**) with corresponding diagram (**b**) (from Morvan [1] with permission)

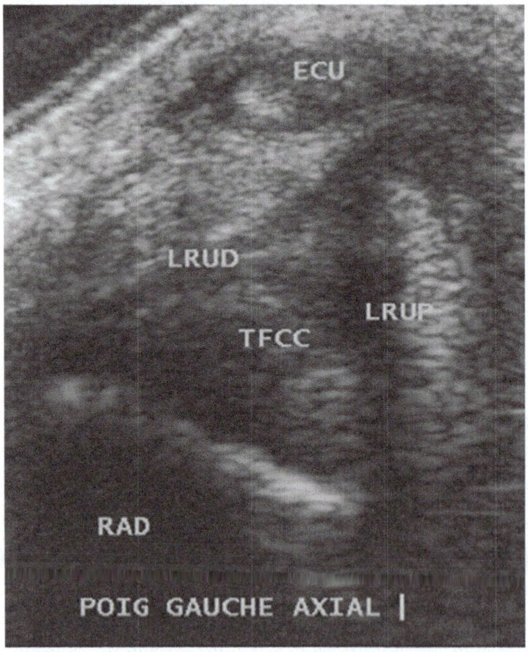

Fig. 15.3 Axial section showing the disc surrounded by the palmar and dorsal radioulnar ligaments

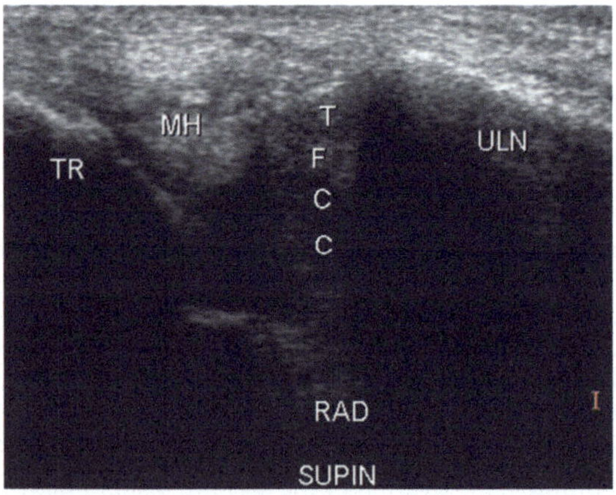

Fig. 15.4 Frontal section of TFCC showing only an unanalyzable hypoechogenic rectangle distinct from the homologous meniscus (HM)

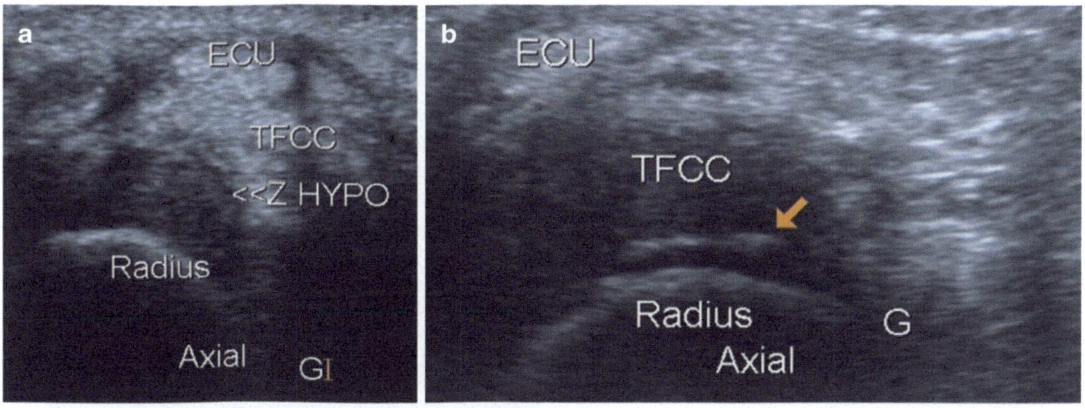

Fig. 15.5 Hypoechoic range of disinsertion of the radial attachment of TFCC (**a**); other patient in whom disinsertion is accompanied by corticoperiosteal detachment (**b**)

15.2 Pathological Ultrasound Appearances

Publications devoted to TFCC ultrasound are rare, and the authors insist on the low interest of ultrasound in the study of TFCC [1–3]; only to our knowledge, one study shows "amazing" performance [6].

The pathology of the attachment of TFCC to the ulnar styloid cannot be visualized, and only disinsertions of radial insertion (Fig. 15.5) and central perforations (Fig. 15.6) can be detected. When the frequency of these lesions is known from 40 years of age [7], a correlation with clinical exam is essential [8], but the comparative study here is a favorable element for ultrasound, whose study is systematically bilateral.

If such a lesion is discovered, confirmation by MRI or arthroCT is indispensable to assess it [1, 7, 9] because only these two techniques can make a correct analysis.

In case of pain in the ulnar side of the wrist, ultrasound will help guide the diagnosis by showing an injury to the tendon of the extensor carpi ulnaris or its retinaculum (see this chapter) but also by detecting distal radioulnar swelling (Fig. 15.7), a lesion of the pisotriquetral interval (Fig. 15.8), ligament lesion (Fig. 15.9), or hamate hamulus damage (Fig. 15.10).

In addition, ultrasound detects the subluxations and instabilities of the distal radio-ulna through supination (Fig. 15.11) or other dynamic test [10].

Another indication is the search for calcification in case of chondrocalcinosis [5] (Fig. 15.12). Ultrasound detects them as well as standard X-rays, but these are indispensable in case of damage to the ulnar slope of the carpus; this indication seems unimportant.

15.3 Conclusion

Ultrasound therefore has little interest in the study of TFCC. It may suspect certain lesions in a study for ulnar side pain and must systematically "switch the hand" to another technique if an anomaly is detected.

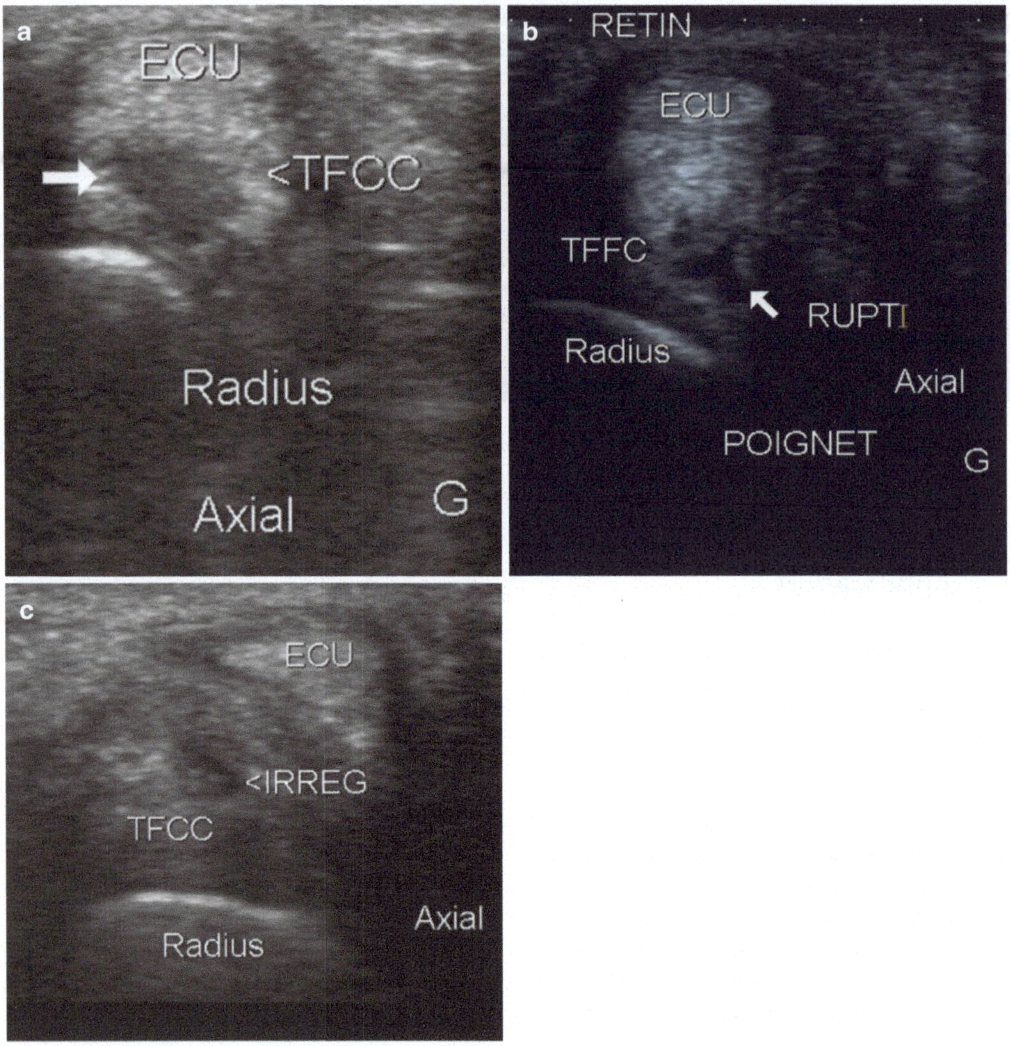

Fig. 15.6 Rupture (arrow) of the central portion of TFCC (**a**); other patient with a rather cracked lesion (RUPT) (**b**); third patient with minimal perforation (IRREG) but very painful (**c**)

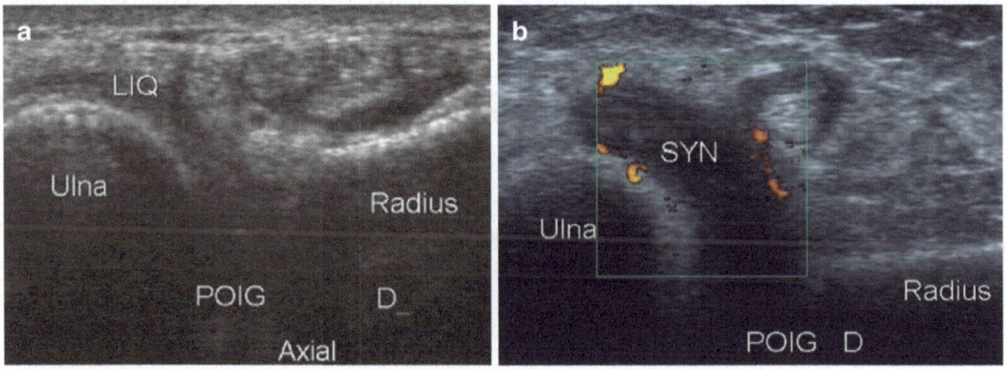

Fig. 15.7 Minimal distension of distal radio-ulna (**a**); other patient with major synovitis of this interval (**b**)

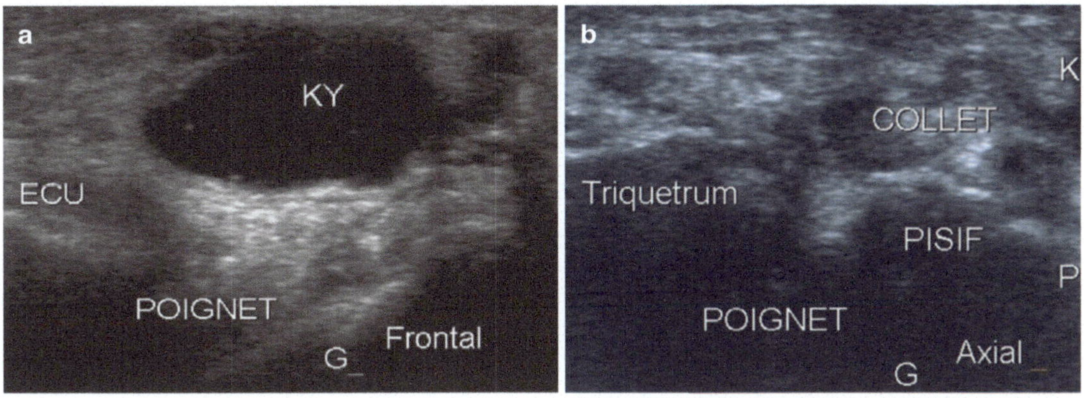

Fig. 15.8 Painful cyst of the ulnar side of the carpus (**a**) with neck showing pisotriquetral origin on an ulnar axial section (**b**)

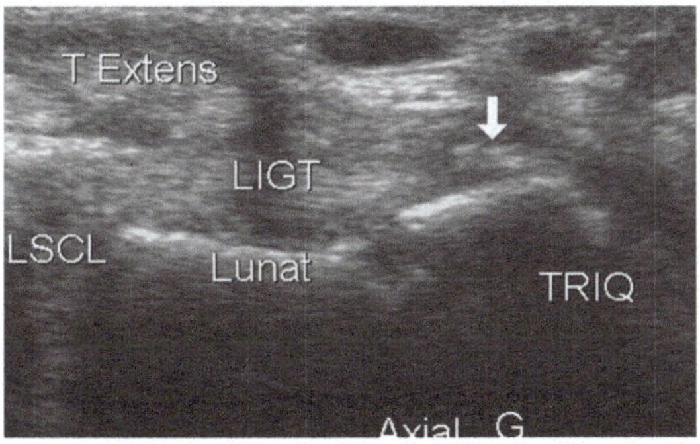

Fig. 15.9 Sequellary tearing of ligament strap from dorsal surface of triquetrum

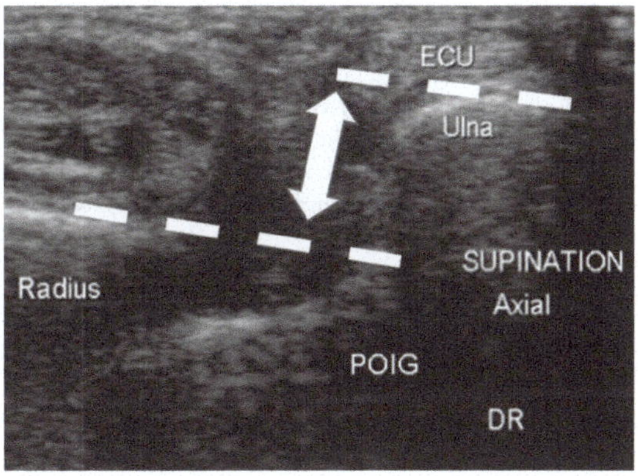

Fig. 15.11 Dorsal subluxation of the distal ulnar epiphysis on an axial view in supination (patient with a rupture of the TFCC)

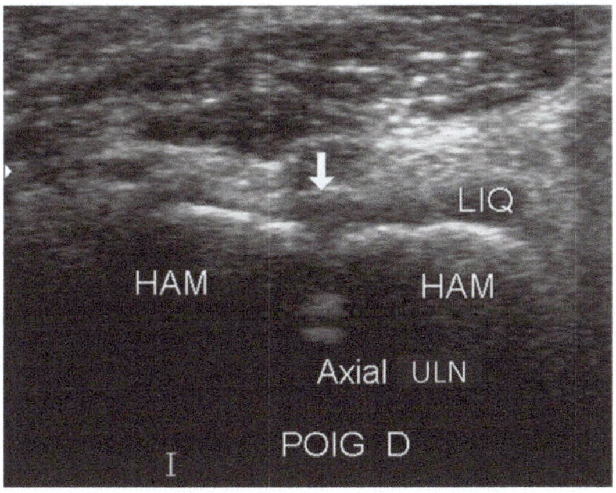

Fig. 15.10 Fracture of hamulus of hamatum on ulnar axial view

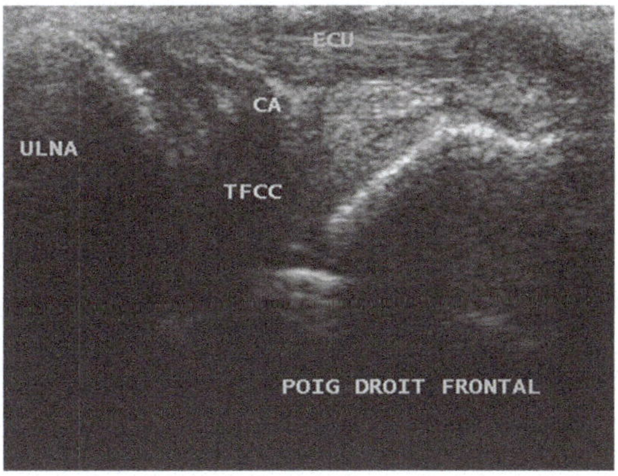

Fig. 15.12 Calcification of TFCC in chondrocalcinosis

References

1. Morvan G, Vuillemin V, Guerini H. Ultrasound of wrist and hand. Montpellier: Sauramps Médical. 2017, 358pp.
2. Bianchi S, Martinoli C. Wrist in ultrasound of the musculoskeletal system. Springer; 2007. pp. 425–94.
3. Renoux J, Demondion X, Zeitoun-Eiss D, Brewer JL. Echo-MRI correlation of the triangular complex. In: News in ultrasound of the musculoskeletal system, vol. 4. Montpellier: Sauramps Médical; 2007. p. 109–18.
4. Chen JH Sr, Huang KC, Huang CC, Lai HM, Chou WY, Chen YC Sr. High power Doppler ultrasound score is associated with the risk of triangular fibrocartilage complex (TFCC) tears in severe rheumatoid arthritis. J Investig Med. 2019;67(2):327–30. https://doi.org/10.1136/jim-2018-000821. Epub 2018 Aug 29.
5. Di Matteo A, Filippucci E, Salaffi F, Carotti M, Carboni D, Di Donato E, Grassi W. Diagnostic accuracy of musculoskeletal ultrasound and conventional radiography in the assessment of the wrist triangular fibrocartilage complex in patients with definite diagnosis of calcium pyrophosphate dihydrate deposition disease. Clin Exp Rheumatol. 2017;35(4):647–52. Epub 2017 Mar 23.
6. Lee SH, Yun SJ. Point-of-care wrist ultrasonography in trauma patients with ulnar-sided pain and instability. Am J Emerg Med. 2018;36(5):859–64. https://doi.org/10.1016/j.ajem.2018.01.005. Epub 2018 Jan 4.
7. Levy SM, Reid M, Montgomery AM, Botterill E, Kovalchik SA, Omizzolo M, Malara F, Wood TO, Hoy GA, Rotstein AH. Do magnetic resonance imaging abnormalities of the non-dominant wrist correlate with ulnar-sided wrist bread in elite tennis players? Skeletal Radiol. 2020;49(3):407–15. https://doi.org/10.1007/s00256-019-03285-y. [Epub ahead of print].
8. Watanabe A, Souza F, Vezeridis PS, Blazar P, Yoshioka H. Ulnar-sided wrist bread. II. Clinical imaging and treatment. Skeletal Radiol. 2010;39(9):837–57. https://doi.org/10.1007/s00256-009-0842-3. Epub 2009 Dec 10.
9. Treiser MD, Crawford K, Iorio ML. TFCC injuries: meta-analysis and comparison of diagnostic imaging modalities. J Wrist Surg. 2018;7(3):267–72. https://doi.org/10.1055/s-0038-1629911. Epub 2018 Feb 14.
10. Hess F, Farshad M, Sutter R, Nagy L, Schweizer A. A novel technique for detecting instability of the distal radioulnar joint in complete triangular fibrocartilage complex lesions. J Wrist Surg. 2012;1(2):153–8. https://doi.org/10.1055/s-0032-1312046.

Ultrasound of De Quervain's Tendonitis

16

P. Croutzet

De Quervain's tendonitis is the main tendonitis of the wrist [1]. It is a tenosynovitis, progressing to stenosing of the tendons of the first extensor compartment: the abductor pollicis longus (APL) and the extensor pollicis brevis (EPB).

The diagnosis is first and foremost clinical based on pain in the radial side of the wrist radiating on the column of the thumb and altering the constrained pollici digitalis forceps. Clinical examination finds elective pain in the radial styloid, sometimes swelling, and Finkelstein's maneuver is positive. This tendonitis is more common in diabetic patients and during the peripartum period.

In the majority of cases, clinical examination is sufficient for diagnosis. Paraclinical examinations, especially ultrasound, will help confirm the diagnosis, clarify anatomy, and guide treatment.

Ultrasound is the best and most accessible paraclinical examination. It allows bilateral analysis. The diagnosis is confirmed by various positive elements:

- *Thickening of the first compartment of the retinaculum of the extensors* is the cardinal sign that is confirmed by ultrasound by thickening, the threshold value often used is greater than 2 mm. It is also possible to compare the thickness of the retinaculum of the first compartment with the thickness of another compartment or the contralateral side.
- *Peritendinous synovitis of the first compartment*, a true synovial development having the appearance of *hyperechogenic granulations surrounded by* an exudate (liquid effusion) forming a *hypoechogenic halo* in the periphery. This exudative synovial development is regularly associated with peritendinous *hypervascularization* which results in Doppler hyperemia.
- *Tendon remodeling*, resulting in tendon thickening sometimes associated with signal changes in tendon fibers including hypoechogenic areas (Figs. 16.1, 16.2, 16.3, 16.4, 16.5, 16.6, 16.7, 16.8, and 16.9)

Ultrasound also has an interventional planning function, whether for infiltration or intervention:

- *Identification of a septum* that is sometimes present (30–70% depending on the populations studied) between the 2 APL and EPB tendons, which may or may not be affected by thickening. The identification of this septum according to the Hiranuma classification will guide the implementation of the infiltration and/or intervention.

P. Croutzet (✉)
Conservative and Traumatological Surgery Department, Union Clinique, Saint-Jean, France

T. Apard, J. L. Brasseur (eds.), *Ultrasonography for the Upper Limb Surgeon*,
https://doi.org/10.1007/978-3-030-84234-5_16

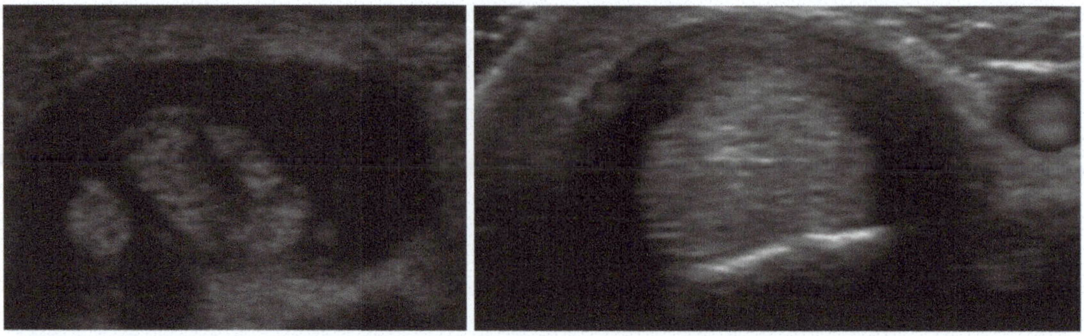

Fig. 16.1 Cross sections showing a significant thickening of the retinaculum

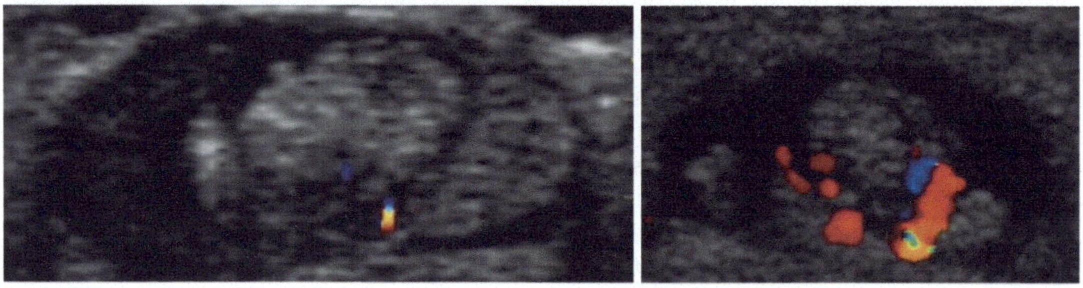

Fig. 16.2 Transverse sections showing exudative synovitis with hypervascularization

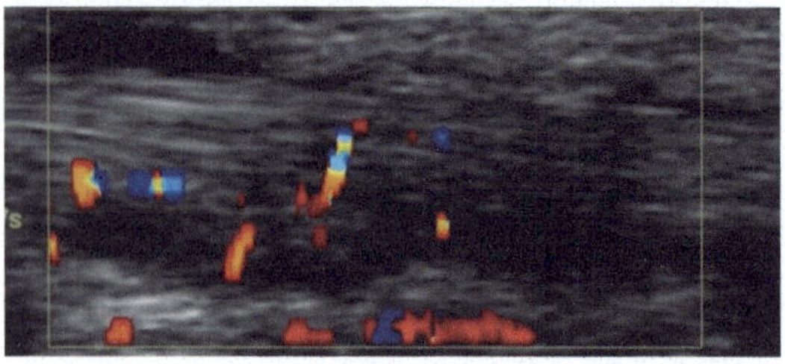

Fig. 16.3 Longitudinal section showing exudative synovitis with hypervascularization

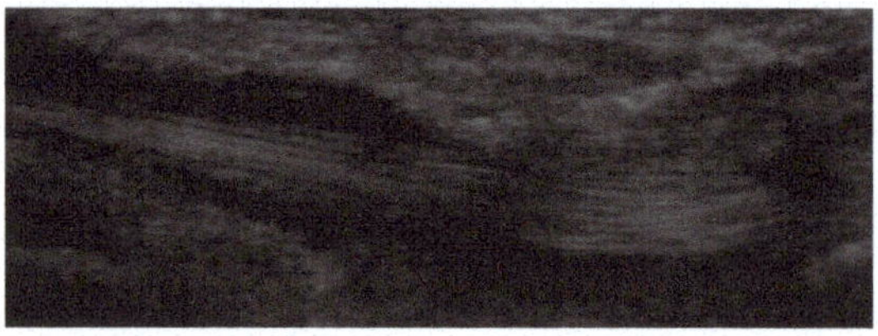

Fig. 16.4 Longitudinal section showing tendon remodeling with hypoechogenic areas within a tendon bulge

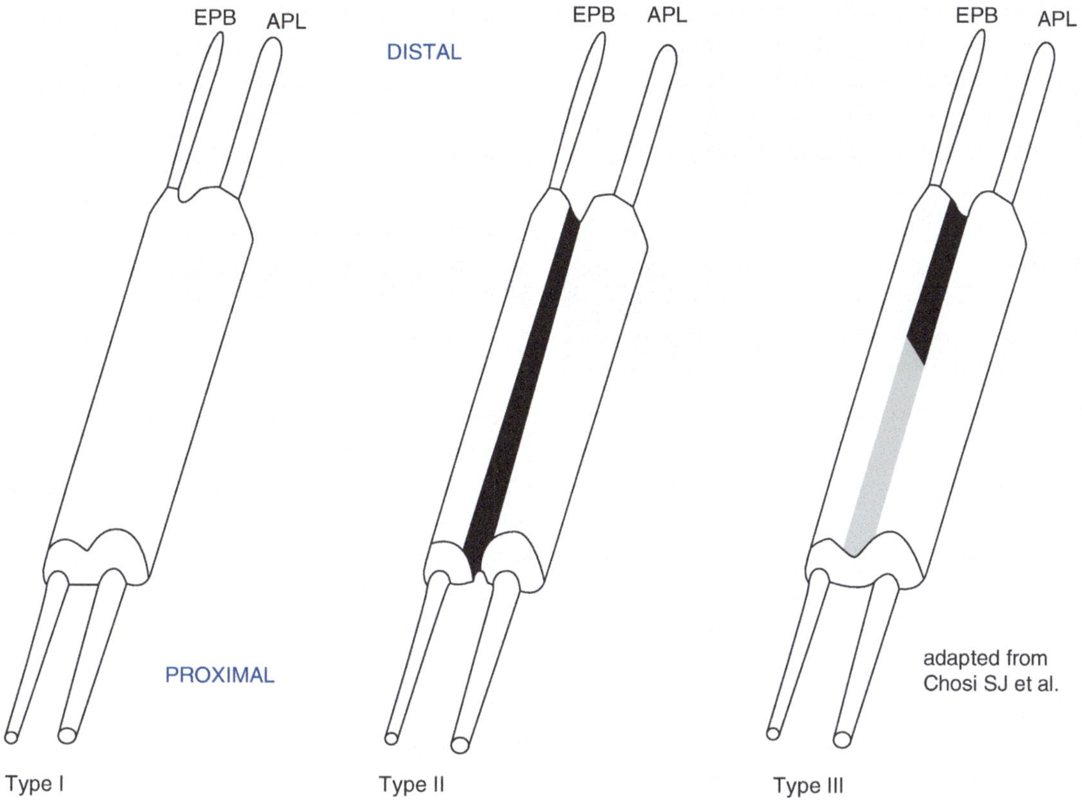

Fig. 16.5 The different types of sheaths according to their sub-compartmentalization (septation): Hiranuma classification (adapted from Choi et al. [2])

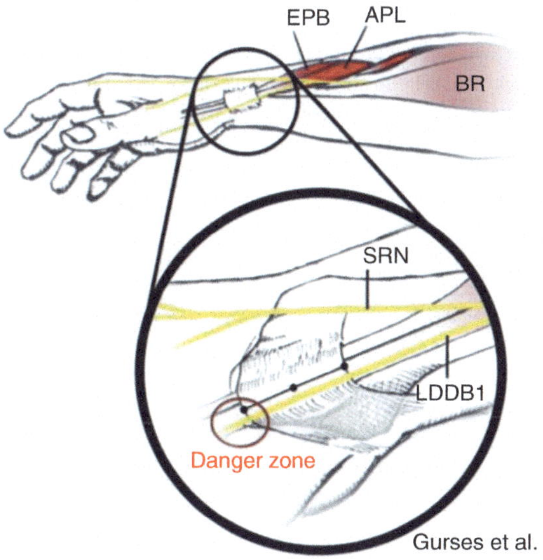

Fig. 16.6 Relationship of radial nerve to first extensor compartment (from Gurses et al. [3])

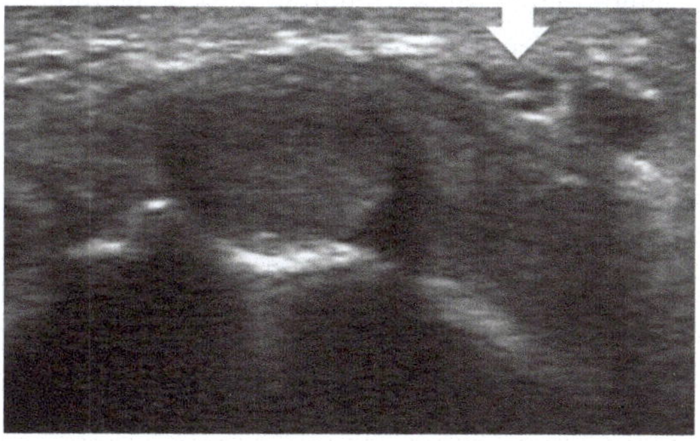

Fig. 16.7 Cross section showing the dorsolateral digital branch of the thumb

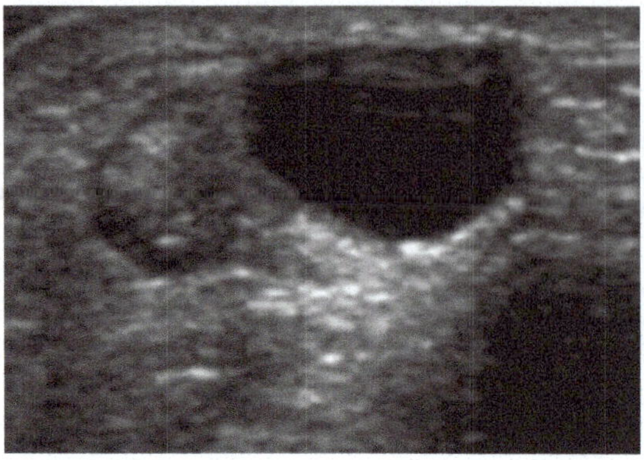

Fig. 16.8 Cross section showing a cyst of the first compartment

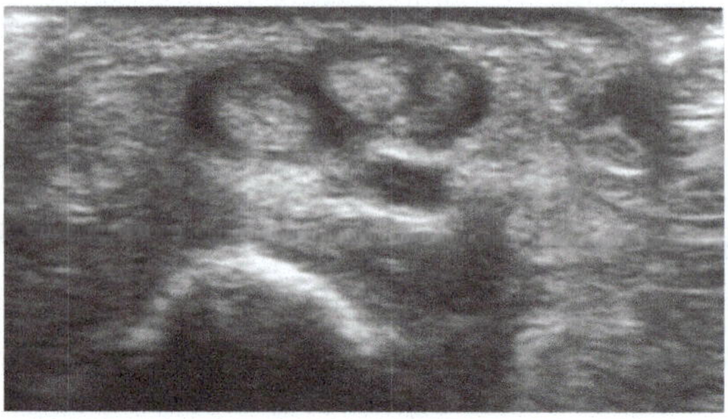

Fig. 16.9 Cross section showing a two-pennate LPA

- *Mapping of the superficial sensory branches of the radial nerve* that is made possible by the advent of high-frequency probes. The precise anatomy of the radial sensory branches has been perfectly described by Gurses et al. [3]: the sensory branch of the radial nerve gives its first division to the thumb 5 cm above the radial side of the wrist (the dorsolateral digital branch of the thumb) with a variation ranging from 26 to 72 mm.
- *Identification of a synovial cyst*: indeed a peritendinous cyst is sometimes present, developed depending on the first compartment.
- The APL tendon is regularly multipennate, and ultrasound allows the identification of the different tendon strips.

In conclusion, while ultrasound is not indispensable for the positive diagnosis of de Quervain's tendonitis, it is the first-line examination in case of doubt. It is very useful for therapeutic orientation in particular by identifying a septum and securing an interventional sign by identifying with precision the sensory branches of the radial nerve.

References

1. Adams JE, Habbu R. Tendinopathies of the hand and wrist. J Am Acad Orthop Surg. 2015;23(12):741–50.
2. Choi S-J, Ahn JH, Lee Y-J, et al. Quervain disease: US identification of anatomic variations in the first extensor compartment with an emphasis on subcompartmentalization. Radiology. 2011;260(2):480–6.
3. Gurses IA, Coskun O, Gayretli O, Kale A, Ozturk A. The relationship of the superficial radial nerve and its branch to the thumb to the first extensor compartment. J Hand Surg. 2014;39(3):480–3.

Ultrasound of Rhizarthrosis

17

Thomas Apard and Jean Louis Brasseur

17.1 Introduction

The development of high-frequency ultrasound now allows real-time, fast, cheap, comparative, dynamic, and noninvasive exploration of the surface structures of the hand and wrist [1]. Ultrasound is the ideal examination of hand arthritis in addition to X-ray and MRI to assess synovial tissue, cartilage, effusion, chondrocalcinosis deposits, or erosions [2].

The radiological and rheumatological literature is very poor regarding the ultrasound data of rhizarthrosis [3–6].

17.2 How to Carry Out an Ultrasound of Rhizarthrosis?

17.2.1 Mode B

The wrist is placed under a block (e.g., the gel box) for a slight extension and supination of the wrist. Ultrasound is always comparative so as not to ignore anatomical variation or congenital hyperlaxity. The trapeziometacarpal joint (TM) is simple to see if we place the probe longitudinally on the first metacarpal and then follow the diaphysis (hyperechogenic) proximally up to the palmar face of the joint (hypoechogenic edge of the cartilage and separation between trapezius and the first metacarpal). In the same and more proximal axis, we observe the palmar face of the scaphotrapeziotrapezoidal joint (STT) and finally the palmar face of the S-shaped scaphoid.

At the longitudinal section of the TM, the examiner can then gently press the first metacarpal and open the joint space (fish mouth) to make an injection or to explore the cartilage of the first metacarpal (Figs. 17.1 and 17.2).

Osteophytosis appears as irregular hyperechogenic bone attached to the cortex of healthy bone. The posterior shadow cone prevents seeing underneath (the bone stops ultrasonic waves), and the examiner is forced to mobilize the probe for correct overview (lift maneuver).

The dorsal face of the TM joint explores the dorso-oblique ligament [7]. Just medially, the trapezius bone is an extension of the second metacarpal.

Adduction of the first metacarpal can be painful and detect a dorsal impingement with hyperechogenic synovitis (Fig. 17.3).

The flexor carpi radialis tendon (FCR) is located on the palmar face on the scaphoid tubercle. It is easy to locate it in the cross section of the

T. Apard (✉)
Hand Sonosurgery Center, Versailles, France

J. L. Brasseur
G.H. Pitié-Salpêtrière, Service de Radiologie, Paris, France

T. Apard, J. L. Brasseur (eds.), *Ultrasonography for the Upper Limb Surgeon*,
https://doi.org/10.1007/978-3-030-84234-5_17

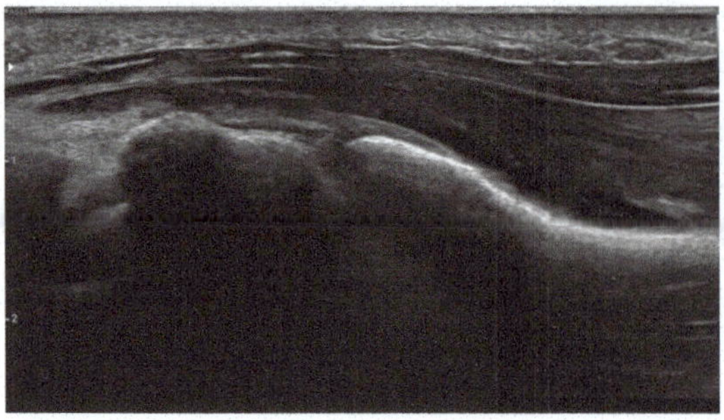

Fig. 17.1 Longitudinal view of the trapeziometacarpal joint

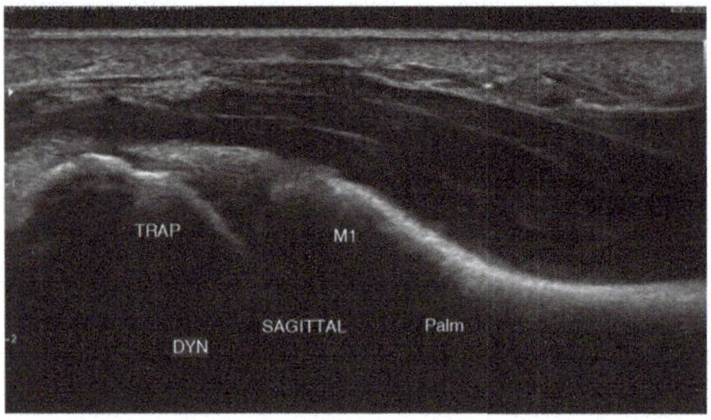

Fig. 17.2 Palmar view of the trapeziometacarpal joint with the image in "fish mouth"

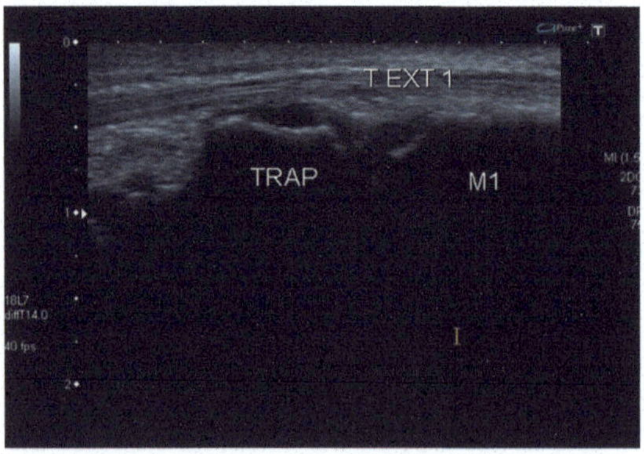

Fig. 17.3 Longitudinal view of the dorsal face of the trapeziometacarpal joint

carpal canal. In longitudinal section, it dives just before the trapezius and disappears in the image (anisotropic artifact). To follow it, it is necessary to tilt the probe forward and inward (like a car gear shift) [8]. Its enthesis is located at the base of the second metacarpal just below a transverse artery that is easy to spot.

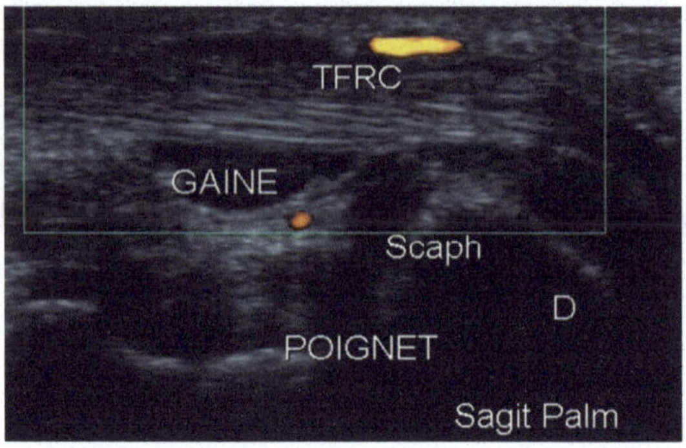

Fig. 17.4 Tenosynovitis of the flexor carpi radialis in Doppler mode

17.2.2 Doppler Mode

The power Doppler mode identifies the red blood cells under the probe: their direction and speed of propagation are not specified, but it is possible to tell if there is an inflammatory tissue (do not press with the probe). The patient warns if they feel pain.

17.3 Differential Diagnosis of Rhizarthrosis Pain

17.3.1 De Quervain's Tendonitis

The peritendinous anechogenic border around the tendons of the first extensor compartment indicates De Quervain tenosynovitis. The patient experiences pain under the pressure of the probe, and usually the painful area corresponds exactly to the pathological area in the image. The central crest on the dorsal cortex of the radius should search for a septum between the long abducting tendon of the thumb and the short extensor tendon of the thumb. The latter is easily identifiable by asking the patient to extend the metacarpophalangeal joint [9].

17.3.1.1 Tendonitis of Flexor Carpi Radialis (Fig. 17.4)

Tenosynovitis of the tendon of the flexor carpi radialis is often unknown because its clinic examination is difficult [8]. Wrist pain against

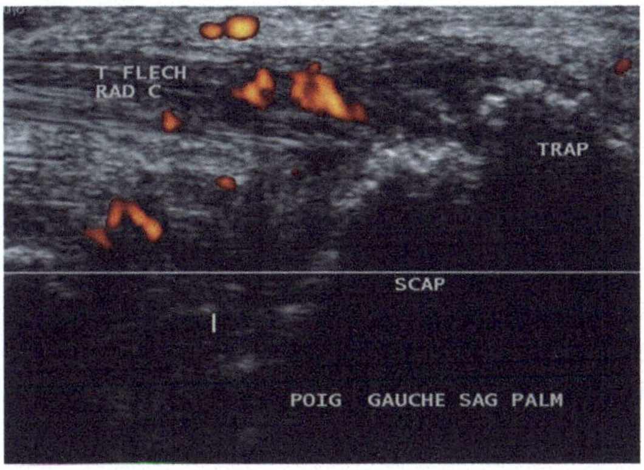

Fig. 17.5 Synovitis of the scaphotrapeziotrapezoidal joint in the palmar longitudinal view with Doppler mode

resistance is not obvious from interpretation. Cross-sectional ultrasound is easy: it is necessary to put the wrist flat on the table and not in extension so as not to expel the liquid.

17.3.1.2 Scaphotrapeziotrapezoidal Osteoarthritis (Fig. 17.5)

STT osteoarthritis is often associated with TM osteoarthritis [6]. Ultrasound shows synovitis and trapezius osteophytosis (it is rare on the scaphoid side). The patient then reports that his/her pain is more likely to be under the wrist probe. The mobilization of the first metacarpal does not mobilize the STT. Thus ultrasound exploration will be more useful than clinical examination to prescribe a first-line wrist orthosis without thumb immobilization, a wrist orthosis with thumb immobilization, or a gauntlet orthosis.

17.3.2 Trapeziometacarpal Instability

Ultrasound is a dynamic imaging examination without adverse effects. TM instability is often observed: it can be lateral, vertical, or in all planes. The examination must be bilateral for congenital instability, Ehlers-Danlos disease, or posttraumatic instability. The main stabilizing element is the dorsal TM ligament [10].

17.3.3 Trapeziometacarpal (Osteo) chondral Fracture

A chondral or osteochondral fracture is easy to see because of its hyperechogenic appearance within the hypoechogenic area. It is necessary to search for it by gently mobilizing the thumb without too much pressure on the probe. Note that this appearance of foreign body is not accompanied by a cone of posterior shadow because the bone fragment is too small.

In these rare and often unrecognized cases, the X-ray is constantly taken in default and sometimes even the scanner. Only a TM arthroCT could detect it, but this examination is minimally prescribed, invasive, and painful.

17.4 The Patient Looks at the Ultrasound Screen

17.4.1 Echo-pedagogy

The patient is participatory. The patient feels the probe exploring his hand, does not move, and enjoys participating in the investigation of the causes of his/her problem. It is thus nice to explain this image to patients by comparing it with the other hand.

17.4.2 The Medicolegal Interest

Each annotated image can be recorded and given to the patient for analysis by another doctor (e.g., medical expert). The image proves the examination, the care given, and the explanations given.

17.5 Postoperative Ultrasound of Rhizarthrosis

17.5.1 Scaphometacarpal Impingement After Trapeziectomy

This impingement is difficult to see on an X-ray or scanner for three reasons:

1. Impingement is often dynamic.
2. Impingement is often painless (rare synovitis).
3. The cause of pain is often elsewhere (tenosynovitis of the flexor carpi radialis or scapho-trapezial impingement).

For these three reasons, ultrasound is the best examination in case of post-trapeziectomy pain.

17.5.2 Aseptic Tenosynovitis of FCR

Low and Hales have shown the high frequency of this complication after trapeziectomy and suspensionplasty along the abductor of the thumb [11]. This diagnosis is unrecognized by surgeons who do not do ultrasound and by radiologists who do not have the operating report (specifying the type of graft used for ligamentoplasty and/or suspensionplasty).

17.5.3 Ultrasound of TM Implants

Surgeons can use several types of implants: coupled total prosthesis (single or double mobility) and interposition implant (PLA, pyrocarbon implant).

- In the case of a coupled prosthesis, it is impossible to explore polyethylene in the cup. The synovial membrane of the neo-capsule must be analyzed. A thickened anechogenic synovium should suspect an infection. Mobility of the cup or too good vision of the polyethylene in circumduction of the thumb should make it possible to suspect a loosening or mobilization of the cup.
- In the case of an interposition implant, ultrasound must be dynamic to confirm its stability. Similarly, a thickened anechogenic synovium should cause an infection to be suspected.

17.5.4 Neuroma of the Dorso-radial Branch of the Radial Nerve

This branch may be injured during surgery or compressed by postoperative immobilization by the splint [12]. This nerve branch is easy to follow from the radial edge of radius and is followed to the dorsal face of the first commissure until you see a pathological picture or see the patient report exquisite pain under the probe.

17.6 Conclusion

Ultrasound provides valuable information on preoperative and postoperative rhizarthrosis. It can guide orthotic treatment and correct diagnosis. Finally, it allows the patient to participate in the examination and understand the pathology.

References

1. Sivakumaran P, Hussain S, Ciurtin C. Comparison between several ultrasound hand joint scores and conventional radiography in diagnosing hand osteoarthritis. Ultrasound Med Biol. 2018;44(3):544–50.
2. Hazani R, Engineer NJ, Elston J, Wilhelmi BJ. Anatomic landmarks for basal joint injections. Eplasty. 2012;12:e2.
3. Kroon FPB, van Beest S, Ermurat S, Kortekaas MC, Bloem JL, Reijnierse M, Rosendaal FR, Kloppenburg M. In thumb base osteoarthritis structural damage is more strongly associated with pain than synovitis. Osteoarthr Cartil. 2018;26(9):1196–202.
4. Kortekaas MC, Kwok WY, Reijnierse M, Watt I, Huizinga TW, Kloppenburg M. Pain in hand osteoarthritis is associated with inflammation: the value of ultrasound. Ann Rheum Dis. 2010;69(7):1367–9.
5. Lee JC, Healy JC. Normal sonographic anatomy of the wrist and hand. Radiographics. 2005;25(6):1577–90.
6. Morvan G, Vuillemin V, Guerini H. Mechanical arthropathies. In: Brasseur JL, Morvan G, editors. Ultrasound of wrist and hand. Montpellier: Sauramps Medical; 2017. p. 231–3.
7. Morvan G, Vuillemin V, Guerini H. Trapezometacarpal joint. In: Brasseur JL, Morvan G, editors. Ultrasound of wrist and hand. Montpellier: Sauramps Medical; 2017. p. 43–5.

8. Luong DH, Smith J, Bianchi S. Flexor carpi radialis ultrasound tendon pictorial essay. Skelet Radiol. 2014;43(6):745–60. Review.
9. Kwon BC, Choi SJ, Koh SH, Shin DJ, Baek GH. Sonographic identification of the intracompartmental septum in Quervain's disease. Clin Orthop Relat Res. 2010;468(8):2129–34.
10. Lin JD, Karl JW, Strauch RJ. Trapeziometacarpal joint stability: the evolving importance of the dorsal ligaments. Clin Orthop Relat Res. 2014;472(4):1138–45.
11. Low TH, Hales PF. High incidence and treatment of flexor carpi radialis tendinitis after trapeziectomy and abductor pollicis longus suspensionplasty for basal joint arthritis. J Hand Surg Eur Vol. 2014;39(8):838–44.
12. Morvan G, Vuillemin V, Guerini H. Radial nerve. In: Brasseur JL, Morvan G, editors. Ultrasound of wrist and hand. Montpellier: Sauramps Medical; 2017. p. 196–200.

Part V
Finger

Ultrasound of the Flexor Tendons of the Fingers

18

Thomas Apard

Ultrasound is the ideal examination for exploring the anatomy and pathologies of the flexor tendons from the palm to the tip of the finger: it is the only dynamic, comparative examination available.

We will approach the technique of ultrasound examination and its various indications for the orthopedist.

18.1 Installation

The hand and fingers are laid in supination on the table, fingers stuck together so that the gel does not fall between the fingers. Enough gel should be put on to fill the flexion folds of the fingers.

A high-frequency linear probe of at least 13 MHz (ideally 15–18 MHz) should be selected. Short hockey-stick probes are ultimately of little use because the wide probes allow to visualize all the fingers at the same time in cross section (comparative examination with the neighbor finger). The pulleys are thus visualized by the "quilt" artifact.

In cross section, the lift technique must be practiced by sweeping the finger from proximal to distal.

In longitudinal section, the flexor system must be clearly displayed on the entire screen. It can be noted that the long flexor of the thumb (LFT) tendon is not in the axis of the thumb, and the flexor tendons of the index finger and the fifth finger are not in the axis of their finger. The cartilage of the head of the metacarpal and the heads of the phalanges is well visualizable in the form of an anechogenic crescent (the cartilage at the base of the phalanges is not visible). Palmar plates are thick, isoechogenic ligament reinforcements at the joint level and at the deep common flexor (DCP) level.

Underwater examination is useful in case of a probe less than 13 MHz or within 15 postoperative days. Check that the probe is waterproof.

Technical tip for the thumb: if the patient does not have shoulder pain or stiffness, he/she can place his/her thumb flat, in maximum pronation, which facilitates ultrasound examination.

18.2 Dynamic and Comparative Review

In passive mobilization, tendons slide into the digital canal normally without impingement. The sliding must be harmonious: a tendon rupture should be suspected if the tendon moves less quickly than the passive mobilization of the third phalanx.

In active mobilization, the tendon must enter the digital canal after a tense suture. It is useful to

T. Apard (✉)
Hand Sonosurgery Center, Versailles, France

T. Apard, J. L. Brasseur (eds.), *Ultrasonography for the Upper Limb Surgeon*,
https://doi.org/10.1007/978-3-030-84234-5_18

spot the knots of the threads and follow them during the test.

In mobilization against resistance (the examiner puts his finger on the fingertip of P3 or the patient can grab a horizontal stick), a tendon detachment will be sought by the removal of the first phalanx (pathology of the A2 pulley) or the second phalanx (pathology of the A4 pulley).

18.3 Trigger Finger

In the case of a trigger finger, the superficial common flexor (SCF) lifts the A1 pulley, which is thickened and slightly hypoechogenic (Fig. 18.1) when the examiner mobilizes the finger. The slippage of the DCF is not disturbed in this pathology. The patient sometimes reports pain under the probe in front of the A1 pulley. Ultrasound allows to confirm the diagnosis, the main differential diagnosis being the rupture of the intertendinous junction of the extensors because the patient also complains of a snap, and to appreciate the tenosynovitis of the flexors, which is marked by a peritendinous anechogenic halo in the longitudinal section (Fig. 18.2) and sometimes intertendinous in cross section (perfect visualization of the chiasma of the SCF around the DCF). Sometimes there is a cyst of the pulley A1 or more rarely A2 in addition to the trigger finger. This clinical swelling can be perceived as a nodule and simulate the impingement of the SCF. The difference is visible in clinical and ultrasound examination since the cyst does not move with the tendon in dynamics.

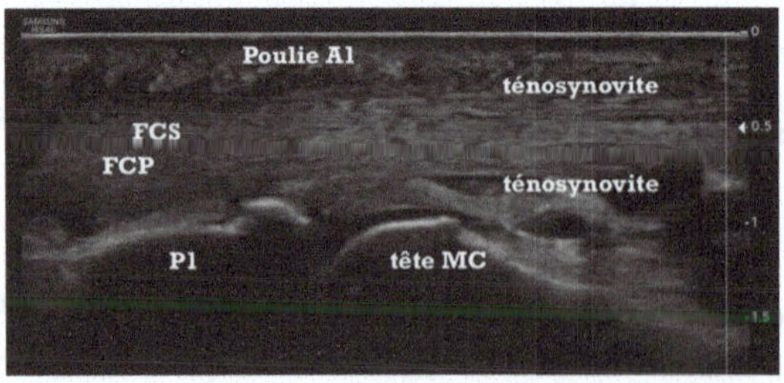

Fig. 18.1 Longitudinal cut of the painful flexors of a trigger finger. *P1* first phalanx, *MC* metacarpal

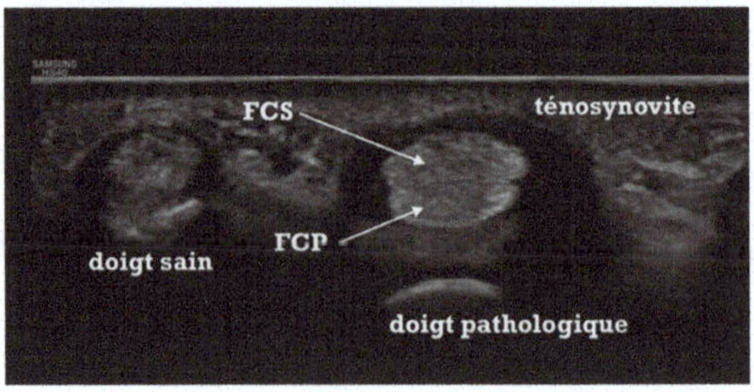

Fig. 18.2 Cross section of the same finger as Fig. 18.1

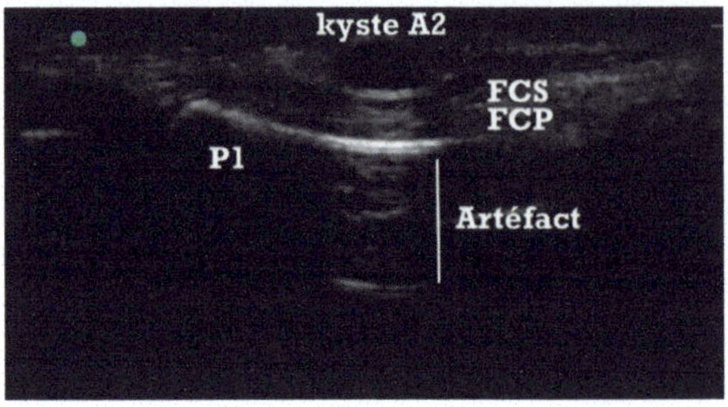

Fig. 18.3 Dr. Bouyer's device for testing pulleys against resistance with submerged probe *(courtesy Dr. Michael Bouyer)*

The association between Dupuytren's fibromatosis and trigger finger is classic: Dupuytren's disease is not diagnosed under ultrasound. If thick, the examiner observes a vague isoechogenic or slightly hypoechogenic range.

18.4 Cyst of the A1 Pulley

This is a mucoid process due to friction of the flexor tendons in its digital canal. It is not very painful on palpation or under the probe. It becomes very uncomfortable when it presses on a digital nerve.

It does not mobilize itself in active and passive mobilization.

The difference in contrast between the anechogenic cyst and the hyperechogenic tendon apparatus creates an artifact of "posterior acoustic shadow" under the cortex of the first phalanx (Fig. 18.3).

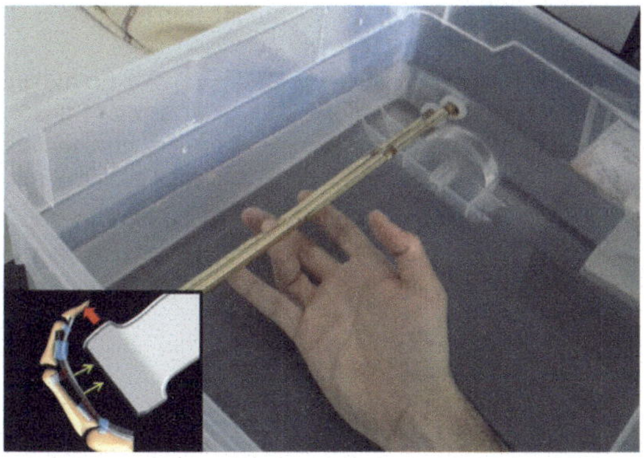

Fig. 18.4 A2 pulley cyst with posterior reinforcement artefact. *P1* first phalanx

18.5 Pulley Rupture

Ultrasound is the best examination because the tendon actively takes hold of the antagonized flexion cord: it has a sensitivity of 98% and a specificity of 100% for the diagnosis of pulley ruptures according to Klauser. In case of a recent rupture, the ruptured area is painful on palpation and under the probe, the tendons are thickened like tenosynovitis (anechoic halo), and the comparative examination with a neighboring finger shows the difference in course [1]. The minimum distance between the anterior cortex of the phalanx and the deep surface of the DCF (bowstring effect) must be measured.

Mr. Bouyer has developed a device to combine ultrasound in water [2] and flexion against resistance of the finger for exploration of broken or repaired pulleys (Fig. 18.4).

18.6 Distal Rupture of the FDP Tendon ("Jersey Finger")

The combination of clinical examination (inability to bend the distal interphalangeal joint actively) and radiography makes it possible to diagnose the type of jersey finger [3]. The interest of ultrasound is to identify the distal stump of the torn tendon and thus appreciate the injury of the vascular attachments (vincula) necessary for its healing. Preoperatively, this makes it possible to explain to the patient their pathology (visualization of the detached stump). When operating, this avoids systematically opening the entire finger. It is not possible with the Doppler to explore the vincula by seeing blood flow to the tendons (certainly because of the traction exerted).

In case of jersey finger more than 3 weeks old, its repair is possible if the stump is not retracted in the palm. Local anesthesia allows to test the strength of the suture in full active flexion of the finger and the muscular flexibility of the flexors in full active extension.

18.7 Operative Suites After Tendon Suture

The issue of the sore finger a few days after tendon suture is a challenge for the surgeon: Infection? Algodystrophy? Edema? Tendon rupture? Ultrasound allows to answer these questions. Sterile gel should be used if healing is not complete.

Infection results in tenosynovitis of the sheath (phlegmon) and pain under the probe along the entire length of the finger. A biological assessment will be requested as a supplement.

Edema of the finger shows a healthy digital canal with hypoechogenic swelling of the soft parts.

Tendon rupture is easy to diagnose in longitudinal section by mobilizing the distal phalanx.

Algodystrophy is a diagnosis of elimination often associated with a mixture of nociceptive pain (tendon surgery and scar pain), neuropathic pain (in case of associated nerve suture), and mental pain (misunderstanding of the problem, poor contact with the healthcare team). Ultrasound reassures the patient by visualizing their tendon repair by gentle maneuvers of passive mobilization.

References

1. Klauser A, Frauscher F, Bodner G, Halpern EJ, Schocke MF, Springer P, et al. Finger pulley injuries in extreme rock climbers: depiction with dynamic US. Radiology. 2002;222(3):755–61.
2. Blaivas M, Lyon M, Brannam L, Duggal S, Sierzenski P. Water bath technical evaluation for emergency ultrasound of painful superficial structures. Am J Emerg Med. 2004;22(7):589–93.
3. Ravnic DJ, Galiano RD, Bodavula V, Friedman DW, Flores RL. Diagnosis and localization of flexor tendon injuries by surgeon-performed ultrasound: a cadaveric study. J Plast Reconstr Aesthet Surg. 2011;64:234–9.

Ultrasound Extensor Tendons of the Fingers

19

G. Morvan, V. Vuillemin, and J. -L. Drapé

19.1 Introduction

The human hand is made to grasp, in different ways. To grasp, you need to bend your fingers. In order to flex them, it is essential that they are previously extended, hence the essential role of the extensor tendons [1].

The specifications of these, terribly restrictive, explain their anatomical characteristics, directly related to this biomechanical requirement:

- Extensor tendons are born from a single muscle, the common extensor muscle of the fingers whose role is to extend long fingers [2]. Its terminal tendon is divided into four strips, one for each finger. In addition, the second and fifth fingers also have a small, proper extensor muscle whose tendon doubles the strip of the common extensor. This arrangement, the most common, is subject to very many variations [3], much more common than in flexor tendons.
- While flexor tendons can afford to be massively thick, the slimming space between the skin and the dorsal surface of the hand skeleton through which the extensor tendons pass requires that the thickness of the tendons be reduced to the strict minimum, hence a slender and flattened morphology.
- A relaxed tendon loses all its power. However, each tendon has exactly the length necessary to travel its anatomical path. If it cuts a bend, the path shortens: the tendon becomes proportionally too long, flabby, and without force. The extensor tendons must therefore remain clad against the dorsal surface of the skeleton, including during dorsal flexion and lateral tilt movements of the wrist, which requires a strong tendon fastening system to the underlying skeleton.
- In contrast to flexor tendons, which follow hollow paths where stability is natural, the extensors take naturally unstable ridge paths: the dorsal surfaces of the wrist, hand, metacarpophalangeal joint, and finger hence the need for a series of stabilizing mechanisms (Fig. 19.1).
- The biomechanical role of extrinsic and intrinsic flexor tendons of the fingers is closely related to that of the extensor tendons, resulting in the necessary and subtle anatomic relationships between these two systems.
- To meet these biomechanical requirements of anchoring, stabilization, and coordination nature has designed five formations placed in series on the path of the extensor tendons.

G. Morvan (✉) · V. Vuillemin
Centre d'imagerie médicale Léonard de Vinci, Paris, France

J. -L. Drapé
Radiology Department B, Cochin Hospital, Paris, France

T. Apard, J. L. Brasseur (eds.), *Ultrasonography for the Upper Limb Surgeon*,
https://doi.org/10.1007/978-3-030-84234-5_19

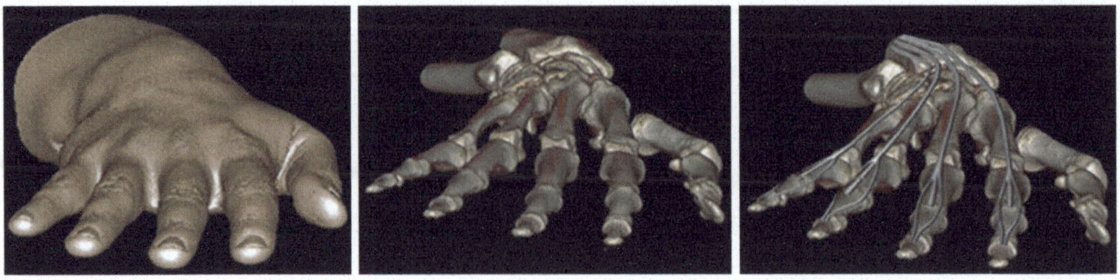

Fig. 19.1 Back of the hand; skeleton; splitting branches of the common extensor tendon of fingers

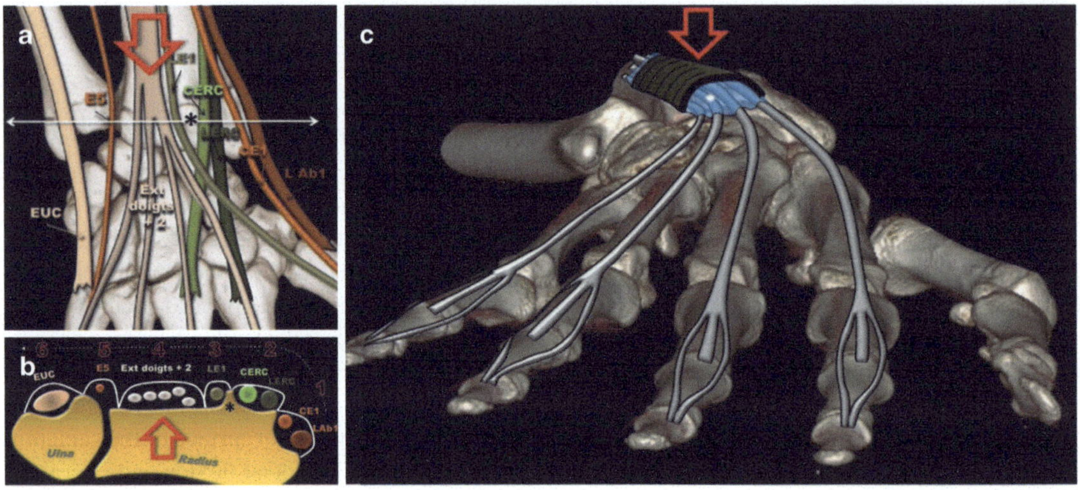

Fig. 19.2 The retinaculum of the extensor tendons and the fourth compartment (red arrow). (**a**) Scheme in dorsal view. (**b**) Axial cut according to the arrow; (**c**) extensor tendons in their retinaculum and synovial sheath (blue)

- These characteristics: small size, the presence of different stabilization and anchoring structures and frequent variants make the imaging of extensor tendons more delicate than that of flexor tendons.
- The purpose of this work, limited to this aspect of the extensor tendons of the fingers, is to try, by explaining their anatomy, to simplify their imaging. Indeed, the morphology of each region of the extensor tendons, of each of their anchoring or stabilization structures obeys an unstoppable logic. Their appearance in ultrasound (E°) or MRI is characteristic, and their pathologies are most often summed up to a unique condition with the typical appearance [4].

19.2 Normal and Pathological Imaging of the Five

19.2.1 Anchoring and Stabilization Formations of the Extensor Tendons

The retinaculum of the fourth dorsal compartment of the wrist provides a particularly strong first proximal anchor.

The function of the dorsal retinacular complex of the wrist is to secure to the antebrachial skeleton the twelve tendons that manage the extension of the wrist, long fingers and thumb, divided into six compartments.

The fourth of these compartments (Fig. 19.2), that of the extensor tendons of the fingers, contains the dividing strips of the common extensor tendon of the fingers as well as, usually, the proper extensor tendon from the index finger, which travels along the ulnar edge of the common extensor tendon of that finger. The proper extensor tendon of the fifth finger occupies the fifth compartment alone.

The retinaculum in the fourth compartment is wider and stronger than its neighbors. It firmly plates the extensor tendons of the fingers against the skeleton, including during dorsal flexion or lateral inclination of the wrist. Under the retinaculum of the fourth compartment, the extensor tendons of the fingers are surrounded by a common synovial sheath. It is limited to the length of the retinaculum and only slightly overflows upstream and downstream. There is no synovial sheath on the back of the hand nor on the back of the finger.

19.2.1.1 Normal Imaging

On an E° or MRI axial section, extensor tendons are flattened oval structures arranged between skin and skeleton. In E°, each tendon, hyperE° and subject to anisotropy, can be detected by mobilizing the corresponding finger in isolation. All these extensor tendons have the same appearance and more or less the same size.

The retinaculum that straps them is a hyperE° or hypointense band, slightly thicker than the neighbors. In the normal state, no peritendinous effusion or synovial membrane is visible.

Frequent anatomical variants are visible in E° or MRI.

19.2.1.2 Main Pathologies

They are not specific:

- Microtraumatic or rheumatic tenosynovitis can be complicated by intratendinous cysts or even ruptures.
- Ectopic muscular body descending too low (especially that of the extensor of the index finger) causing a congestion that hinders the functioning of the compartment.
  - Direct tendon trauma.
  - Fracture sequelae of the distal end of the radius that can transform the dorsal cortex of the radius, normally smooth, into a fractured surface that grates the tendons.

19.2.2 On the Back of the Hand, Intertendinous Connections Transform Four Independent Strips into a Plexiform Structure

At the exit of the retinaculum, the extensor tendons continue on the back of the carpus and then the metacarpals.

Just upstream of the metacarpophalangeal joints, three intertendinous fibrous connections, each called "juncturae tendinum" or "connexus intertendinei," anatomically and functionally unite the extensor tendons (Fig. 19.3). These junctions coordinate the action of the tendons, redistribute their forces, and contribute to their steady stabilization when flexing the fingers (Figs. 19.3 and 19.4) [2, 5]. It is understood that a plexus is inherently more stable than four independent tendons.

Like the tendons they unite, the junctions are subject to many anatomical variations. Usually, the one that connects the tendons of the second and third finger is flattened, a kind of membrane leaving the proper extensor of the index finger free. Those that connect the common extensor tendons of the third and the fourth fingers and those of the fourth and fifth fingers are ligamentous and most often concern the proper extensor tendon of the fifth finger, when it exists.

The juncturae tendinum which, with extended fingers, sit upstream of the metacarpophalangeal joints, move distally during flexion and come onto the back of the latter, thus contributing to the stability of the tendons [2].

These fibrous junctions are of great importance in the clinic: they can mask a tendon lesion or even be a source of snap by subluxation on a MCP [3].

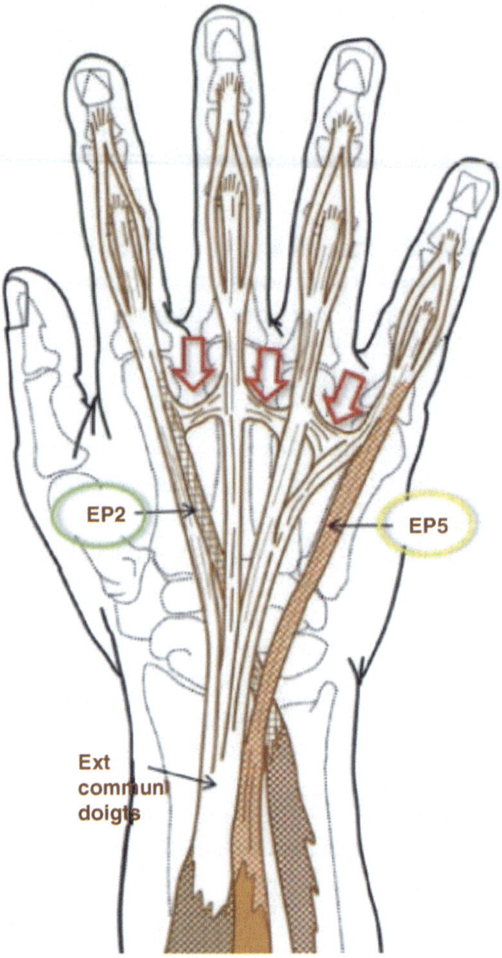

Fig. 19.3 Common and proper extensor tendons of fingers and their *juncturae tendinum* (red arrows)

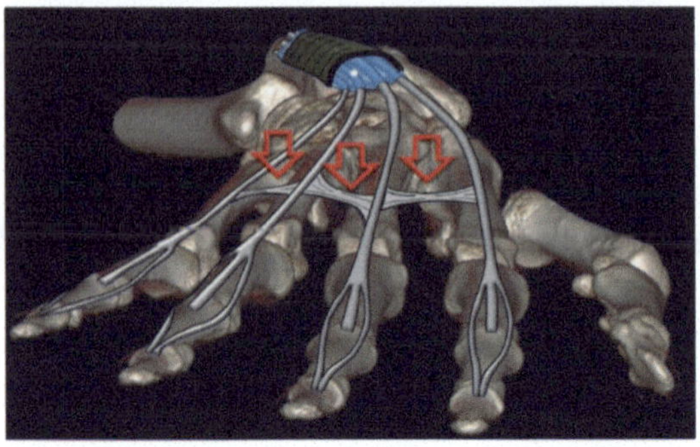

Fig. 19.4 The *juncturae tendinum* (gray, red arrows)

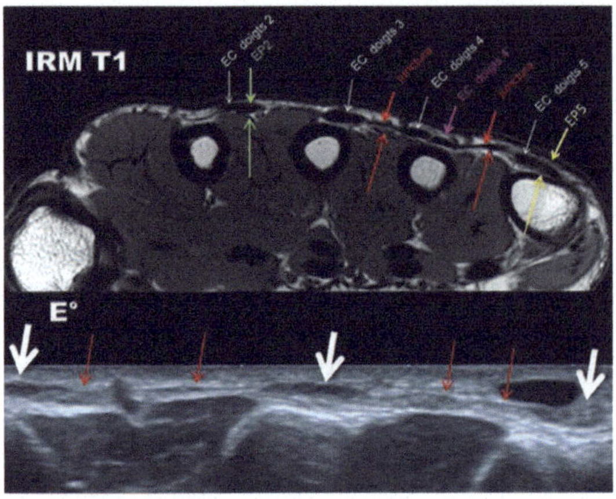

Fig. 19.5 Normal appearance of juncturae tendinum in axial sections MRI T1 and E° (white arrows)

19.2.2.1 Normal Imaging

With current devices, the MRI or E° axial analysis of these structures has reached a high degree of accuracy but not yet the absolute character of direct vision. Normal juncturae tendinum are presented as thin linear structures parallel to the skin, stretched obliquely between extensor tendons, immediately upstream of the MCP (Fig. 19.5).

19.2.2.2 Main Pathologies

- These are ruptures, tears or traumatic sections. They are characterized by thickening and irregularity of the fibrous junction (Fig. 19.6).

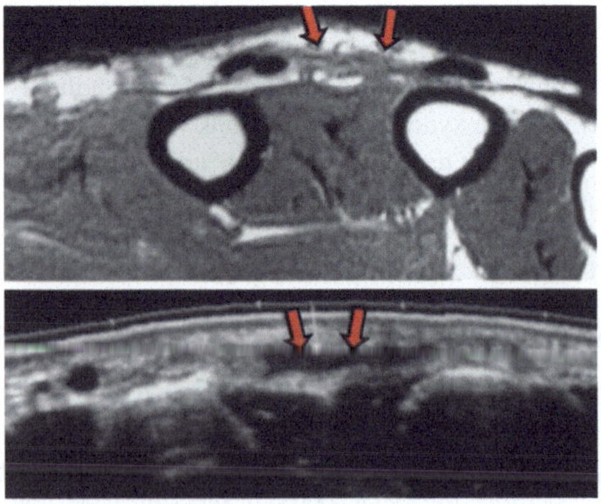

Fig. 19.6 Tear of the intertendinous junction between the second and third extensor tendons in axial section E° and MRI T1 (red arrows)

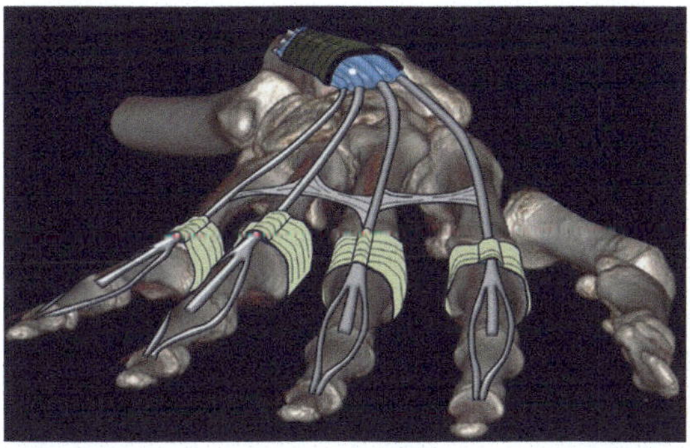

Fig. 19.7 Sagittal bands (pale green)

These tears are rarely isolated. They most often accompany a lesion of the following anchoring system, placed more distally: the sagittal bands.

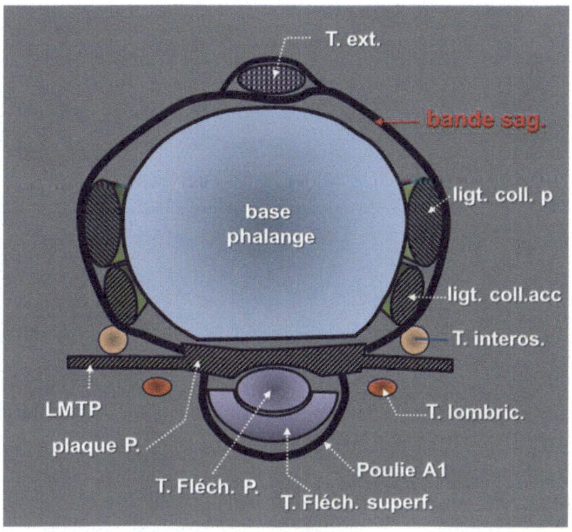

Fig. 19.8 Sagittal bands (red arrows). Axial cut through MCP

19.2.3 Sagittal Bands Are a Powerful Strap that Keeps the Extensor Tendons on the Back of the MCPs

The crossing of MCP is a critical area for extensor tendons. To remain tense and effective, they must remain in equilibrium at the top of the peak represented by the back of the metacarpal heads, especially when flexing the fingers (Fig. 19.9). A simple system of bands: the sagittal bands allow this tour de force. These are two fibrous bands that are born from the palmar plate. They rise in a sagittal plane on either side of the metacarpal head which they flank laterally. On the dorsal side of this, each band is split into two layers: a superficial layer that passes over the extensor tendon and a deep layer that passes underneath. By joining, these layers tie the extensor tendon [6, 7] and fix it at the top of the head forming an arch, a periarticular circular shroud (Figs. 19.7 and 19.8) [6, 7]. If there are two extensor tendons, these, united by a small fibrous tract, are both covered by the sagittal bands [6].

19.2.3.1 Normal Imaging

The dorsal part of the sagittal bands is perfectly visible on current E° and MRI in the form of two thin hypoE° (anisotropy) or hypointense bands that run along the back of the metacarpal head and surround the tendon (Fig. 19.9). Their deep, intermetacarpal part is difficult to see in E° but better visible in MRI.

In dynamic E°, when the patient strongly flexes his/her metacarpophalangeal joint and/or when the operator's finger or probe pushes the tendon laterally, the tendon should remain firmly encamped at the top of the peak (Fig. 19.9), without falling into the adjacent valley.

19.2.4 Main Pathologies

The tearing or distension of a sagittal band as a result of repeated microtrauma (sometimes on an underlying osteophyte) or a single macro-trauma (punch) sums up the essence of their pathology.

This rupture allows the contralateral (sub) luxation of the extensor tendon, usually on the ulnar side ("boxer's knuckle") (Fig. 19.10). Clinically, an MCP (usually the third or fifth) has a bulky dorsal face and its full extension is impossible. The injured sagittal band (usually the radial) is thickened, disorganized, hypoE°, and hyperemic to Doppler. The extensor tendon dis-

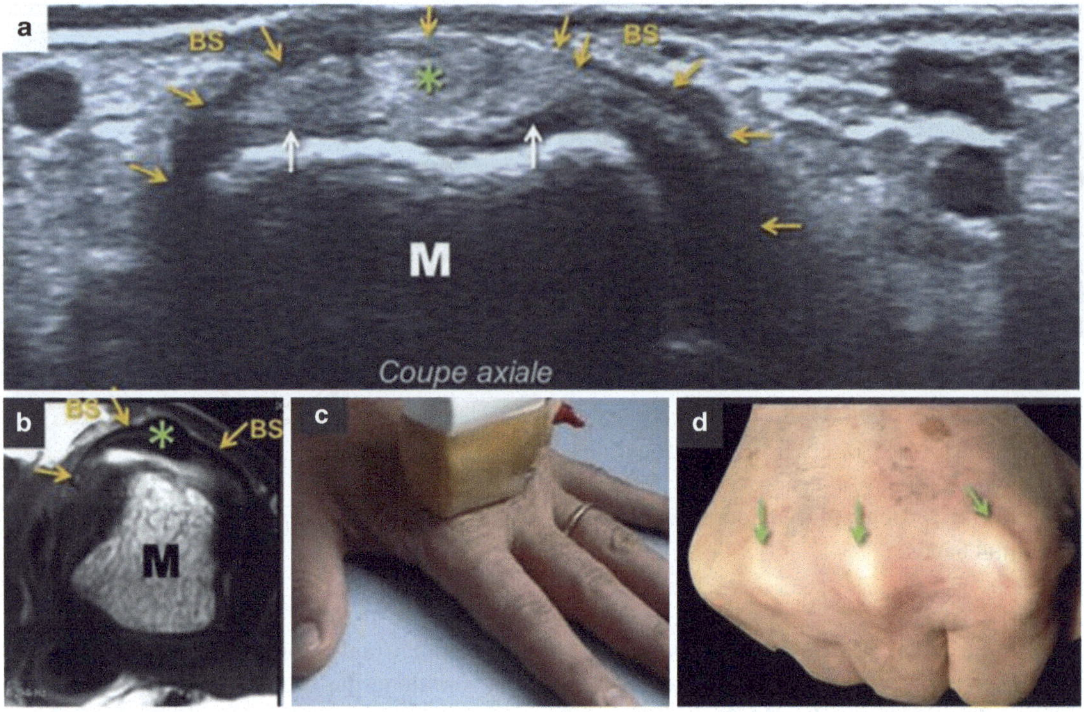

Fig. 19.9 Normal sagittal bands (yellow arrows). Axial cuts E (**a**) and MRI T1 (**b**); (**c**) position of the E° probe. (**d**) Protrusion of tendons with a closed fist (green arrows)

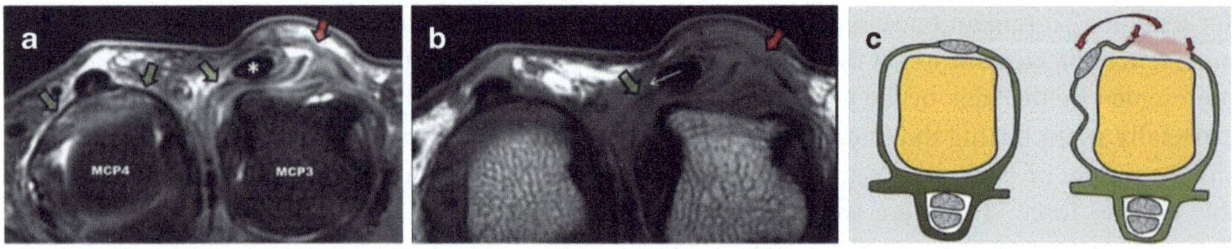

Fig. 19.10 "Boxer's knuckle" by rupture of the radial sagittal band (red arrow), with ulnar subluxation of the extensor tendon (asterisk). Axial MRI T1 and T2 (**a**, **b**); (**c**) diagram

located on the opposite side when flexing the fingers and falls into the valley that separates two metacarpal heads (Figs. 19.10 and 19.11).

If there are two extensor tendons, there may be rupture of the fibrous tract that connects the two tendons, each of them dislocated on either side of the head.

In case of incomplete or chronic lesion of a sagittal band, there is no dislocation of the tendon, and the damage is reduced to swelling of the dorsal surface of the MCP ("preboxer's knuckle").

19.2.5 The Interosseous Hood Is a Delicate Shroud that Covers the Base of P1 and the Extensor Tendon by Connecting the Dorsal and Palmar Tendon Apparatus

The distal insertion of the interosseous muscles is twofold:

- Lateral part of the base of P1 by a small tendon that serves to spread and bring fingers closer.

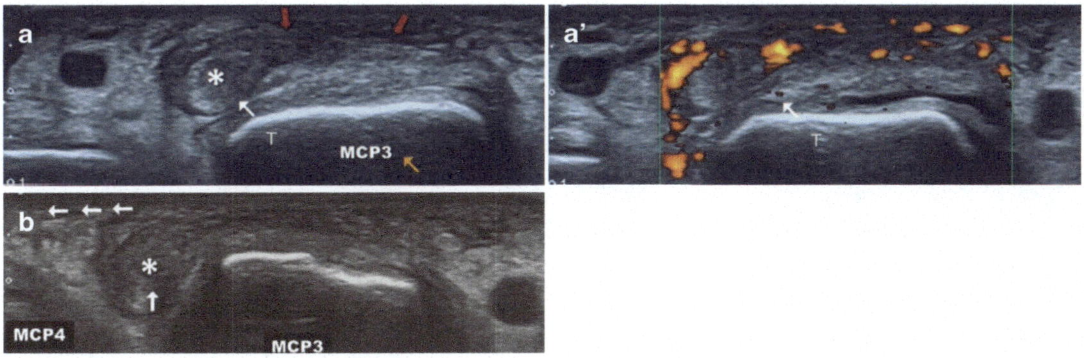

Fig. 19.11 Analogous case of "boxer's knuckle" in another patient. Axial E° at rest (**a**, **a'**) and closed fist (**b**). Thick radial sagittal band, hypoechoic and hyperemic (red arrow). Subluxation of the tendon (asterisk) becomes complete with a closed fist

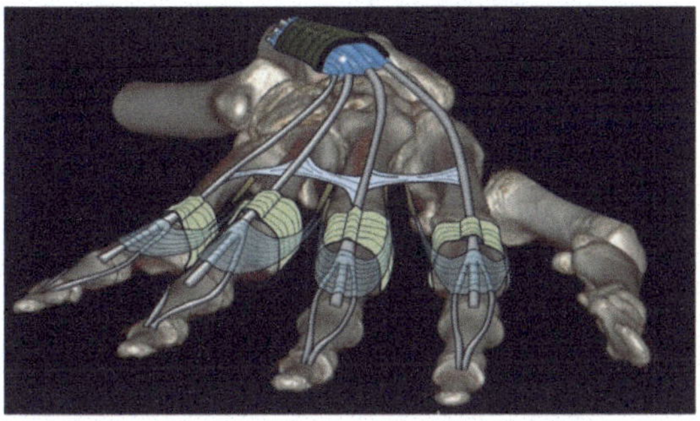

Fig. 19.12 The interosseous hood (in pale blue)

- Extensor tendon by two fibrous lamina, one of which is inserted on the median strip of this tendon, the other a little more distally on its lateral band. Both rejoin their counterpart on the back of the extensor tendon: this set, called the "interosseous hood," extends the sagittal lamina forward (Figs. 19.12, 19.13, and 19.14).

The lumbrical tendons also emit a small fibrous lamina that joins that of the interosseous and participates in the hood (Fig. 19.12).

19.2.5.1 Normal Imaging

The back, very thin, is visible on an MRI of very good quality or on an E° made with a high-performance material: very thin line HypoE° or hypointensity extending the extensor tendon laterally at the height of P1.

19.2.5.2 Pathology

This is a partial or complete rupture, usually associated with a lesion of the sagittal band.

These stabilizing systems mean that, in the event of rupture, the retraction of the extensor tendons remains moderate, unlike the flexor tendons (Fig. 19.15).

19.2.6 A Sophisticated Enthesis Consisting of a System of Bands

When we imagine an extensor system of one finger, we readily see an extensor tendon that runs straight ahead to the base of P3, in the process leaving behind a deep strip for the base of P2.

As with flexor tendons nature has retained a less simplistic model, quite similarly for reasons of mechanical efficiency and/or overcrowding [4]: at the height of P1, the extensor tendon splits into three strands:

- A median strip that fits on the back of the base of P2.
- Two side strips that bypass the distal interphalangeal joint by the sides to join on the back of P2 and then merge into a terminal strip that fits on the base of P3 (Fig. 19.16).

This anatomical layout explains the two main pathologies encountered at this level : the "mallet finger" and the "boutonniere finger."

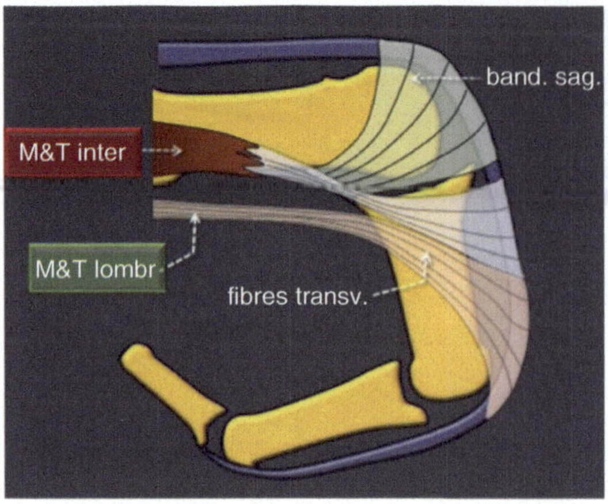

Fig. 19.13 The interosseous hood (in purple and beige). Diagram in side view *(inspired by 6)*

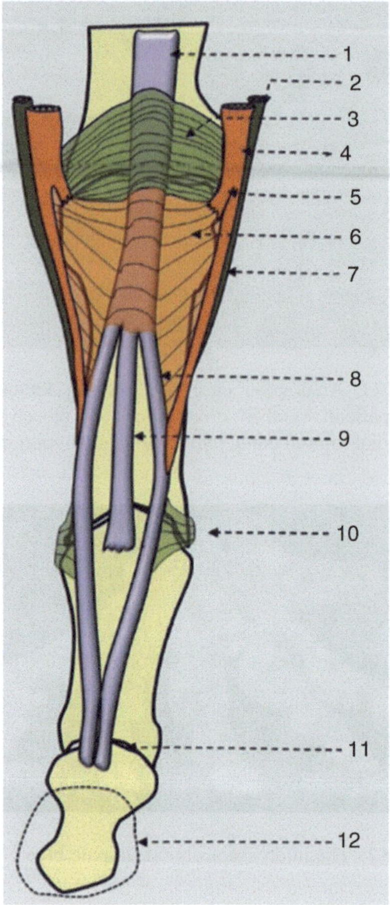

Fig. 19.14 The interosseous hood (in orange). Dorsal view. (1) extensor tendon; (2) lumbrical tendon; (3) sagittal band; (4) distal interosseous tendon (IOT); (5) division of the IOT going toward the lateral process of the phalangeal base; (6) interosseous hood; (7) division of the IOT going toward the lateral strip of the extensor tendon; (8) lateral strip of the extensor tendon; (9) median strip of extensor tendon; (10) transverse retinacular ligament; (11) extensor tendon terminal strip

19.2.6.1 Normal Imaging

Despite their small size, these strips are currently visible on good ultrasonography and MRI in the form of flattened structures in axial section and fine tracts in longitudinal sections.

19.2.6.2 Main Pathologies

"Mallet Finger"

The "mallet finger" (so called because of its shape) corresponds to the closed traumatic rupture of the terminal strip of the extensor tendon or the avulsion of its bone insertion on the dorsal surface of P3 (Fig. 19.17). Imbalance of forces to the benefit of flexor tendons leads to a flexion of the distal interphalangeal joint (hence the mallet shape) and a deficit of its active extension [8]. Diagnosis of this condition is clinical. An X-ray of the profile finger looks for bone tearing (Fig. 19.17). The E°, not always indispensable, shows a complete or partial discontinuity of the distal strip of the extensor, replaced by a hypoE° area and a retracted and thickened tendon stump (Fig. 19.17) [9]. Treatment is conservative.

19.2.6.3 "Boutonniere" Finger

This is the rupture of the median strip of the extensor or the tearing out of its insertion on the dorsal side of P2 (Fig. 19.18). This solution of continuity of the medial band causes a transfer of the force of the extensor tendon onto the lateral bands. As a result, they tend to take the cord and migrate to the palmar region of the proximal interphalangeal joint [7], resulting in a flexion blockage of the proximal interphalangeal joint (Fig. 19.18). This vicious attitude is quickly fixed by the retraction of transverse and oblique retinacular ligaments (Fig. 19.14), small fibrous structures connecting the lateral strips of the extensor tendon to the palmar face of the joint and comparable to the sagittal bands of

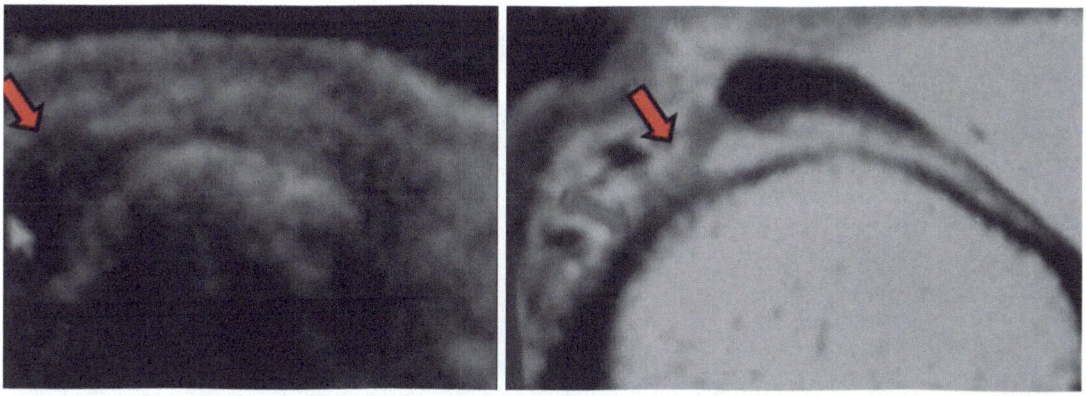

Fig. 19.15 Rupture of the backrest of the interosseous. E° and MRI T1 axial (red arrow)

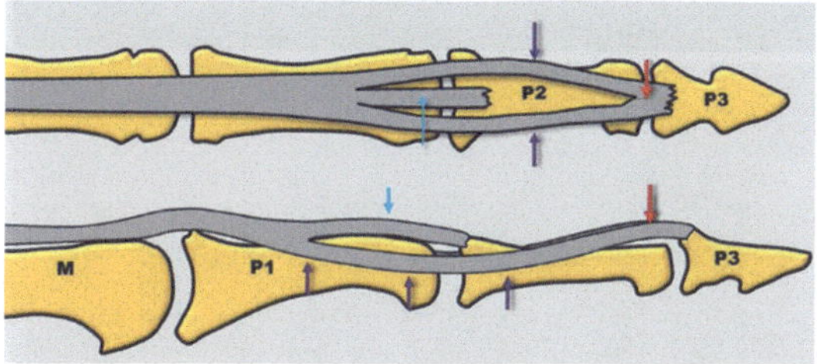

Fig. 19.16 Anatomic disposition of extensor tendon termination. Middle strip: blue arrow; side strips: purple arrow; terminal strip: red arrow

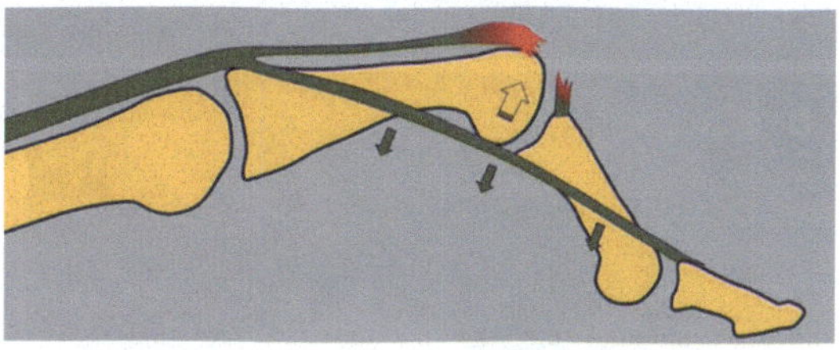

Fig. 19.18 "Boutonniere" finger mechanism

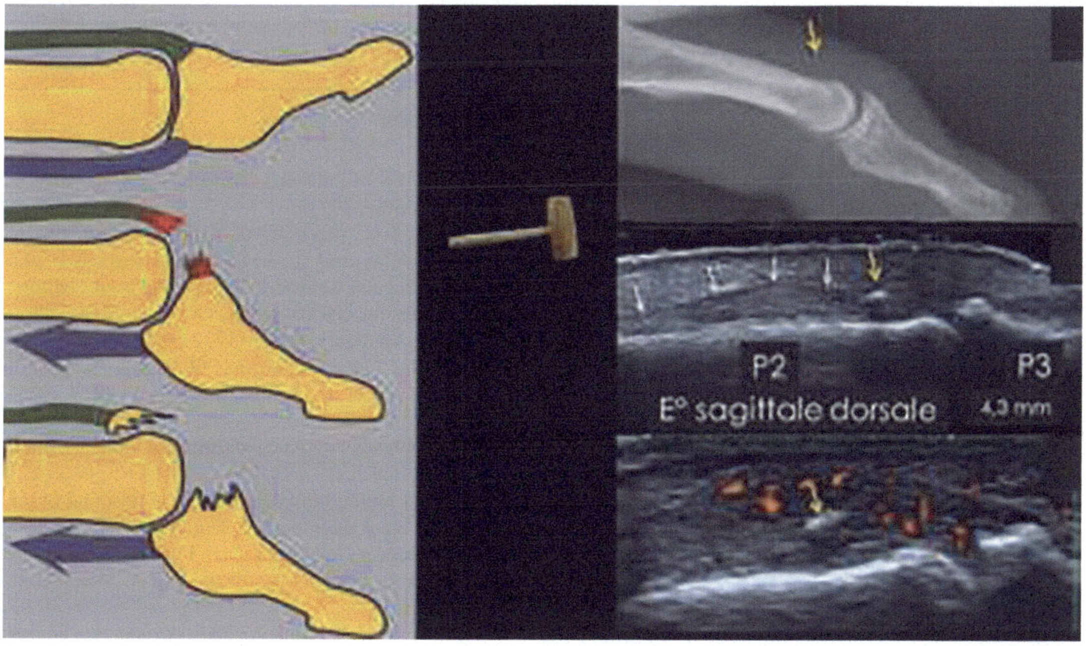

Fig. 19.17 On the right: "mallet finger" and its two varieties: pulling the tendon or avulsion of a bone fragment. Left: X-ray and sagittal ultrasonography of a case with avulsion (yellow arrow). Tendon retracted stump: white arrows

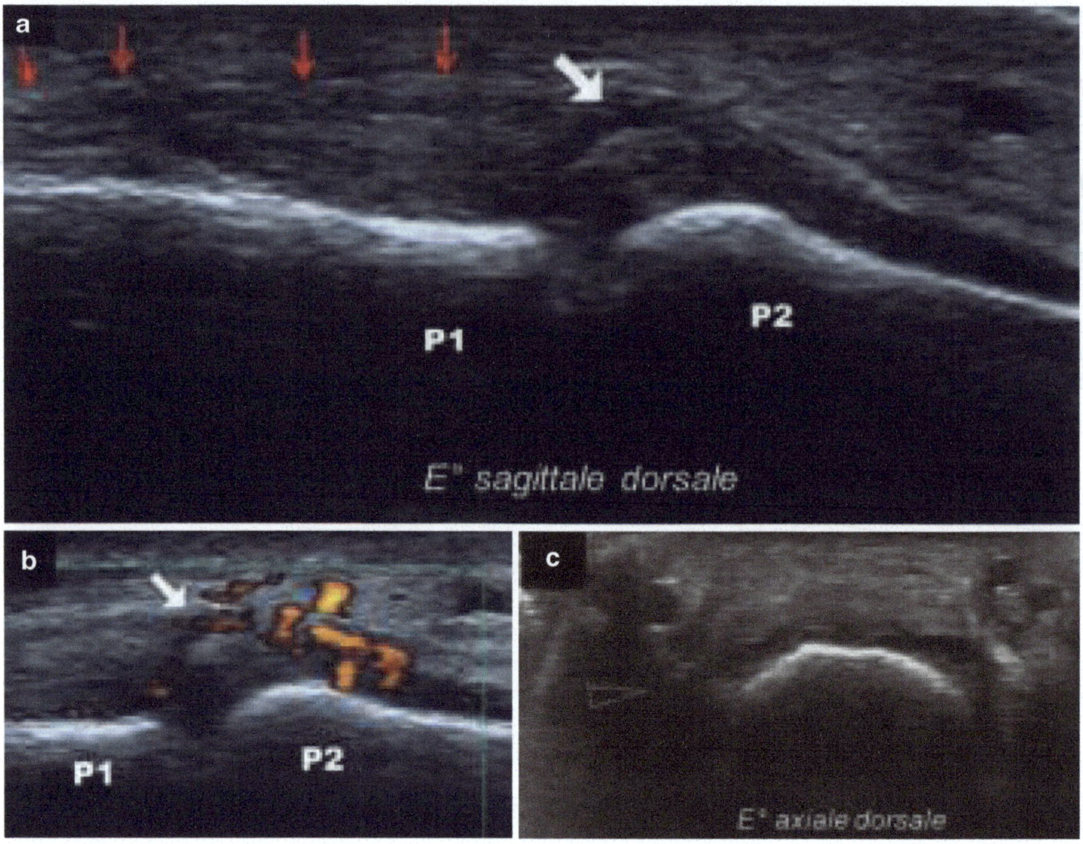

Fig. 19.19 (**a**) Boutonniere finger by breaking the median band. (**b**) E° sagittal. Thickened median strip, hypoechoic and hyperemic. (**c**) E° axial. Disappearance of the median strip. Palmar migration of the lateral bands (arrows heads)

MCP. Objective imaging shows a complete or partial discontinuity of the median strip of the extensor to the dorsal face of P1, replaced by a hypoE° area and a retracted and thickened tendon stump. The palmar migration of the side strips can be seen in ultrasonography or in MRI (Fig. 19.19).

19.3 Conclusion

A series of five anatomical structures in series was nature's elegant, efficient, and aesthetic response to the delicate biomechanical problem of the balance of extensor tendons.

Each of the structures which constitute it has a logical purpose and anatomy, a known semiology and a limited pathology that is characteristic and easy to search in E° or MRI.

References

1. Kapandji IA. Joint physiology, fascicle 1. 4th ed. Paris: Maloine; 1973.
2. Demondion X, Wavreille G, Canella C, Budzik JF, Fontaine C, Cotton A. Anatomy and variants of the appareil finger extensor. In: Drapé JL, et al., editors. Wrist and hand, Getroa-gel opus XXXVI. Montpellier: Sauramps Medical; 2009. p. 17–23.
3. Clavero JA, Golanó P, Fariñas O, Alomar X, Monill JM, Esplugas M. Extensor mechanism of the fingers: MR imaging—anatomic correlation. Radiographics. 2003;23:593–611. https://doi.org/10.1148/rg.233025079.
4. Morvan G, Vuillemin V, Guerini H. Ultrasound of the wrist and hand. Montpellier: Sauramps; 2017.
5. Von Schroeder HP, Boot MJ. Functional anatomy of the extensor tendons of the digits. Hand Clin. 1997;13:51–62.
6. Theumann NH, Pfirrmann CWA, Drape JL, Trudell DJ, Resnick D. MR imaging of the metacarpophalangeal joints of the fingers. Part I. Conventional MR

imaging and MR arthrographic findings in corpses. Radiology. 2002;222:437–45.
7. Without N, Lapègue F, Jacob D. Musculoskeletal ultrasound. Paris: Elsevier Masson; 2014.
8. Alla SR, Deal ND, Dempsey IJ. Current concepts: mallet finger. Hand. 2014;9:138–44. https://doi.org/10.1007/s11552-014-9609-y.
9. Kleinbaum Y, Heyman Z, Ganel A, et al. Sonographic imaging of mallet finger. Ultraschall Med. 2005;26:223–6.

20 Ultrasound of the Metacarpophalangeal Joint of the Thumb

B. Bordet, J. Borne, A. Ponsot, P. -F. Chaillot, and O. Fantino

20.1 Introduction

Sprain of the metacarpophalangeal joint (MCP) of the thumb is common. The "gamekeeper thumb" of the Anglo-Saxons today also called "skiing thumb" accounts for 6% of the skier's trauma.

In case of rupture of the ulnar collateral ligament (UCL) of the thumb, the presence of a Stener effect prevents effective healing, which progresses to chronic instability and long-term osteoarthritis [1, 2].

Stener's lesion requires surgical repair, and its diagnosis is therefore essential to guide management [3–6].

20.2 Anatomopathological Reminders, Classification, and Treatment

20.2.1 Anatomy and Stener Lesion

The ulnar collateral ligament of the thumb consists of two bundles:

B. Bordet (✉) · J. Borne · A. Ponsot · P. -F. Chaillot
O. Fantino
Imaging Service, Clinique du Parc, Lyon, France

- Metacarpophalangeal main ligament
- Sesamoid phalangeal accessory ligament

The adductor muscle of the thumb has a main distal enthesis on the medial sesamoid. From there it also gives a thin aponeurotic band, the aponeurotic expansion of the adductor of the thumb (AEA), which comes to cross the UCL at its surface and end in a fan on the long extensor of the thumb (Fig. 20.1).

During the flexion-extension maneuvers of the MCP of the thumb, the AEA glides freely in contact with the UCL. In a sprain with ligamentous rupture, the AEA may be incarcerated under the proximal ligament stump and pushed back to prevent possible healing. This is the Stener lesion (Fig. 20.2) [2].

20.2.2 Lesion Classification of Ulnar Sprains of MCP [7, 8]

- Type I: fracture of ulnar edge of undisplaced P1 base
- Type II: fracture of the ulnar edge of the displaced P1 base (displacement of more than 2 mm, joint incongruence, and/or rotation of the fragment)
- Type III: stable ligament rupture
- Type IV: unstable ligament rupture. Stener effect

T. Apard, J. L. Brasseur (eds.), *Ultrasonography for the Upper Limb Surgeon*,
https://doi.org/10.1007/978-3-030-84234-5_20

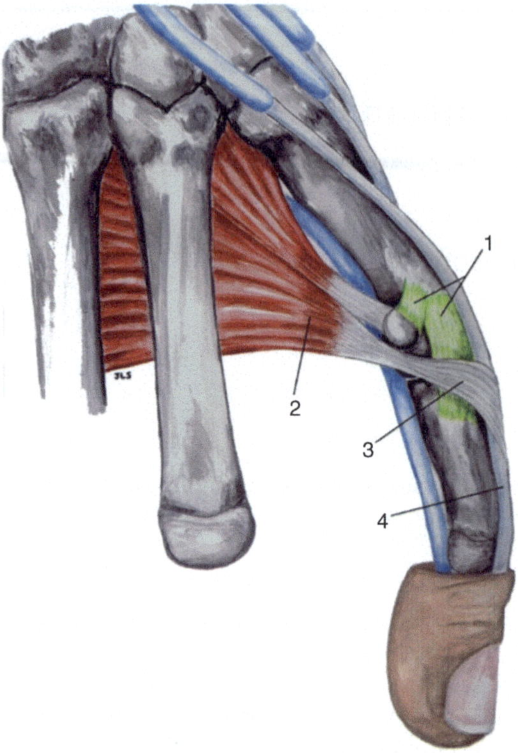

Fig. 20.1 Back view of the hand: deep dissection. (*1*) Ulnar collateral ligament (UCL) with a metacarpophalangeal main bundle and a sesamoid metacarpal accessory bundle. (*2*) Adductor muscle of the thumb. (*3*) Aponeurotic expansion adductor (AEA). (*4*) Long extensor tendon of the thumb

- Type V: fracture of P1 at the enthesis of the palmar plate
- Type VI: fracture of ulnar edge of base P1 (displaced or not) and ligamentous rupture

20.2.3 Cure

Conservative treatment is the rule in case of a mild sprain; it consists of 4 weeks of immobility in a thermomoulded splint [9].

Surgical treatment is conventionally indicated in the presence of major laxity or if X-rays detect a displaced bone fragment [10, 11].

However, these concepts are sometimes discussed; in fact several studies have shown that conservative treatment achieves good results even in case of severe sprain with or without displaced fracture [12, 13], and the only formal surgical indication would be the Stener lesion.

20.3 Imaging

20.3.1 Simple X-Rays

They remain indispensable and must include a workup of the thumb column of the front and profile.

The classical avulsion fracture of the ulnar edge of the phalangeal epiphysis at the distal enthesis of the UCL (Fig. 20.3) will be investigated.

If surgical treatment is indicated, then the imaging workup is sufficient, the ligament status being specified by the surgeon. It should be borne in mind that a fracture does not eliminate ligament rupture (type VI). A fracture with good prognosis that is not or is slightly displaced may be associated with a Stener lesion [8].

In the acute stage, valgus X-rays remain unreliable given the patient's apprehension and pain and potentially harmful [14, 15] in the literature.

20.3.2 Magnetic Resonance Imaging [13, 16–18]

MRI is able to show whether the ligament rupture is displaced; it identifies a nodular image in hyposignal T2 applied in contact with the ulnopalmar side of the metacarpal head. Often compared to a "yoyo on its string" or "cauliflower," this rounded structure corresponds to the proximal stump pushed back by the AEA and indicates the presence of a Stener effect (Fig. 20.4).

In practice, MRI, although effective, is still not widely used in France at the acute stage given the examination time.

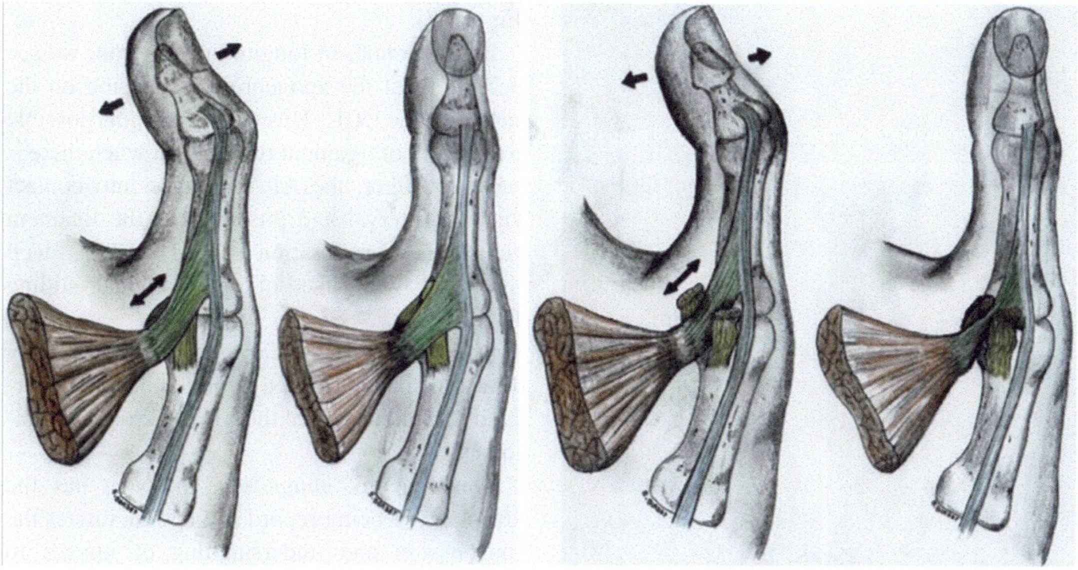

Fig. 20.2 Kinematics of aponeurotic expansion adductor (AEA). Flexion-extension of the IP with physiological sliding in healthy subjects from AEA to the surface of the UCL. In the event of rupture of the UCL with Stener effect, the AEA is incarcerated at contact with the interval, loss of physiological sliding; the AEA pushes back the UCL

20.3.3 Ultrasound [19–29]

Ultrasound is a powerful examination for the diagnosis of UCL ruptures and for the identification of a Stener effect.

The examination shall be carried out with a high-frequency probe preferably "golf" type and shall include dynamic maneuvers [25].

Ultrasound examination explores the main beam of the UCL very well in longitudinal sections along the axis of the ligament fibers.

We will look for a thickened, infiltrated hypoechogenic ligament with loss of fibrillar physiological appearance. The operator will look for loss of ligament continuity, bone avulsion at enthesis, and signs of hyperemia at power Doppler mode (Fig. 20.5).

20.3.3.1 Valgus Maneuver

Using their free hand, the operator performs valgus movements of the MCP to test the UCL. In this way, in longitudinal sections, the operator seeks rupture by visualizing the loss of continuity of ligament fibers. If the ligament remains continuous, the operator evaluates its distension, studies its infiltration, and uses the power Doppler to look for signs of pain (Fig. 20.6).

20.3.3.2 Flexion-Extension Maneuver of IP

This is the fundamental maneuver to search for a Stener effect. The operator performs passive flexion-extension movements of the interphalangeal joint of the thumb. The metacarpophalangeal joint of the thumb remains motionless under the probe, but the maneuver sets the AEA in motion

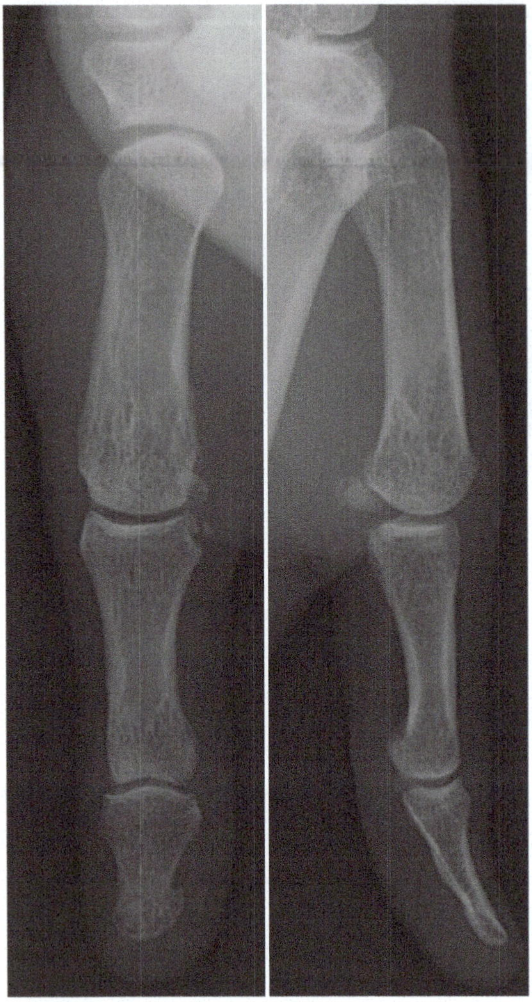

Fig. 20.3 X-ray of the thumb face and profile. Avulsion fracture of ulnar angle of base of P1

via the long extensor tendon of the thumb (Fig. 20.7).

In ultrasound, in longitudinal section, we see the sliding of the aponeurotic expansion on the surface of the UCL. This sliding remains possible in the event of ligament rupture, but when there is a Stener effect, the AEA plunges into contact with the interval and pushes back the ligament stump. Its incarceration in the UCL is well visualized with loss of physiological sliding (Fig. 20.8).

Done well, this specific maneuver very quickly allows an inexperienced sonographer to understand the kinematics of the AEA making exploration easier.

This dynamic diagnostic approach has the advantage of being recordable and facilitates the transmission and understanding of images to correspondents.

20.4 Conclusion

The sprain of the UCL of the thumb is a very common trauma with potentially disabling consequences. In case of a Stener effect, surgical repair is required.

Simple X-rays remain the first-line examination for a fracture. If surgical treatment is indicated, there is no indication of complementary imaging.

It is important to remember that a Stener lesion may be associated with a fracture.

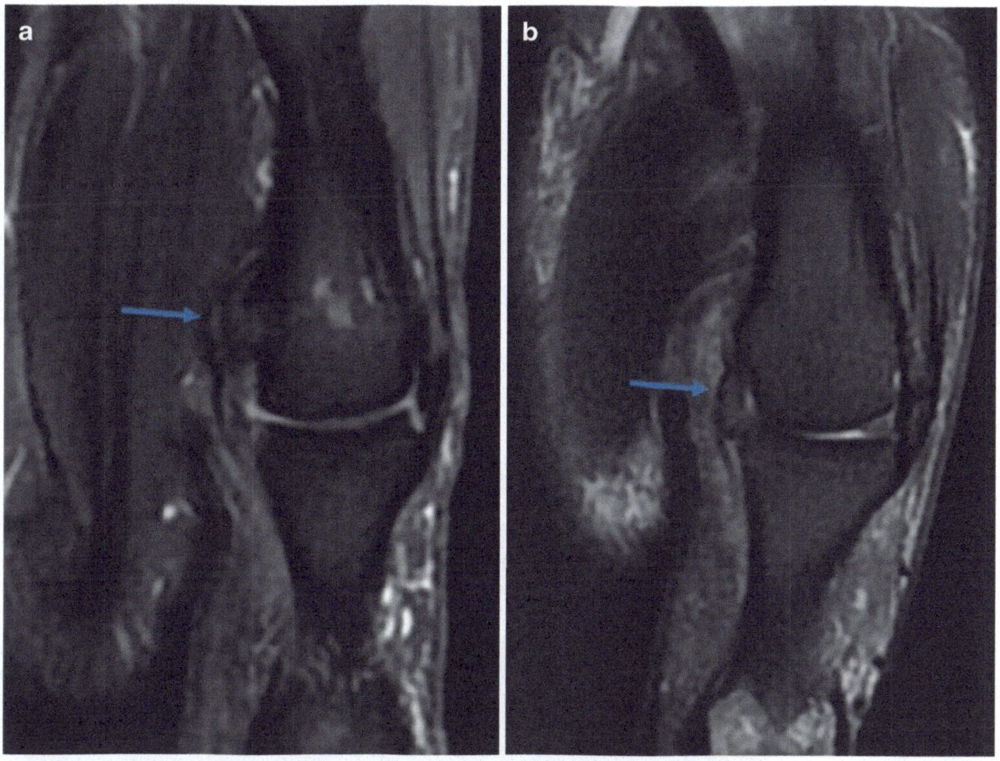

Fig. 20.4 Coronal section MRI of the MCP of the thumb (**a** and **b**). Weighted density of protons with fat erasing technology. Break of the UCL (blue arrow) with retraction of the ligament stump upstream of the line in the example **a**

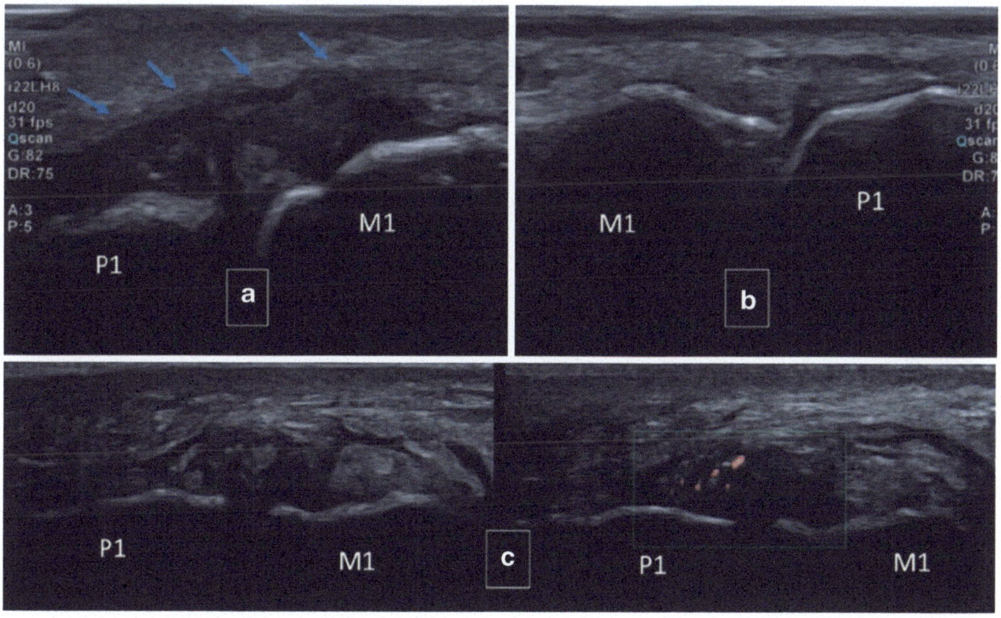

Fig. 20.5 Examples of traumatic injuries of UCL in ultrasound. Thickened, deconstructed, hypoechogenic ligaments with loss of fibrillar appearance (**a**, **c**) compared to normal ligament (**b**). Hyperemia at exploration with power Doppler mode at phalangeal enthesis (**c**)

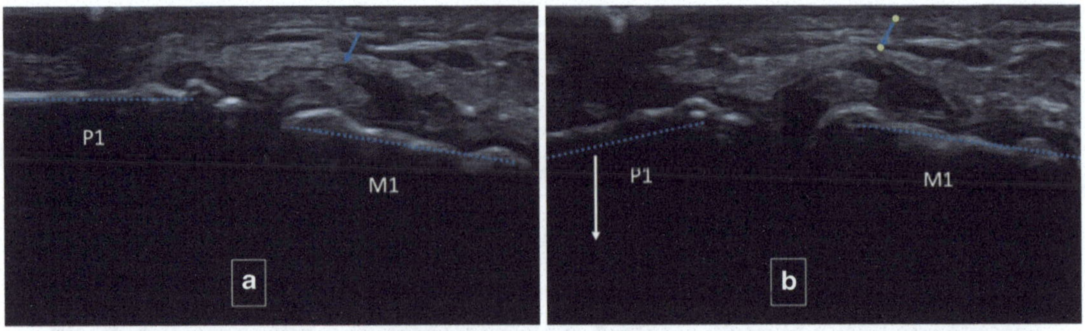

Fig. 20.6 Dynamic valgus maneuver of the MCP. Ligament rupture with retracted ligament upstream of the space. Clear pathological valgus at dynamic exploration (blue lines)

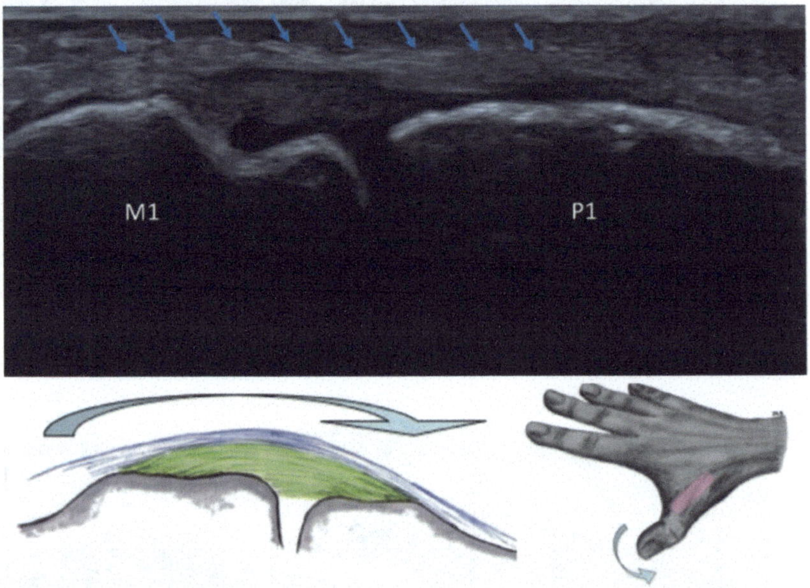

Fig. 20.7 Ultrasound longitudinal section and dynamic flexion-extension maneuver of the IP. The MCP remains motionless. The UCL is stretched from the metacarpal (M1) to the phalangeal base (P1). It is covered on its surface by the AEA (blue arrows). During flexion-extension of the interphalangeal interval (small full arrow), the AEA slides over the ligament (large full arrow)

Dynamic X-rays are poorly performing for fracture diagnosis. Their achievement is often difficult, and they are no longer indicated in the acute stage.

Dynamic ultrasound makes it possible to establish an accurate lesion diagnosis. It evaluates ligament integrity through valgus maneuver and allows the visualization of the Stener effect through the flexion-extension maneuver of the IP. While MRI can also diagnose the presence of a Stener lesion, ultrasound has valuable advantages: its dynamic character, availability, and cost support it as second-line imaging.

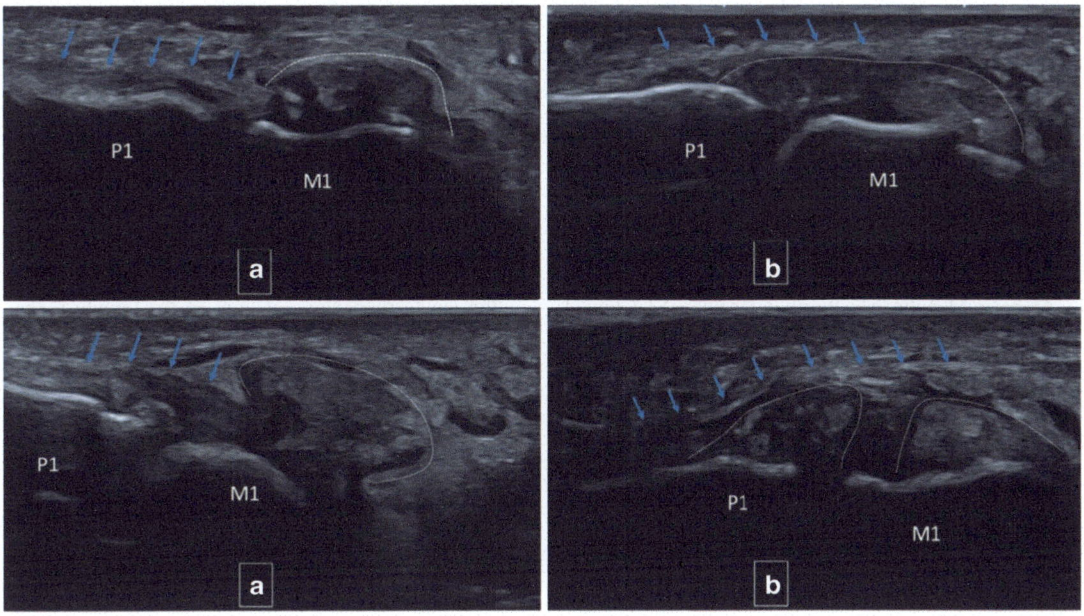

Fig. 20.8 Ultrasound longitudinal cuts. Rupture of the UCL with incarceration of the AEA on the two examples (**a**). The ligament stump is retracted upstream of the interval (white dotted line). Sliding thwarted with the AEA that comes down on the ligament. Severe impairment of UCL (**b**) but without Stener effect. The AEA (blue arrows) remains in physiological position on the surface of the ligament (white dotted line)

References

1. Campbell CS. Gamekeepers thumb. J Bone Joint Surg Br. 1955;37:148–9.
2. Stener B. Displacement of the ruptured ulnar collateral ligament of the metacarpophalangeal joint of the thumb. J Bone Joint Surg Br. 1962;44:869–79.
3. Reikeras O, Kvarnes L. Rupture of the ulnar ligament of the metacarpophalangeal joint of the thumb. Arch Orthop Trauma Surg. 1982;100:175–7.
4. Neviaser RJ, Wilson JN, Leviano A. Rupture of the ulnar collateral ligament of the thumb (gamekeeper's thumb): correction by dynamic repair. J Bone Joint Surg Am. 1971;54:1357–64.
5. Louis DS, Huebner JJ, Hankin FM. Rupture and displacement of the ulnar collateral ligament of the metacarpophalangeal joint of the thumb. J Bone Joint Surg Am. 1986;8:1320–5.
6. Massart P, Bezes H. Severe metacarpophalangeal sprain of the thumb in surgical repairs. In a group of 34 cases of metacarpophalangeal sprains from skiing accidents. Ann Chir Main Memb Super. 1984;3:101–12.
7. Palmer AK, Louis DS. Assessing ulnar instability of the metacarpophalangeal joint of the thumb. J Hand Surg Am. 1978;3(6):542–6.
8. Hintermann B, Holzach PJ, Schütz M, Matter P. Skier's thumb—the significance of bony injuries. Am J Sports Med. 1993;21(6):800–4.
9. Campbell JD, Feagin JA, King P, et al. UinAR collateral ligament injury of the thumb: treatment with glove spica cast. Am J Sports Med. 1992;20:29–30.
10. Heyman P, Gelberman HR, Duncan K, Hipp JA. Injuries of the ulnar collateral ligament of the thumb metacarpophalangeal joint. Clin Orthop. 1993;292:165–71.
11. Moutet F, Lebrun C, Massart P, Guinard D. Sprains of the meacarpophlangian thumb. An experience of more than a thousand cases. Ann Chir Main. 1989:99–109.
12. Kuz JE, Husband JB, Tokar N, McPherson Ltd. Outcome of avulsion fractures of the ulnar base of the proximal phalanx of the thumb treated nonsurgically. J Hand Surg Am. 1999;24(2):275–82.
13. Spaeth HJ, Abrams RA, Bock GW, and *al.* Gamekeeper thumb: differentiation of nondisplaced and displaced tears of the ulnar collateral ligament with MR imaging. Radiology 1993; 188:553–556.
14. Bowers WH, Hurst LC. Gamekeeper's thumb: evaluation by arthroscopy and stress roentgenography. J Bone Joint Surg Am. 1977;59:519–24.
15. Höecker K, Pachucki A. Diagnostik and behandlung der the bandverletzung am daumengrundgetenk. Sportverl Sportschad. 1992;6:165–9.

16. Harper MT, Chandnani VP, Spaeth J, Santangelo JR, Providence BC, Bagg MA. Gamekeeper thumb: diagnosis of ulnar collateral ligament injury using magnetic resonance imaging, magnetic resonance arthrography and stress radiography. J Magn Reson Imaging. 1996;6(2):322–8.
17. Hinke DH, Erickson SJ, Chamoy L, Timins ME. Ulnar collateral ligament of the thumb: MR findings in cadaworms, volunteers, and patients with ligamentous injury (gamekeeper's thumb). RDA Am J Roentgenol. 1994;163(6):1431–4.
18. Mahajan M, Tolman C, Würth B, Rhemrev SJ. Clinical evaluation vs magnetic resonance imaging of the skier's thumb: a prospective cohort of 30 patients. Eur J Radiol. 2016;85(10):1750–6.
19. O'Callaghan BI, Kohut G, Hoogewoud HM. Gamekeeper thumb: identification of the Stener lesion with US. Radiology. 1994;192:477.
20. Jones MH, England SJ, Muwanga CL, Hildreth T. The use of ultrasound in the diagnosis of injuries of the ulnar collateral ligament of the thumb. J Hand Surg (Br). 2000;25(1):29–32.
21. Noszian IM, Dinkhauser LM, Orthner E, Straub GM, Csnady M. Ulnar collateral ligament: differentiation of displaced and nondisplaced tears with US. Radiology. 1995;194:61–3.
22. Ebrahim FS, De Aeseneer M, Jager T, Marcelis S, Jamadar DA, Jacobson JA. US diagnosis of UCL tears of the thumb and stener lesions: technique, pattern-based approach, and differential diagnosis. Radiographics. 2006;26(4):1007–20.
23. Shinohara T, Horii E, Majima M, Nakao E, Suzuki M, Nakamura R, Hirata H. Sonographic diagnosis of acute injuries of the ulnar collateral ligament of the metacarpophalangeal joint of the thumb. J Clin Ultrasound. 2007;35(2):73–7.
24. Hergan K, Mittler C, Oser W. Ulnar collateral ligament: differentiation of displaced and nondisplaced tears with US and MR imaging. Radiology. 1995;194:65–71.
25. Bordet B, Borne J, Fantino O, Pialat JB. Ultrasound of the ulnar collateral ligament (LCU) sprain of the metacarpophalangeal joint of the thumb: a new dynamic maneuver to visualize the Stener effect. J Radiol. 2009;90:217–20.
26. Hergan K, Mittler C, Oser W. Pitfalls in sonography of the Gamekeeper's thumb. Eur Radiol. 1997;7(1):65–9.
27. Melville DM, Jacobson JA, Fessell DP. Ultrasound of the thumb ulnar collateral ligament: technique and pathology. RDA Am J Roentgenol. 2014;202(2):W168.
28. Melville D, Jacobson JA, Haase S, Brandon C, Brigido MK, Fessell D. Ultrasound of displaced ulnar collateral ligament tears of the thumb: the Stener lesion revisited. Skeletal Radiol. 2013;42(5):667–73.
29. Bordet B, Fantino O, Borne J. Dynamic ultrasound of the Stener lesion. In: Drape JL, et al, editors. Wrist and hand. Getroa-Gel Opus XXXVI. Montpellier: Sauramps Médical; 2009. pp. 491–500.

Ultrasound of the Nail

21

Thomas Apard and R. Baran

The diagnostic approach in onychology is always fundamentally based on anamnesis (professional activity, medication intake, systemic disease) and clinic examination (general nail shape, nail surface, subungual fasteners, perionychium, chromonychia) [1]. Medical imaging is always made up of the standard radiography of the distal phalanx. MRI is now the examination of choice because the nail does not need a dynamic and comparative examination, two of the main qualities of ultrasound. However, ultrasound is still cheaper and more accessible than MRI and can thus allow immediate diagnosis in consultation. The advent of ultrahigh-frequency probes allows the complete examination of the ungual complex.

21.1 Ultrasound Anatomy of the Nail (Fig. 21.1)

The nail is visualized in its entirety in ultrasound [2]: from its proximal end that emerges from an invagination that has as its roof the deep surface of the supra-ungual fold that ends with the cuticle at its distal end or free edge.

The nail matrix consists of two parts: the proximal part that produces the superficial layers of the nail (about 33% of the thickness) and the distal part that ends with the lunule and produces the median layers (about 50% of the thickness). The rest of the layers (27%) come from the nail bed. The thickness of the nail is conditioned by the thickness of the matrix. A large lunule (as physiologically on the thumb or pathologically in onychotillomania) is accompanied by a thicker shelf.

The distal interphalangeal joint is easy to spot. It is limited dorsally by the capsule and the insertion of the extensor apparatus. Passive mobilization of the distal phalanx in flexion allows the tendon fibers to be well identified.

Cortical bone (and osteophytes) stops ultrasound. It is impossible to explore intraosseous pathologies with ultrasound.

Vascularization of the nail is studied in power Doppler mode (Fig. 21.1c) [3]. The two arches under the proximal and distal ungual are perfectly visualized. Hand warmth (heat of the room or vascular pathology such as arteritis or Raynaud's syndrome) is an important factor to consider. Be careful not to press with the probe.

21.2 Ultrasound Examination in Practice

The hand should be flat on a piece of paper (paper from the roll of the examination table) with the fingers stuck together so that the gel

T. Apard (✉)
Hand Sonosurgery Center, Versailles, France

R. Baran
Nail Diseases Center, Cannes, France

T. Apard, J. L. Brasseur (eds.), *Ultrasonography for the Upper Limb Surgeon*,
https://doi.org/10.1007/978-3-030-84234-5_21

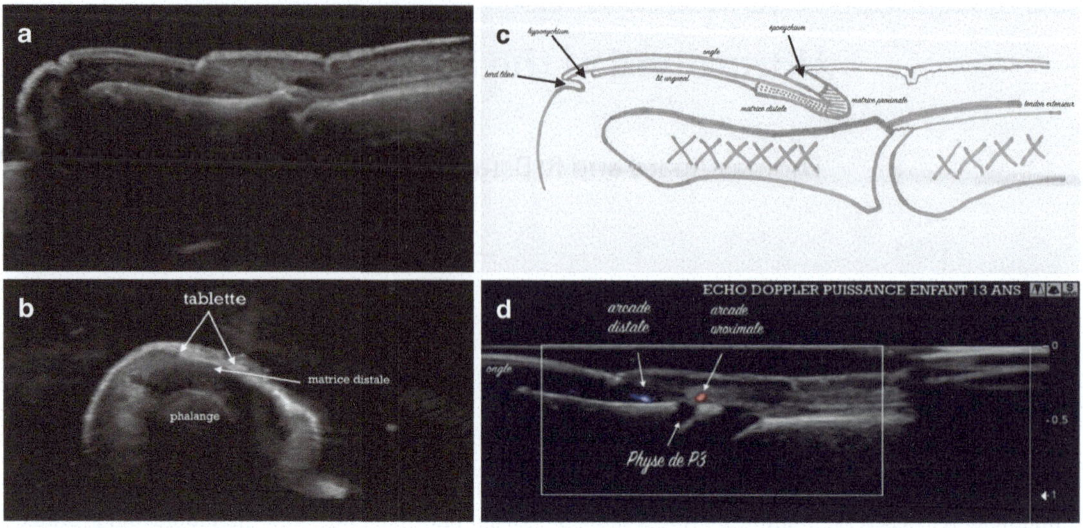

Fig. 21.1 (**a**) Longitudinal cut of fingertip and diagram (**d**). (**b**) Cross section of the tip of the finger. (**c**) Longitudinal cut of the tip of the finger with power Doppler

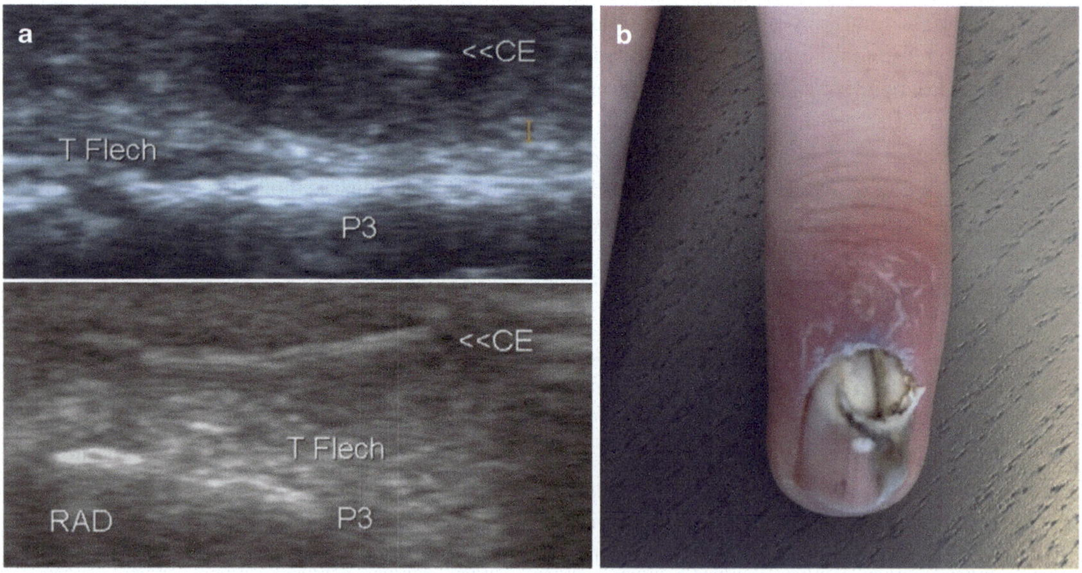

Fig. 21.2 (**a**) Foreign body (CE) in longitudinal and axial view (*collection by Dr. Brasseur with permission*). Note the absence of a posterior shadow cone and the hypoechoic halo around the CE corresponding to the reaction granuloma. Finally, it is interesting to note here the angulation of the foreign body: its preoperative measurement must correspond to the actual length after removal to be sure not to leave a piece in the pulp. (**b**) Plant CE discovered after antibiotic therapy for periungual abscess

does not fall. The analysis is done in longitudinal and cross sections and then in the power Doppler mode.

If the probe is waterproof, the examination in water is very useful so as not to have to use gel.

We will not deal with inflammatory diseases (psoriasis, scleroderma, dermatomyositis, lupus) here which are not the usual reasons for consultation in orthopedics: a dermatological opinion will then be requested.

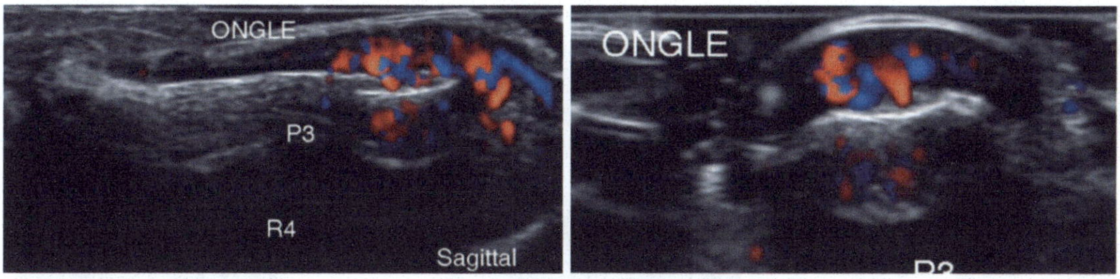

Fig. 21.3 Glomus tumor in longitudinal and axial view with power Doppler mode (collection by Dr. Brasseur with permission)

21.3 Ultrasound of the Pathological Nail

We will study the most common situations where ultrasound is useful.

21.3.1 Foreign Body Search

The penetration of radiotransparent foreign bodies is a frequent reason for consultation (Fig. 21.2a). Patients often try to "crush" the port of entry and put on Dakin's solution, which makes the eponychium and the free edge of the nail inflammatory. The request for radiography is systematic. MRI is rarely accessible in emergency.

Ultrasound will make it possible to locate the foreign body and also to check whether it is single or multiple (classic situation of the broken plant spine).

Joint analysis also makes it possible to check whether or not there is interphalangeal synovitis. Synovitis is examined in power Doppler with the joint in slight hyperextension.

Figure 21.2b illustrates the case of a periungual infection treated medically and leaving an 11 mm plant foreign body revealed 1 week later.

21.3.2 Solid Tumor Search

The glomus tumor (Fig. 21.3) is usually small in size hypoechoic or anechogenic at the level of the bluish spot on the nail. This is the differential diagnosis of subungual hematoma.

Giant cell tumors are isoechogenic or weakly hypoechogenic and originate from the deep joint flexor tendon sheath of the finger. It can mark an imprint on the cortex, but in practice the asymmetry of curvature of the phalanx is not detected by ultrasound. The interest of ultrasound is to identify the tumor that can wrap the bone or be bilobed. Its en bloc ablation is necessary, and the surgeon will always prefer to incise on the less sensitive pulp surface.

Osteoid osteoma is visible in case of presentation in subperiosteal form. It is then associated with macrodactyly with digital pseudo-hippocratism of the nail (Fig. 21.4a and b). Its removal allows the phalanx to regain its original shape. Cortical and medullary forms with the typical roundel image in the scanner are not seen on ultrasound.

Granuloma is a slightly hyperechogenic or isoechogenic solid tumor. It is necessary to search for a hyperechogenic foreign body without a posterior shadow cone. It can be silicic, talcous, etc.

Keratoacanthoma is a rare and benign epithelial tumor. Ultrasound shows a very limited heterogeneous area with erosion of the phalangeal cortex and a cone of posterior shadow. Differential diagnosis is basal cell carcinoma.

Subungual melanoma is the most feared malignant tumor. Ultrasound features of melanoma are unspecific: hypervascularization with Doppler in relation to the part of the nail without melanoma; there is no identifiable mass on

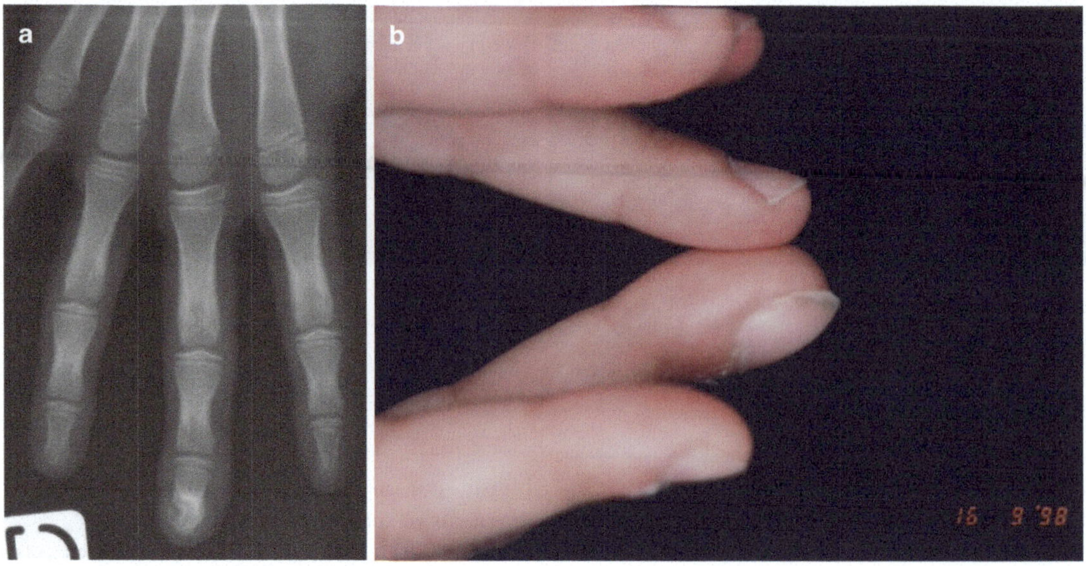

Fig. 21.4 (**a**) Frontal radiography of osteoid osteoma of P3 cortical type (collection by Pr Dautel with permission). (**b**) Digital pseudo-hippocratism from osteoid osteoma (collection by Pr Dautel with permission)

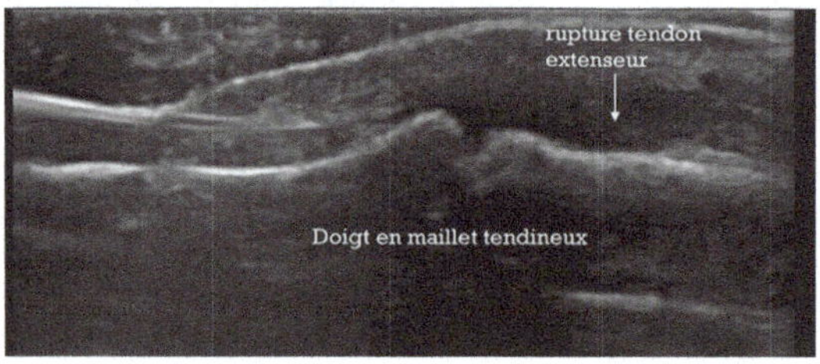

Fig. 21.5 Mallet finger lesion

ultrasound. Biopsy is recommended at the slightest doubt.

21.3.3 Analysis of the Distal Interphalangeal Joint

The insertion of the extensor apparatus and the joint capsule should be analyzed.

- The extensor apparatus is broken in case of a mallet finger. Its diagnosis is then clinical, and the interest of ultrasound is only intended to detect bone tearing from the cortex (Fig. 21.5). In the case of a chronic mallet finger, the attachment of the "neo-tendon" is hypoechogenic, and the flexion of the phalanx causes only a slight movement on the extensor tendon (comparative analysis with the neighboring finger). The matrix is never affected with this type of trauma.
- The joint capsule can cause a tumor that compresses the matrix. The most frequently encountered is the mucoid pseudocyst, a reaction to chondral pain. Ultrasound confirms by the analysis of the neck the joint origin of the cyst. It is sometimes clinically difficult to distinguish between a small cyst and an osteophyte: ultrasound shows cortical irregularity with posterior shadow cone in case of osteophyte, whereas the cyst is an anechogenic tumor (Fig. 21.6).

In case of hyperechogenic swelling, it is a solid tumor: abscess (paronychia) with septic arthritis, epidermal or foreign body granuloma, gouty tophus (Fig. 21.7), epidermoid carcinoma, melanoma, metastasis, etc.

One of the differential diagnoses is Orf's nodule or epidermal *Parapoxvirus* infection (Fig. 21.8a and b): the patient has no pain, and the tumor does not distort the matrix. Above all, you should not puncture because the risk of bacterial superinfection is high. Treatment is simply regular handwashing and finger protection (spontaneous healing within a month). This virus is

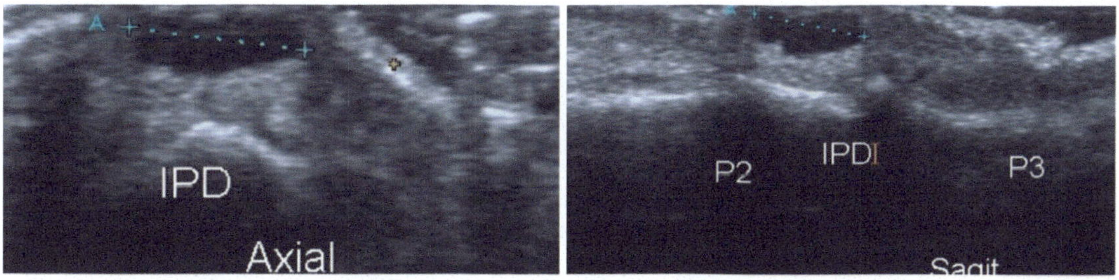

Fig. 21.6 Mucoid cyst in axial and longitudinal view (collection by Dr. Brasseur with permission)

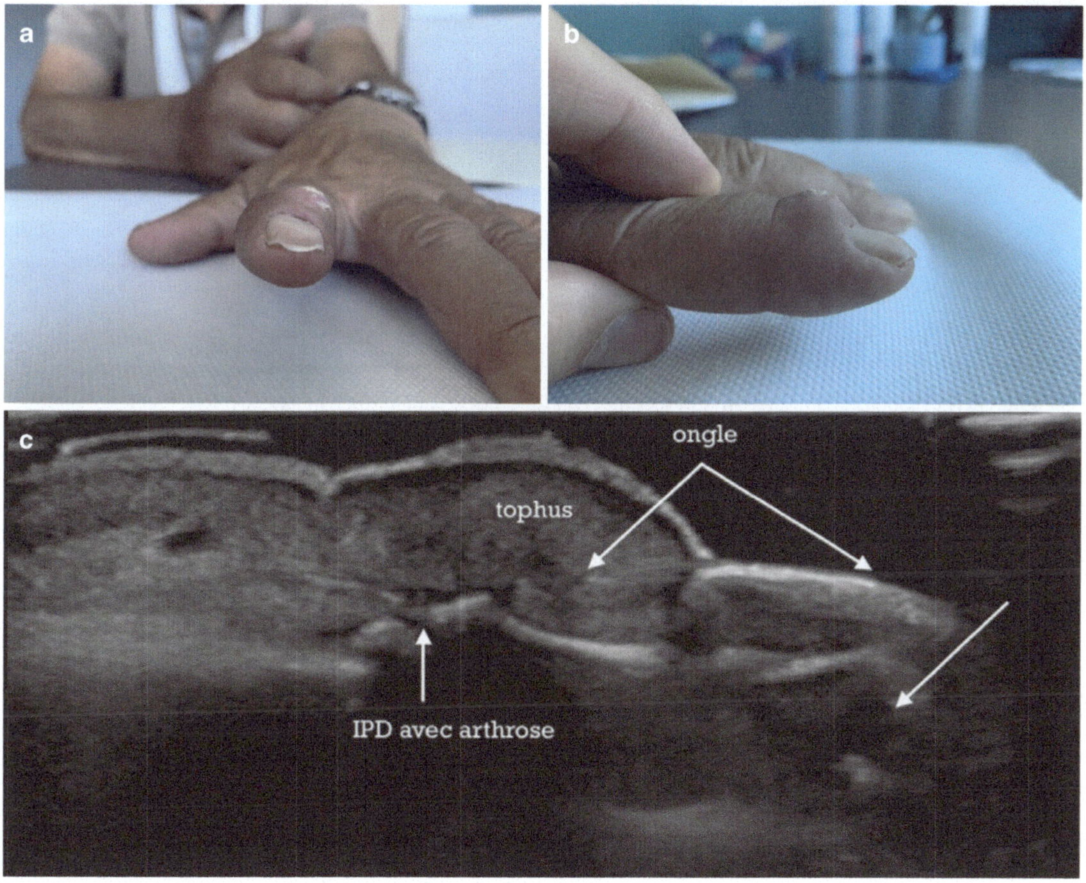

Fig. 21.7 (**a**) Appearance of the concave ungual shelf by compression of the matrix by the gouty tophus. (**b**) Profile appearance of the finger with distal interphalangeal tophus. (**c**) Ultrasound of the tophus (isoechogenic mass)

present on animal fur. The lesion appears 3 weeks from contact. These injuries are most often found in veterinarians or in Muslims 3 weeks after the feast of Eid al-Adha (sheep sacrifice).

In case of microcrystalline pathology, power Doppler mode looks for hematic joint activity. Care should be taken not to place the probe on the finger (leave a large amount of gel or do an examination in water) or be careful that the hands are not too hot or too cold.

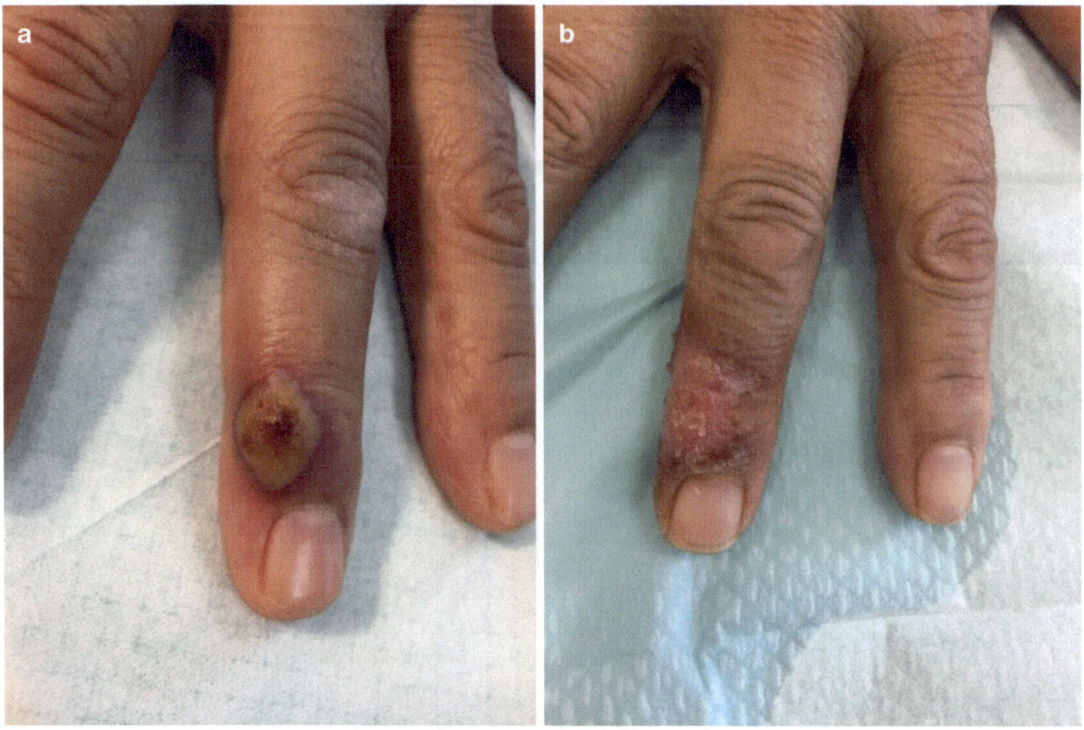

Fig. 21.8 (**a**) Orf nodule at 3 weeks. (**b**) Orf nodule at 6 weeks (after conservative treatment)

21.4 Posttraumatic Nail

Classic finger traumas affecting the nail bed without affecting the matrix are well known to surgeons (door finger, loss of fingertip substance, fracture of the phalanx, etc.): their evolution is conventionally favorable. Ultrasound does not have particular interest in these clinical situations.

- *Retronychia* is the result of an often unrecognized axial trauma in which the nail abruptly recedes under the eponychium and damages the matrix. The delay between trauma and consultation can be significant as the pain fades within a few days. Retronychia is characterized by a triad: discontinuation of ungual-paronychia-xanthonychia growth [1]. The patient often consults for ungual deformation in the form of a staircase with Beau lines. Ultrasound shows a decrease in the distance between the proximal edge of the shelf and the proximal edge of the neighboring phalanx.
- *Onychomadesis* involves proximal detachment of the nail following extensive trauma to the matrix but can also be seen after an episode of severe systemic disease. On ultrasound the ungual shelf appears divided if the regrowth is rapid with often less echogenicity on the distal part (Fig. 21.9).

21.5 Conclusion

Ultrasound is very useful in consultation for ungual pathology due to its availability and noninvasive and comparative nature [4, 5]. It must always be coupled with the radiograph in the imaging workup.

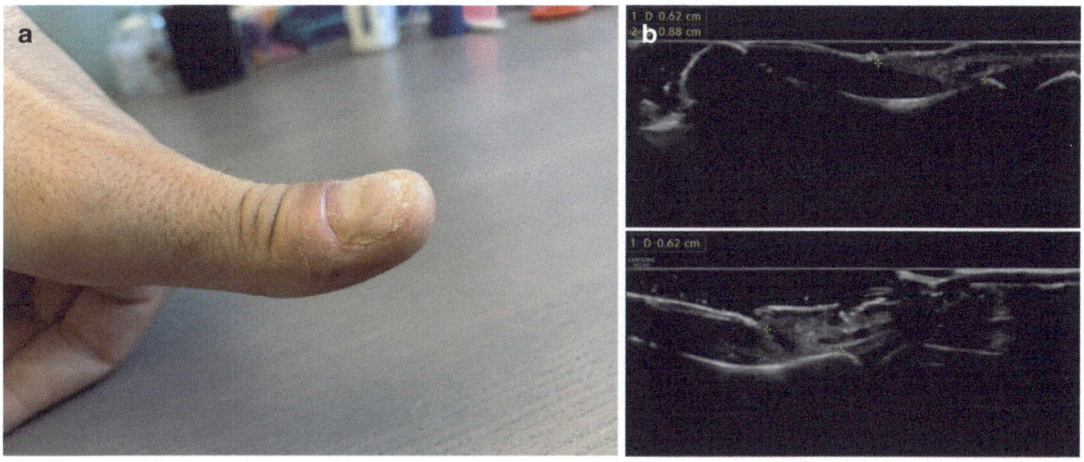

Fig. 21.9 (**a**) Clinical appearance of a retronychia (2 years after trauma). (**b**) Comparative ultrasound showing the retreat from the shelf to the DIP (bottom image) in comparison with the healthy side (top image)

References

1. The Baran-Dawber's nail diseases and their management. Wiley-Blackwell; 2018.
2. Thomas L, Vaudaine M, Wortsman X, Jemec GBE, Drape JL. Imaging the Nail. In: Baran and Dawber's. Diseases of the nails and their management. 4th ed. Hoboken: Wiley Blackwell; 2019. p. 101–82.
3. Bakhach J, Demiri E, Guimberteau JC. Use of the eponychial flap to restore the length of a short nail: a review of 30 cases. Plast Reconstr Surg. 2005;116(2):478–83.
4. Berritto D, Iacobellis F, Rossi C, Reginelli A, Cappabianca S, Grassi R. Ultra high-frequency ultrasound: new capabilities for nail anatomy exploration. J Dermatol. 2017;44(1):43–6.
5. Aluja Jaramillo F, Quiasúa Mejía DC, Martínez Ordúz HM, González-Ardila C. Nail ultrasound unit: a complete guide of the nail diseases. J Ultrasound. 2017;20(3):181–92.

The manufacturer's authorised representative in the EU is Springer Nature Customer Service Centre GmbH, Europaplatz 3, 69115 Heidelberg, Germany. If you have any concerns regarding our products, please contact ProductSafety@springernature.com

Printed and bound by CPI Group (UK) Ltd, Croydon, CR0 4YY
30/09/2026
02225687-0017